Contents

Chapter 6

Tolerance and Dependence   103

Chapter 7

Psychotropic Drug Classification   137

Chapter 8

Sedative-Hypnotics and Anxiolytics   151

Chapter 9

Psychostimulants   191

Chapter 10

Chapter 11

Chapter 12

Chapter 13

Chapter 14

Preface

It is a very rare person who does not, at some time or another, use a psychoactive drug—that is, a drug that alters psychological processes such as mood, thought, and behavior. In fact, some drugs, such as caffeine, nicotine, and alcohol, are so common in our society that we usually do not even think of them as drugs. Although the use of psychoactive drugs has a long history, the actual systematic study of the relationships between drugs and psychological processes—psychopharmacology—is quite new. Therefore, our knowledge about psychoactive drugs is relatively limited. This is rather unfortunate because their use is pervasive in most Western cultures, particularly our own. Drugs are used in a wide variety of social, recreational, and therapeutic settings.

The purpose of this book is to introduce the student to the field of psychopharmacology, with special emphasis on the relationships between drugs, their mechanisms of action in the nervous system, and human behavior. For most students this book will be their first exposure to this diverse field. The text is written for the psychology student who wishes to go into some field of research associated with drugs or into clinical areas where the persons they deal with are taking psychoactive medications or using psychoactive drugs recreationally, and perhaps abusing them. It is also written for nursing students, who will be observing patients who are prescribed psychoactive medication; chemistry students, who may be interested in going into pharmacy; biology students, who may enter the field of medicine and eventually prescribe a number of psychoactive medications for their patients; and any other students interested in the fascinating relationships among drugs, the brain, emotions, mental activities, and behavior.

Because psychopharmacology involves biological functions, chemical reactions, physics, and psychological processes, ideally students reading this book will already have a basic familiarity with each of these areas. The text is not written for the specialist. Therefore, the use of esoteric and specialized jargon to describe the effects of drugs and the psychiatric and psychological conditions they induce or alleviate has been minimized. Key pharmacological terms are set in boldface type and defined the first time they appear. Other scientific and clinical terms which could impede the student's understanding of certain principles are italicized and defined. All definitions in this text are from the following sources: *Stedman's Medical Dictionary*, 25th Edition; *Dictionary of Psychology* by A. S. Reber; *Mosby's Medical and Nursing Dictionary;* and *Webster's Deluxe Unabridged Dictionary*, 2nd Edition.

It is hoped that the information contained in this book will enable the student to appreciate more fully why people use drugs and what the consequences of that use might be. Chapter 1 deals briefly with the field of psychopharmacology from a historical perspective. Chapters 2 and 3 acquaint the student with the principles and mechanisms behind the actions of drugs that can be generalized to all drugs, including those affecting mood, mental functions, and behavior. Chapters 4 and 5 review the nervous system, through which psychoactive drugs induce their effects. All thoughts, emotions, and behaviors are the result of electrical and biochemical activities taking place in the nervous system, and drugs that affect these psychological variables do so by disturbing or altering these activities. Without an understanding of the basic mechanisms behind these electrical and biochemical events, it will be very difficult for the student to appreciate and understand why psychoactive drugs do what they do. These first five chapters contain definitions of psychopharmacological terms and describe concepts necessary for understanding the processes and actions of the drugs to be discussed in the remaining chapters.

Chapter 6 discusses the general processes behind drug tolerance, drug abuse, and drug dependence. Chapters 7 through 11 classify, describe, and discuss the actions and effects of drugs commonly used in our culture for social and recreational purposes, often leading to drug abuse and dependence. Many of these drugs have been or still are being used in a medical or psychiatric context, but their present impact on our society is due primarily to their use in nonmedical settings. These are the drugs with which the students themselves may have direct contact.

Chapters 12 through 14 describe and discuss the actions and effects of drugs used primarily in the treatment of medical and emotional disturbances. Although these drugs are used in a medical context, many students in psychology, biology, chemistry, and nursing will go on to specialize in clinical fields where the patient population has been prescribed such medications. In order to deal fully with the needs of their clients, these clinicians should be aware of what these drugs are capable of doing, what their side effects are, and why they are being prescribed. Even students who do not become clinicians should be aware of these properties because there is a strong likelihood that they will have friends or families who do use these drugs.

I would like to thank the many students I have taught over the years who have provided the inspiration behind this book and whose comments and suggestions on the first edition led to considerable modification in the organization of the second edition. I am most indebted to Barb Simon for her assistance in putting this second edition together and making it more readable from the standpoint of the student. Finally, I would like to thank the reviewers—Helen M. Murphy, Ph.D., John Carroll University; Dr. Mark Masaki, Youngstown State University; Robert W. Bell, Ph.D., Texas Tech University; and John Broida, Ph.D., University of Southern Maine—and also my colleagues, listed here, who read and commented on the manuscript at various stages. Their comments were invaluable. They include Gaylord Ellison, University of California, Los Angeles; Dennis Glanzman, Arizona State University; Carol van Hartesveldt, University of Florida, Gainesville; Keith Jacobs, Loyola University, New Orleans; Frank White, Neuropsychopharmacology Laboratory, Lafayette Clinic; W. Jeffrey Wilson, Purdue University at Fort Wayne.

Chapter One

Psychopharmacology in Perspective

Psychopharmacology is the systematic study of the effects of drugs on behavior, cognitive functioning, and emotions. Drugs that alter behavior, cognitive functioning, or emotions are called **psychoactive** or **psychotropic drugs**. The term "psychopharmacology" is a combination of the terms "psychology" and "pharmacology," which refer, respectively, to the study of the variables affecting behavior and the study of the effects of drugs on biological systems. Originally "psyche" referred to the soul, but lately it has been used to refer to the mind. "Pharmakos" originally meant scapegoat; a pharmakos was a person who was sacrificed as a remedy for whatever maladies another person might have been experiencing. For obvious reasons, there were few volunteers for the position, but I suppose that the procedure worked in roughly a third of the cases—about the same success rate one might get nowadays using a placebo. Later on, around 600 B.C., the term came to refer to a medicine, drug, or poison. Presently, the term "drug" is used in a much more general way to denote chemicals that alter the normal biological functions of the body.

Psychoactive drugs are chemicals that induce psychological effects by altering the normal biochemical reactions that take place in the nervous system. A drug's chemical structure, how much of the drug is taken, how long it has been since it was taken, and how frequently it is taken are important factors that will be discussed in relation to the drug experience. In addition, three other ingredients in the drug experience should always be kept in mind: the **set** (the psychological makeup and the expectations of the individual taking the drug), the **setting** (the social and physical environment in which the drug is taken), and the individual's unique biochemical makeup (Wallace & Fisher, 1991). Factors such as the physical setting and the person's body chemistry, attitudes, emotional state, and previous drug experiences all interact with the drug to alter the person's level of awareness, mood, thought processes, and behavior. When one attempts to describe the effects of a particular psychoactive drug, these factors should always be taken into consideration.

A drug should not be viewed as simply bad or good. Consideration must be given to how much is taken, what it is taken for, and in what context it is taken. For example, heroin can be a very effective drug in the treatment of pain in terminally ill cancer patients, and cocaine is a very effective local anesthetic for use in certain kinds of surgery. However, when injected in unknown quantities for their euphoric properties, these drugs can lead to dependence, economic and social disaster, incarceration, toxic reactions, and death.

A Historical Overview of Psychopharmacology

Ancient records indicate that human beings have been using drugs to alter mood and behavior for a long time. (For fascinating and more detailed versions of this topic, see Brecher, 1972; Caldwell, 1978; and Szasz, 1974.) Considering the thousands of plants available that contain psychoactive substances and the likelihood that our ancestors were just as curious and willing to experiment on themselves as some people are today, this information should not come as any surprise. Substances that can induce mystical experiences and hallucinations are found in cannabis and in numerous herbs, mushrooms, and cacti, all of which grow throughout the world.

In order to enhance their ferociousness, early Viking warriors were said to ingest the mushroom *Amanita muscaria,* which is capable of inducing gaiety, exuberance, and berserk behavior—a term derived from their name, the Berserkers. Some American Indians have used the peyote cactus, which contains the hallucinogen (hallucination-producing substance) mescaline, in their religious ceremonies for centuries. Archaeological findings of "mushroom stones" in Guatemala indicate that a sophisticated mushroom cult existed there some 3,500 years ago. Early Spanish chroniclers wrote of their opposition to the Aztecs' ceremonial eating of the diabolical mushroom *teonanacatl* (food of the gods) for purposes of divination, prophecy, and worship. It is likely that these mushrooms contained the hallucinogenic substances psilocybin and psilocin. Cannabis, which we now call marijuana, was first used more than 4,000 years ago, primarily for its medical value in treating a number of different ailments.

Opium poppies, which contain the narcotics morphine and codeine, were probably used by the ancient Sumerians in Mesopotamia almost 7,000 years ago. Substances that effectively suppress manic symptoms can be found in rauwolfia, a plant common to the Himalayas. Substances that elevate mood and reduce fatigue are found in many plants. For centuries South American Indians have chewed the coca leaf, which contains small amounts of the drug cocaine, to alleviate fatigue, elevate mood, and reduce hunger, and archaeological evidence suggests that early humans may have used coca as far back as 3000 B.C.

The use of tea as a pleasurable stimulant began about A.D. 600 in China. An intoxicating beverage made from coffee beans was introduced to the Arabians in the 13th century. Numerous other plants containing caffeine or similar-acting substances have been used by ancient cultures in Mexico, South America, and Africa, among many others. The use of nicotine-containing tobacco by both South and North American Indians goes back at least 600 years.

In ceremonies during medieval times, witches used various herbs (such as mandrake, henbane, and belladonna) containing scopolamine, hyoscyamine, and atropine to induce hallucinations and the sensation of flying. They also may have thrown in a few toads, whose sweat glands contain the hallucinogenic drug bufotenine, one of the few psychoactive drugs of animal origin. Physicians during this and later periods used the same substances as sleep inducers and analgesics, as well as for other purposes.

Except perhaps for caffeine, the most common psychoactive substance used around the world today is alcohol, and it has been available for thousands of years. There is hardly a culture, primitive or advanced, that does not value its peculiar properties. Alcohol is a simple product of fermentation, which occurs when certain yeasts, molds, and bacteria act upon sugar in a variety of fruits and which is easily produced both accidentally and purposefully. The earliest records of purposeful alcohol production were made by the Egyptians more than 5,500 years ago.

Every culture that we are aware of has used a plant or plants with psychoactive properties at one time or another. In their experimentation over the centuries, human beings must have eaten, drunk, smoked, or rubbed on their bodies thousands of substances. They found that some of these substances nourished them, while others made them ill or killed them, relieved their psychological or physical discomforts, or had extraordinary and incomprehensible effects on mood, consciousness, or behavior.

Even nonhuman animals have been observed to seek out substances with mood-altering properties (Siegel, 1989). Elephants, chimpanzees, baboons, and horses have been noted to prefer water containing a small percentage of alcohol over pure water. Some birds prefer fermented berries over unfermented berries. Goats nibble coffee berries; some species of bees guzzle stupefying nectars of specialized flowers; llamas chew coca leaves (which contain cocaine); and some species of ants maintain "herds" of beetles, apparently for their intoxicating secretions.

These observations have led Siegel to propose the intriguing—and controversial—hypothesis that intoxication is a universal "fourth drive," as natural as the innate drives of hunger, thirst, and sex.

Predecessors to Modern Pharmacotherapies

During the 1800s a number of psychoactive drugs were isolated or distilled from plants or developed from nonplant sources. Morphine was isolated from opium in 1805 and was viewed as a most effective treatment for periodic insanity. Cocaine was extracted from the coca leaf in 1857 and was suggested as a potential treatment for depression. Bromine, discovered in 1826, and chloral, discovered in 1832, were used as sedatives and sleep-inducing agents. The anesthetic gases chloroform and nitrous oxide were suggested as potential treatments for insanity. Compounds such as cannabis, hemlock, strychnine, and *Datura stramonium*—used for centuries to treat a variety of disorders—were still viewed as valuable psychiatric tools, although we realize today that they probably did more harm than good. The first phenothiazine (a type of antipsychotic discussed in Chapter 12), methylene blue, was developed in 1883. A few years later, it was reported to have calming effects on manic and hallucinating patients. Despite its apparent effectiveness, it would take another 50 years before the closely related compound chlorpromazine would revolutionize the treatment of the severely mentally disturbed. Drug-induced sleep therapy, where emotionally disturbed patients were kept unconscious for several days, became popular toward the end of the 19th century.

It was during the 1800s that investigations of the formal relationships between drug variables and psychological processes, particularly those involved in mental illness, began. The first of these investigations was probably that conducted by Jacques-Joseph Moreau de Tours, a highly respected physician in France. In the mid-1800s he published a book, for which he is most noted, called *Hashish and Mental Illness*. After taking a hashish-laced concoction (hashish is a concentrated form of marijuana) on numerous occasions and observing others who volunteered to ingest his concoction, he compared the drug-induced symptoms with the mental symptoms that occur spontaneously in psychoses. Moreau was one of the first to emphasize that the person's particular or immediate context greatly influenced both the quality and intensity of the drug experience. He also observed the effects of hashish on some of his patients with mental disorders and suggested that hashish-induced excitement may be beneficial in treating depressed patients. He reported that some depressed individuals, after taking his hashish concoction, chatted, laughed, and acted silly all evening. Unfortunately, however, those effects were transitory, and the patients relapsed. He also found that occasionally manic patients improved after taking hashish.

Moreau also studied the psychoactive effects of opiates, nitrous oxide, and a number of sedative-hypnotic drugs. Unfortunately, his work in this area went largely unrecognized by his contemporaries, but shortly after *Hashish and Mental Illness* was published, a few American psychiatrists who read of his work tried cannabis preparations in the treatment of insanity. Despite the lack of recognition during his time, today some people view Moreau as the first psychopharmacologist.

However, the very first book in modern experimental psychopharmacology, as well as the first book solely devoted to drugs and animal behavior, was published in 1826 by A. P. Charvel, a young medical student (Siegel, 1989). Charvel studied the effects of opium on a variety of animals, including water beetles, crayfish, snails, fish, toads, birds, and various mammals (including himself and other medical students). Like Moreau, Charvel discovered that a drug's effects depend on numerous factors, such as the individual's past history, tolerance to the drug, dose, and method of administration. But like the observations of Moreau, Charvel's discoveries were largely ignored by his contemporaries.

During the late 1800s and early 1900s, some of psychology's most famous forefathers were also some of the first to explore systematically the relationship between various drugs and psychological variables. Early in his career, Sigmund Freud spent three years investigating the effects of cocaine on fatigue, depression, strength, and morphine addiction, among other things. In many of these studies, he was the test subject. Until recently, many of the most comprehensive, up-to-date descriptions of cocaine's effects were contained in Freud's 25-page essay "Über Coca" (On Coca) published in 1884. However, a growing number of reports critical of cocaine at that time, as well as Freud's own dismal failure in treating a good friend's morphine addiction with cocaine (the friend turned from morphine to heavy cocaine use), led him to direct his scientific interests into very different areas. However, Freud retained an interest in drugs and behavior throughout his lifetime. Curiously, although Freud was able to give up cocaine, apparently with very little discomfort, he remained a nicotine addict who chain-smoked cigars despite suffering from angina (chest pain) and having had multiple operations for oral cancer (Brecher, 1972). Even the man who discovered the ego-defense mechanism of "denial" was unable to avoid its consequences.

Ivan Pavlov, best known for his work in the conditioning of reflexes, attempted to treat schizophrenics by using some of his conditioning techniques and inducing long periods of sleep with bromides. However, it is doubtful that he was very successful with this technique, because bromides tend to accumulate in the body and can reach levels that can induce toxic symptoms such as headache, sedation, violent delirium, mental confusion, and gastric distress. In some cases, these symptoms are very similar to those of a psychosis. Pavlov's work in the area of conditioning reflexes led some of his colleagues to use drugs like morphine as potential stimuli for the induction of new reflexes. These researchers probably did not realize just how important the Pavlovian process is in what we now refer to as drug dependence.

William James, the first American-born psychologist, wrote about some of his fascinating experiences while under the influence of nitrous oxide, sometimes known as "laughing gas" (Leavitt, 1982). He found that consciousness, in which he was very interested, could be profoundly altered by nitrous oxide, although not necessarily for the better. It seems that while he was under the influence of nitrous oxide (the effects last but a few minutes) he was capable of very mystic revelations. Unfortunately, though, he could never remember what the revelations were when the effects wore off. It is reported that upon one occasion while under the influence he was able to quickly jot down one of these profundities. It read:

> Hogamous, higamous
> Man is polygamous
> Higamous, hogamous
> Woman is monogamous   (Gibbons & Connelly, 1970, p. 77).

The first half of the 20th century was accompanied by the synthesis or clinical use of a wide variety of new psychoactive substances with potential therapeutic value. Barbiturates were introduced in 1903 and helped sustain interest in sleep therapy for various mental ailments. Amphetamine, first synthesized in the 1800s, came into clinical use in 1927 in the treatment of narcolepsy and mild depressive states. Albert Hofmann first synthesized lysergic diethylamide (LSD) in 1938. Five years later, when he accidentally ingested LSD during one of his experiments, he discovered that it was one of the most potent psychoactive substances known to humankind. LSD would be used a few years later as a psychedelic (mind-manifesting) adjunct to psychotherapy and as a means of inducing what many people believed to be a model psychosis.

Despite the extensive history of drug use and these early investigations, there was no real interest in studying drugs and their influence on cognition, emotions, and behavior until about the early 1950s. During the 1950s a drug previously used in France as a preanesthetic was tested on some schizophrenic patients and was found to induce a dramatic reduction in their symptoms. Previously, many different drugs had been used in treating schizophrenia, all of which simply put the patients to sleep or made them so drowsy or sedated that they could not do anything. This particular drug, however, did more than simply calm the patients; it worked by reducing the core symptoms. The drug was known as chlorpromazine, and, as we will see shortly, it was this discovery that led to the formation of the formal and distinct discipline known as psychopharmacology.

One of the first antihistamines was developed in 1937. Although antihistamines were initially used in the treatment of allergies, their sedative properties, viewed by those taking them for allergic conditions as an undesirable side effect, were suspected as being beneficial in the treatment of other clinical conditions. The antihistamine promethazine was introduced in 1949 as an adjunct to surgery. It was found to reduce surgical shock, to calm patients both before and after major surgery, and to reduce the emotional suffering associated with surgery. A year later it was used by a psychiatrist in the treatment of schizophrenia, primarily for its hypnotic effects. Although promethazine calmed his patients, the psychiatrist apparently saw it as just another sedative. In the same year another psychiatrist noted similar calming effects in schizophrenic patients with a related compound, but the manufacturer was not interested in developing such a drug. However, reports of these effects in surgical patients and schizophrenics eventually led to the evaluation and development of compounds with similar structures with even more specific actions.

One of these compounds, initially called 4560 RP, was found to have some interesting pharmacological properties. It had minimal antihistaminic action, but it reduced both sympathetic and parasympathetic activity, abolished conditioned reflexes, and had a host of other desirable properties. In clinical trials it abolished preoperative anxiety, reduced surgical stress, and eliminated the postoperative consequences of stress. Here was a drug that could turn off the world and its harrowing stress without inebriating the patient or putting the patient to sleep. The surgeon who attempted these clinical tests closed his report with the suggestion that 4560 RP, now called chlorpromazine, be used in treating psychiatric conditions. The first report on chlorpromazine treatment of psychosis was published in France in 1952. In 1953 chlorpromazine was tried more extensively in psychiatric wards in Paris.

It could be said that at that time chlorpromazine started the pharmacological revolution in psychiatry. Although it did not cure mania and schizophrenia, chlorpromazine did suspend their symptoms with great efficacy and much less toxicity than any previous drug. Chlorpromazine was used immediately in Italy and Switzerland, and shortly thereafter in the United States. Its use spread to England and South America in 1954 and to Australia, Japan, and the Soviet Union in 1955. Its trade name in Europe was Largactil, because of its *large* spectrum of therapeutic *activity*. In the United States it was marketed as Thorazine, perhaps after the powerful god of thunder, Thor (although this derivation is purely speculative).

The pharmacological revolution expanded. Between 1952 and 1954, chlorpromazine monopolized drug therapy for all mental diseases. It stirred the ambitions of drug manufacturers and researchers. New drugs were developed, and drugs that had been abandoned were clinically tested again. In India as early as 1931 it was suggested that the rauwolfia plant, which contains reserpine, had some beneficial effects in the treatment of mental disorders, but it was not introduced to the Western world until 1954. Meprobamate, the first of the so-called anxiolytics (anxiety reducers), was first used clinically in 1955 and became as popular for the treatment of neuroses as chlorpromazine was for psychoses. The treatment of depression with a monoamine oxidase inhibitor became acceptable in 1957, five years after its antidepressant action was noted in tuberculosis patients who were administered the drug for its antituberculosis properties. A drug developed in 1948, with properties that did not generate any enthusiasm on the part of its manufacturer, was again tested clinically in 1957 because of its molecular resemblance to chlorpromazine. Unlike the phenothiazines, however, the drug was relatively ineffective in quieting agitated psychotic patients. Instead, it seemed to have remarkable mood-lifting properties in severely depressed patients. Thus was born the first tricyclic antidepressant, imipramine (Tofranil).

The enthusiasm created by chlorpromazine led to one oversight with respect to a drug that would later take the place of chlorpromazine as one of the most valuable treatments for cyclical mood disorders. As early as 1870, it was suggested that, in one of its salt forms, lithium, an alkali metal, had mood-altering effects. It wasn't until 1949, however, that the Australian psychiatrist John Cade discovered, quite fortuitously, that lithium had profound mood-stabilizing effects in manic patients. Despite verification of his findings in studies conducted one or two years later, the vast majority of psychiatric practitioners remained unimpressed with his findings. Lithium was believed to be too toxic. It also had minimal marketability because it was unpatentable as a natural substance. In addition, chlorpromazine suppressed the symptoms of mania much more quickly than lithium did and had a much lower potential for toxicity. It took almost 10 years for the medical community, at least in the United States, to recognize the true value of lithium and to rectify the oversight.

Even LSD research advanced because of chlorpromazine and the interest stimulated between brain biochemistry and psychosis. Because chlorpromazine could readily block the effects of LSD, it made research and psychotherapy with LSD safer. LSD psychosis became the model with which other potential antipsychotic drugs could be tested, and with LSD inducing a model psychosis, it became a tool in exploring the etiology (the science of causes or origins of diseases) of schizophrenia. Unfortunately, we now know that the LSD psychosis is considerably different from the psychoses that occur "naturally" in humans.

Beginning in the early 1950s, a multitude of drugs were developed that revolutionized the treatment of major mental and emotional illnesses. Despite the increase in the general population, the number of schizophrenics hospitalized in the United States dropped from around 600,000 in 1954 to less than 200,000 today. The goal of the community mental health movement—to deinstitutionalize patients and allow them to function successfully in the community—became a reality. Many patients who were totally refractory to behavioral therapy and psychotherapies became more amenable to these treatments with these drugs. The new pharmacotherapies also encouraged practitioners to become more rigorous in their diagnoses. The drugs stimulated interest in the relationships between brain biochemistry and behavior.

Since the 1950s psychopharmacologists have made great strides in understanding and treating virtually every affliction of the human mind. Many, if not most, mental disorders are now viewed as having a biochemical basis and can often be treated as such. (It should be not be inferred from this statement that environmental events such as stress, conflict, and inappropriate parental activities are not important factors in these biochemical disturbances or that psychologically based therapies are inappropriate in treating many forms of mental dysfunctions. But we will leave these issues for others to discuss in textbooks more suited for those purposes.)

With new techniques, such as magnetic resonance imaging, computerized axial tomography, and positron emission tomography, researchers are now able to look at the machinery and workings of the living brain. Molecular biologists are even beginning to relate abnormal behavior to specific parts of chromosomes. The specific actions of new drugs like clozapine (Clozaril), fluoxetine (Prozac), and buspirone (BuSpar) are giving us a better understanding of the relationship between moods and feelings, and the action of specific chemicals in the brain. Drugs with greater degrees of specificity and effectiveness have been developed for treating schizophrenia and depression. Symptoms of disorders such as Tourette's syndrome, panic and phobic disorders, and obsessive-compulsive disorder, which were formally treated with ineffective psychoanalytic talk therapy, can now be reduced or eliminated with newly developed drugs. Different methods of delivering old drugs, like morphine, into the body have been developed that have enhanced their effectiveness or reduced their side effects. More information about these drugs, disorders, mechanisms of action, and methods will be presented in subsequent chapters.

Unfortunately, however, psychotherapeutic drugs do not cure mental disorders nor suppress their symptoms in all individuals. Sometimes they cause toxic or irreversible side effects. The potential for such side effects brings out a number of ethical questions about the right of a society to control the behavior of individuals with substances that might do them harm. Although drugs allow patients to leave hospitals, the communities to which the patients return are often poorly prepared to provide continuing care. In other cases practitioners rely solely on medications to deal with their patients' problems, without looking into other psychological or socioeconomical interventions that might be available and beneficial for their patients. In spite of the fact that the prognosis for mentally and emotionally ill people is much better now than it was 35 years ago, we as a society must continue searching for drugs with greater specificity and for other interventions that will help us deal with these problems and allow these individuals to lead happier and more productive lives.

Recreational and Social Drug Use

Many individuals who exhibit the normal range of moods, emotions, cognitive activity, and behavior willingly administer drugs to themselves to alter their emotional experiences, consciousness, or behavior in recreational, social, or religious settings. Such phenomena are of particular interest to psychopharmacologists. Very few individuals in modern cultures do not, at some time or another, use a psychoactive drug for such a purpose. Even caffeine, nicotine, and alcohol, which we often do not even think of as drugs, are psychoactive drugs. In many cases, taking these drugs is explicitly (in advertisements) or implicitly indicated as having positive or beneficial effects. For example, smoking cigarettes and drinking alcohol are often portrayed in fiction as beneficial tools for coping with emotionally stressful situations (Kushnir, 1986). As a whole the mass media reflect the national culture and have conditioned Americans to accept drug use as part of daily life (Gitlin, 1990). (With all the references to drugs that occur—many of them uncritical, to say the least—it is reasonable that questions should be raised about the media's contributions to drug use.)

Over the past several years, Americans have spent approximately $45 billion a year on alcoholic beverages. That amounts to approximately 40 gallons a year (or 2.5 gallons of pure ethyl alcohol) for the average American drinker (Barnes, 1988). In 1990 almost 530 billion nicotine-containing tobacco cigarettes were sold in the United States; the good news is that this figure represents approximately 20% fewer cigarettes consumed than in 1980. The average American adult consumes approximately 5.2 ounces of caffeine a year; most of this amount comes from drinking coffee or tea, but in young adults up to 50% of dietary caffeine may come from soft drinks (Weidner & Istvan, 1985).

In addition to these socially accepted drugs—caffeine, nicotine, and alcohol—Americans are heavy consumers of numerous illicit substances (Stephens, 1987). Because of its nature, the extent of illicit drug use in the United States is difficult to estimate, but it is clearly pervasive. Estimates from the office of National Drug Control Policy indicate that, during the late 1980s, approximately $40–50 billion was spent every year on illicit drugs in the United States. Approximately 20% was for marijuana and hashish; just over 40% was for cocaine; and just over one-third was for narcotics or other illicit drugs, such as black-market amphetamines and barbiturates and illicitly manufactured hallucinogens. Over 20% of the population has tried marijuana. The Drug Enforcement Administration (DEA) has estimated that on a yearly basis Americans consume around 200 tons of hashish (a highly concentrated form of marijuana) and 15,000 tons of marijuana. This tonnage estimate for marijuana represents almost two joints per user per day! In 1984 the National Organization for the Reform of Marijuana Laws (NORML) claimed that marijuana was the number-two cash crop in the United States—behind corn and ahead of soybeans. In 1987, NORML claimed it was the number-one cash crop. The number of cocaine users is smaller, but the DEA estimated that in 1985 they consumed 70 tons of cocaine a year (or over 10 grams per user per year) at around $100 a gram (Barnes, 1988). Nine tons of heroin worth $9 billion are used per year, but because of its low purity when it finally reaches the streets, pharmaceutical narcotics that are channeled into the illicit market are becoming more and more popular.

It is clear that those who engage in recreational or social use of drugs may eventually cause functional or physical damage to themselves or others around them. For as long as humankind has been using drugs for such purposes, there have been concerns over drug abuse and attempts to restrict it (Szasz, 1974). As far back as 2000 B.C., an Egyptian priest attempted to proselytize alcohol users, suggesting that they were degraded like the beasts. In the 17th century a prince in England paid money to people to denounce coffee drinkers, and the Russian tsar executed those found to possess tobacco (after torturing them into divulging the names of their suppliers). A similar penalty was levied by the sultan of the Ottoman Empire.

In 1736 the Gin Act of England was passed, making alcohol so expensive that the poor could not use it excessively. In 1792 the first prohibitory laws against opium in China went into effect; the punishment for possession was strangulation. Similar draconian attempts to reduce drug use have been made around the world. The United States passed the Harrison Narcotic Act in 1914 and the Marijuana Tax Act in 1937, among others, which basically outlawed the nonmedical (or untaxed) possession or sale of a number of drugs, including opium, morphine, heroin, and marijuana. In addition, prohibition of alcoholic beverages was in effect in the United States from 1920 to 1933. In 1921 cigarettes were illegal in 14 states.

Unfortunately, however, drug use did not decline in most cases (Brecher, 1972). One of the fundamental reasons restrictions have failed is that it is not clear to many users why they must stop using the drugs, since they feel their drug consumption affects only themselves. Society as a whole might agree that there are certain forms of drug consumption that should be avoided and that can be called drug abuse, but there is no universal agreement as to what these are. The criteria for what constitutes drug abuse are heavily dependent on one's culture and the time period. Generally, the term "drug abuse" refers to the self-administration of any drug in a manner that deviates from the approved medical or societal patterns within a given culture. A more operational definition might be the use of any drug that causes functional or structural damage to the users or to others, or that results in the users' inability to voluntarily control their social or drug-taking behavior. Unfortunately, human beings are excellent at self-deception and rarely recognize instances in their own lives when these criteria apply.

Thus it is clear that psychotropic drugs are used widely in a nonmedical context and that this use is fraught with many problems. In 1988 the Alcohol, Drug Abuse, and Mental Health Administration (ADAMHA) estimated that the annual cost to U.S. society of substance abuse reached $144.1 billion, with alcohol abuse alone accounting for $85.8 billion. In addition to the cost of treatment (24% of the total), these figures include costs related to lost productivity, law enforcement, crime, traffic accidents, and fires. Cigarette smoking is the leading cause of lung cancer and a key component of other cancers, cardiovascular disease, and other disorders, which end up shortening the lives of more than 300,000 people every year.

Use of other psychotropic drugs, and the rapid development of new ones, can only worsen the situation. The question frequently asked is, What can be done about it? Some people rely on the legislative process, whereby certain drug-taking practices are declared illegal. Unfortunately, though, history reveals that the legislative approach has rarely had much impact on these practices except to make them less safe than they were originally, and it has numerous other repercussions (Stephens, 1987).

Since the passage of the Harrison Narcotic Act in 1914, the United States has engaged in a war on drug abuse. This and subsequent legislation have done little to dampen the desire for or use of drugs (Marshall, 1988a). Traditionally, around 70% of the money appropriated for drug control has gone toward interdiction of supply, and only 30% has gone toward manipulating the demand for drugs (Jarvik, 1990). Because of difficulties in smuggling and concealment of drugs, less bulky, more potent drugs became preferred (e.g., heroin instead of morphine or opium), and more hazardous methods of administering drugs came into use (e.g., injecting or smoking instead of oral administration). Drug prices skyrocketed, and drug quality declined. Sellers willing to take high risks for lucrative financial gain began to engage in violence to settle disputes over drug trading, and users began committing crimes to help in buying their drugs. In response, federal antidrug expenditures continued to grow (e.g., from around $130 million in 1970 to around $3 billion in 1988), with most of this paying for catching and jailing of drug law violators. In the mid-1980s drug violations accounted for more than half of all felony prosecutions and one-third of all new prisoners sentenced. Meanwhile, prisons were so packed to capacity that convicts had to be released early to make room for new arrivals. Despite these efforts, the illicit drug business continued to grow.

In recognition of these phenomena, in the 1980s a number of political and academic leaders raised a provocative alternative—drug legalization (Marshall, 1988b). They argued that the cheapest and cleanest way to reduce drug-related crime and the hazards of drugs of unknown quality and quantity would be to do away with the laws that make drug use a crime. Their assumption was that society would be better off if it did not stand in the way of the drug users and their habit. Less tax money would be needed for interdiction, prosecution, and imprisonment of illicit drug suppliers; in fact, legalization would enhance tax revenues. Users would not be submitted to the hazards of unknown drug quality or quantity or the disastrous consequences of imprisonment. Violent crimes against property and people would be significantly reduced. Urban street gangs and organized crime, now sustained by the illegal drug trade, would be severely weakened.

Critics of this idea (Jarvik, 1990; Goldstein & Kalant, 1990) were quick to point out that it would likely have some potentially disastrous outcomes. It would probably increase the number of new addicts. Some drugs, such as cocaine and phencyclidine (PCP), have properties that are potentially hazardous to users and society no matter how they are used. Other drugs would likely be developed that produce faster and more intense effects, and thus be more addictive, than currently available ones. Finally, even with legalization, there would have to be age restrictions, as with alcohol, for legally obtaining drugs; consequently, there would still be a group of individuals for which a black market would likely exist. So, at the present time, we are at a stalemate, with minimal prospects for moving away from the legal approaches for dealing with drug abuse.

Another unsuccessful approach has been to tell exaggerated stories about the potentially harmful effects of particular drugs. For example, in the 1930s authorities indicated that even occasional use of marijuana commonly led to permanent insanity, excessive violence, criminal activities, and sexual depravity. Such stories are quickly recognized by the potential drug users for their hypocrisy and misrepresentation, and before long warnings about drugs are no longer heeded, no matter what the truth is (Newcomb & Bentler, 1989).

Unfortunately, drug prevention programs targeted at young people, which have attempted to provide correct information on the long-term consequences of drug use, provide general skills useful in resisting drugs, or provide peer models of not using drugs, have produced minimal benefits in altering drug-taking patterns of behavior (Ellickson &

Bell, 1990; Wallack & Corbett, 1990). It is likely that truly effective prevention efforts will require numerous (and in many cases, politically difficult) strategies and approaches. Because use of alcohol and tobacco by adolescents has been so strongly associated with the subsequent use of illegal drugs (e.g., marijuana, cocaine, heroin), and because alcohol and tobacco themselves may produce more adverse consequences than many illegal drugs, approaches focusing on the demand for and acceptability of these substances may be the most fruitful approach to decreasing all forms of drug abuse (Goldstein & Kalant, 1990; Wallack & Corbett, 1990). For example, we could (1) increase the price of alcohol and tobacco through taxes; (2) be more careful in monitoring age restrictions on their purchase; (3) increase restrictions on their use in public settings; (4) provide alternative forms of recreation; (5) make drug abuse treatment more accessible; (6) increase public warnings of their negative health consequences (e.g., by providing more noticeable warning labels on these products); (7) decrease their promotion through advertising; (8) reduce modeling of their use in television and films; (9) enhance the civil liability of producers and suppliers for harm caused to users; and (10) decrease their general availability (e.g., sell them through special outlets rather than grocery stores). Numerous studies have noted that each of these approaches, by itself, has a small impact on alcohol and tobacco use. If all of these approaches were combined, it is likely that they would have a much greater impact than they have had in the past (Jarvik, 1990; Mosher, 1990; Wallack & Corbett, 1990).

Over the years, there have been numerous attempts to curtail the positive image of tobacco and alcohol use by the mass media and increase the knowledge of their harmful consequences. Unfortunately, the hundreds of billions of dollars a year earned by the tobacco and alcohol industries is a tremendous incentive for them to fight most of these proposals with every legal recourse available to them, and they have done so fairly successfully. They also spend more than $4 billion a year ($2.8 billion for tobacco, $1.3 billion for alcohol) to promote and advertise their products and continue to be a major promoter of sports events and of youth- and sports-oriented programs and media (Gerbner, 1990).

Despite the mass media's glaring headlines, national surveys have revealed that over the past 15 years nonprescription drug use in the United States has stabilized and, in many cases, has declined (Kozel & Adams, 1986; Johnston et al., 1991). Furthermore, most drug use by young adults appears to be experimental or occasional. Alcohol use is the most common (caffeine use may be more common, but most surveys do not ask about it) and has been stable. Cigarette use is next but has been declining at a rate of 1.1% a year since 1987, more than double the rate of decrease from 1965 to 1985. Much of this reduction may be related to recent policies that ban or restrict smoking in public places and work sites (Davis, Boyd, & Schoenborn, 1990); these policies, although not making smoking illegal per se, consistently reinforce the view that smoking is an unhealthy practice. Use of marijuana, PCP ("angel dust"), LSD-like drugs, and sedatives peaked between 1975 and 1980 and has gradually declined. There has generally been a low rate of narcotic use that has not changed, although, as noted earlier, a decline in heroin use has been compensated for by an increase in pharmaceutical narcotic use.

According to data from sequential National Institute on Drug Abuse (NIDA) household surveys (Johnston et al., 1991), use of cocaine rose rapidly in the 1970s, reaching a peak in 1979. It then remained relatively stable until 1985, at which point use declined, from 5.8 million users in 1985 to 2.9 million in 1989. On the other hand, the proportion of heavy users increased by 37%, and the number of emergency room episodes increased dramatically from 1985 to 1990, most likely as a consequence of cocaine being marketed and administered in a form called **crack.**

Finally, although multiple illicit drug use increased from the 1960s to the 1970s, there was a concomitant decrease in the proportion of both exclusive and multiple psychotherapeutic drug users (Smart & Adlaf, 1986). Thus it appears that what has changed is not the extent of drug use, but the types of drugs used.

The approach to drug abuse taken in this book is an educational one. In order to combat drug abuse people need to be educated as to what drugs are and what their effects are. People should know under which circumstances drugs may be beneficial and under which they may be detrimental. The information given must have validity and must not be hypocritical. A person sipping on a martini cannot give a very convincing argument against marijuana use. Unfortunately, as just discussed, information alone will not necessarily stop, or even decrease, drug use. But it is hoped that individuals reading this book will adopt safer drug-taking practices, at the very least.

Bibliography

Barnes, D. M. (1988). Drugs: Running the numbers. *Science, 240,* 1729–1731.

Brecher, E. M. (Ed.). (1972). *Licit and illicit drugs.* Boston: Little, Brown.

Caldwell, A. E. (1978). History of psychopharmacology. In W. G. Clark & J. Del Giudice (Eds.), *Principles of psychopharmacology* (pp. 9–40). New York: Academic Press.

Davis, R. M., Boyd, G. M., & Schoenborn, C. A. (1990). "Common courtesy" and the elimination of passive smoking. *Journal of the American Medical Association, 263,* 2208–2210.

Ellickson, P. L., & Bell, R. M. (1990). Drug prevention in junior high: A multi-site longitudinal test. *Science, 247,* 1299–1305.

Gerbner, G. (1990). Stories that hurt: Tobacco, alcohol, and other drugs in the mass media. In H. Resnick (Ed.), *Youth and drugs: Society's mixed messages* (pp. 53–127). Rockville, MD: U.S. Department of Health and Human Services.

Gibbons, D., & Connelly, J. (Eds.). (1970). *Selected readings in psychology* (p. 77). St. Louis: Mosby.

Gitlin, T. (1990). On drugs and mass media in America's consumer society. In H. Resnick (Ed.), *Youth and drugs: Society's mixed messages* (pp. 31–52). Rockville, MD: U.S. Department of Health and Human Services.

Goldstein, A., & Kalant, H. (1990). Drug policy: Striking the right balance. *Science, 249,* 1513–1521.

Jarvik, M. E. (1990). The drug dilemma: Manipulating the demand. *Science, 250,* 387–392.

Johnston, L. D., O'Malley, P. M., & Bachman, J. G. (1991). *Drug use among American high school seniors, college students and young adults, 1975–1990.* Rockville, MD: National Institute on Drug Abuse.

Kozel, N. J., & Adams, E. H. (1986). Epidemiology of drug abuse: An overview. *Science, 234,* 970–974.

Kushnir, T. (1986). Smoking and drinking as psychological tools in stressful social situations: Assumptions of fiction writers. *International Journal of the Addictions, 21,* 1119–1123.

Leavitt, F. (1982). *Drugs and behavior.* New York: John Wiley & Sons.

Marshall, E. (1988a). Flying blind in the war on drugs. *Science, 240,* 1605–1607.

Marshall, E. (1988b). Drug wars: Legalization gets a hearing. *Science, 241,* 1157–1159.

Mosher, J. F. (1990). Drug availability in a public health perspective. In H. Resnick (Ed.), *Youth and drugs: Society's mixed messages* (pp. 129–168). Rockville, MD: U.S. Department of Health and Human Services.

Newcomb, M. D., & Bentler, P. M. (1989). Substance use and abuse among children and teenagers. *American Psychologist, 44,* 242–248.

Siegel, R. K. (1989). *Intoxication.* New York: Pocket Books.

Smart, R. G., & Adlaf, E. M. (1986). Patterns of drug use among adolescents: The past decade. *Social Science and Medicine, 23,* 717–719.

Stephens, R. C. (1987). *Mind-altering drugs.* Newbury Park, CA: Sage.

Szasz, T. (1974). *Ceremonial chemistry.* New York: Anchor Press/Doubleday.

Wallace, B., & Fisher, L. E. (1991). *Consciousness and behavior* (3rd ed.). Boston: Allyn & Bacon.

Wallack, L., & Corbett, K. (1990). Illicit drug, tobacco, and alcohol use among youth: Trends and promising approaches in prevention. In H. Resnick (Ed.), *Youth and drugs: Society's mixed messages* (pp. 5–30). Rockville, MD: U.S. Department of Health and Human Services.

Weidner, G., & Istvan, J. (1985). Dietary sources of caffeine. *New England Journal of Medicine, 313,* 1421.

Chapter Two

Basic Principles of Pharmacology

Before getting into the "psycho" part of psychopharmacology, it might be useful to become familiar first with the "pharmaco" part—that is, the drug component. There are some basic pharmacological principles that all drugs share and that influence the action of psychotropic drugs. This chapter will briefly describe these principles and define many terms that will be used in subsequent chapters.

The first term that should be defined is **drug**. This might appear to be a simple task, but in fact there is no legal or commonly accepted definition of "drug." As indicated in Chapter 1, a drug originally referred to any substance used in chemistry or medical practice. Gradually, the term was restricted to any agent used in medicine or any ingredient in medicines. Today many people use the term as a synonym for a narcotic agent or illicit substance. None of these definitions is of much value. Each one defines the term in a highly restrictive way, defines it by using a synonym that itself is undefined, or fails to define it in terms of function.

What is a drug then? In general, it is a chemical that affects one or more biological processes. However, not all chemicals that affect biological processes are considered drugs. Substances that are commonly used for nutritional purposes, such as salt, water, proteins, fats, carbohydrates, vitamins, and minerals, are not generally considered drugs, because they are necessary for carrying out the normal biological functions of the body. However, certain vitamins and minerals that might be found in our diet, if isolated and used in certain quantities, might also be thought of as drugs.

For example, not long ago, *starch blockers* were in vogue. Manufacturers of these substances claimed that they prevented the absorption of starches, like pasta and bread, by blocking the action of certain enzymes needed to digest the starch. Because these substances were simply extracts made from beans, the manufacturers claimed they were not drugs.

The Food and Drug Administration (FDA) disagreed, claiming that by altering the digestive process by manipulating enzymes, these substances were drugs. After a lengthy court battle and after millions of tablets containing these substances had been purchased by the public, the FDA finally won. (Eventually it was found that starch blockers did not do what they were supposed to do in the body, and in some cases caused gastrointestinal disturbances, so interest in them quickly died out.)

Chemicals originating or produced within an organism that are used to carry out the normal biological functions in the body are also not usually thought of as drugs. Such chemicals are referred to as *endogenous* substances, as opposed to drugs, which are *exogenous* substances. However, biochemists and neuroscientists have isolated a variety of substances found to be important in the functions of the body, have extracted or synthesized them, and have administered them in purified form to reverse neurological deficits. The use of L-dopa, a chemical necessary for the production of an important brain chemical, in the treatment of Parkinson's disease is one example, and it is viewed as a drug.

In short, chemicals used in the normal biological processes of the body are generally not viewed as drugs. However, what is considered normal? As an example, consider aspirin, which is an effective treatment for several kinds of pain. It is believed that most of its action is due to its ability to inhibit the activity of prostaglandins, a class of chemicals found throughout the body that play a vital role in almost every life process, including respiration, reproduction, and circulation. Unfortunately, their presence can also be painful, presumably because they induce swelling of the sensory nerve tips responsible for detecting painful stimuli. If one thinks of the pain as the result of excessive prostaglandin activity, is this considered an abnormal condition that is restored to normal with a chemical, or is it a normal condition that is altered through the action of aspirin?

In this context, it would seem most appropriate to define a **drug** as a nonfood chemical that alters one or more normal biological processes in living organisms. However, as already noted, there are several potential exceptions to this definition.

Aside from the actual molecular structure of a drug, the most important factors in determining a drug's effect are the concentration of the drug at its site(s) of action and the rate of accumulation there. These factors, in turn, can be affected by many other factors, most commonly the drug **dose**—that is, the quantity of drug administered at one time. Often, particularly under experimental conditions in psychopharmacology, drug dose is expressed in terms of unit of drug per unit of body weight of the organism, such as milligrams per kilogram (mg/kg). (Drug **dosage** refers to administrations of the drug per unit of time, such as 10 mg/kg four times a day for three days.) That is, we would clearly expect

10 mg of a drug to result in much higher concentrations in a rat than in a human, and therefore to be capable of exerting a much greater effect in that rat than in the human. Unfortunately, equivalent units of drug per unit of body weight do not usually translate into equivalent effects, either across species or within species. As we will see, there can be large differences in the rate and degree of a drug's absorption, distribution, metabolization, and excretion across species and in different ages. Also, animal species differ with respect to the amounts of tissue for drug storage. The fact that drugs are not generally dispersed evenly throughout the body and are usually taken up in tissues other than the site of drug action can affect the drug's action.

Drugs and Receptors

The study of the biochemical and physiological effects of drugs and their mechanisms of action is termed **pharmacodynamics** (Ross, 1990). The vast majority of drugs act at very specific sites throughout the body. These interaction sites are referred to as *receptors.* They are fairly large molecules (usually protein) which comprise the sites where biologically active chemicals of the body, often called **ligands**, induce their effects. (Most of the ligands you are probably familiar with are hormones, such as insulin, testosterone, estrogen, and adrenaline. Later on you will become familiar with the ligands known as neurotransmitters, neurohormones, and neuromodulators.) When a chemical occupies a receptor, it is referred to as being "bound" to it. If the receptor then starts some biological activity, it is said to be "activated." In most cases, binding is temporary, or, reversible, and when the chemical leaves the receptor, it is said to "dissociate" from the receptor. **Affinity** refers to the capacity of a compound to maintain contact with or be bound to a receptor. **Intrinsic activity** refers to the relative capability of a compound to activate the receptor after being bound to it.

Compounds with both an affinity for and a capability of activating a receptor are referred to as **agonists**. If the compound activating the receptor is endogenous (naturally synthesized in the body), it is called a ligand. If it is exogenous (produced outside the body), it is a drug. Both ligands and some drugs can be called agonists. In some cases, drugs do not combine directly with a receptor, but enhance the amount of the endogenous ligands available for the receptor. In such situations, the drug may be referred to as an **indirect agonist**. Some drugs exert their effects by blocking the action of agonists and are thus called **antagonists**; different types of antagonists will be discussed later in this chapter.

In addition to the preceding classifications, a complicated and sometimes contradictory nomenclature has arisen to describe the effects of some classes of drugs, for example, opiates and benzodiazepines. That is, drugs may produce complex patterns of response that have led to the terms **inverse agonist** and **mixed agonist-antagonist** (Kenakin, 1987). Specifically, an inverse agonist is defined as a drug that appears to act through the same receptor as an agonist but produces effects opposite to those of the agonist; thus it can also be viewed as a type of agonist (e.g., see p. 155). Most notably, a mixed agonist-antagonist is evidenced when a drug acts as an agonist by itself, but blocks the activity of another agonist in the same system (e.g., see p. 236).

Although these scenarios are indeed confusing, the overall picture is not likely to become clearer until we get a better understanding of how receptors and their ligands interact to alter biological systems. For example, one view of the receptor is that it consists of one element comprising a "binding" site and another element comprising an "effector" site (Cooper et al., 1991). This model very easily handles cases in which a drug with a molecular structure compatible with both sites is an agonist and a drug with a structure compatible only with the binding site prevents the agonist from binding and thus prevents its action; that is, the latter drug acts as an antagonist. However, this model has difficulties in explaining some phenomena, most notably inverse agonism and mixed agonism-antagonism. Another model proposes that receptors exist in an active and an inactive configuration, each of which is capable of combining with a drug molecule. Thus, whether a drug acts as an antagonist or agonist will be determined by the ratio of the drug's affinity for the two configurations. For example, a drug may have a higher affinity for the active configuration than the inactive configuration, so that at low concentrations the drug acts as an agonist. However, at higher concentrations the drug may combine with the inactive configuration, preventing the receptor from attaining its active configuration, so that the drug acts as an antagonist. These and other models of receptors are at present purely conjectural and subject to modification as we gain more information on receptor structure-activity relationships. A fuller discussion of the way brain cell receptors are believed to work will be presented in Chapter 4.

It is likely that a critical number of receptors of some specific type have to be occupied by an agonist before a biological response can begin to occur and that once all receptors are occupied no further biological activity is possible. This hypothesis accounts for the typically nonlinear relationship between drug dose and drug effect. An agonist with high intrinsic activity causes a maximal response by activating proportionately fewer receptors. An agonist with low instrinsic activity may fail to elicit a maximal response compared to compounds with higher intrinsic activity.

The interaction between ligands (or drugs, since they operate in much the same way) and receptors is much like that between keys and locks. Just as one may have many keys and many locks, the body has many ligands and many receptors. Not all keys (ligands) fit all locks (receptors), but some keys may fit in several different locks, although one may have to wiggle the key a lot in some cases in order to get it into the lock. It could be said that the keys have different affinities for each lock; in some cases there is no fit at all, in others the fit is poor but adequate, and in others the fit is very good.

Continuing this analogy, note that each lock (receptor) and key (ligand) combination serves a different function; one key may unlock your car door, another may turn on the ignition, another opens your front door, another opens your safe-deposit box, and so on. It could be said that each key has intrinsic activity at its respective lock. However, have you ever driven a car with separate keys for the door and the ignition? If so, have you ever stuck the ignition key in the door lock or vice versa? It fit fine, but you could not turn the key (activate the receptor). The same thing happens with ligands and receptors. Thus a key may have an affinity for a lock but have no effect on it—that is, no intrinsic activity. As is the case with affinity, a key's intrinsic activity may be high, low, or absent; that is, it may open (activate) the lock easily, with difficulty, or not at all.

There are a few basic differences between the ligand/receptor relationship and the key/lock relationship. First, although the receptor fit may be determined by a ligand's molecular shape—that is, the arrangement of its atoms—it may also be determined by the position of the molecule's positive and negative electrical charges. Second, there is no human hand guiding the ligand into the receptor; except for the differential electrical charges on the ligands that allow proper alignment with their receptors, ligands run into receptors pretty much randomly. Therefore, whether ligands come in contact with their receptors or not is heavily dependent on the concentration of the ligands and the number of receptors available.

Dose-Response Relationships

From the previous discussion, you learned that a drug's actions depend upon the amount of drug available, which, in turn, is dependent upon the dose of drug given (Abel, 1974). The usual way of discussing a drug's action is in terms of the **dose-response function**, which expresses the relationship between the dose administered and the response observed. Dose-response functions are determined by taking groups of individuals, which represent a certain population that one is interested in, administering each group a different amount of the drug in question, waiting a sufficient length of time for the drug to act, and assessing the degree of effect or the number of individuals displaying a specified effect of the drug.

For purposes of comparison, one group is administered a substance without any physiological effects, called a **placebo**, instead of the drug, because many individuals display physical or psychological symptoms if they expect to receive a drug (Leavitt, 1982). In animals, a placebo generally consists of **saline** solution (water containing the same amount of sodium chloride as is normally found in the body). In some cases—for instance, with humans who may be knowledgeable about some of the characteristics of a drug they are reportedly taking—it is advisable to administer an **active placebo**. This is a substance that mimics some of the noticeable physiological characteristics of the drug being evaluated but without the effects on the brain that the researcher is interested in. As a final control measure, a **double-blind procedure** is used, whereby neither the subject nor the person administering the preparation knows whether it is a drug or a placebo.

Though proper experimental drug protocols require the use of a placebo, in clinical trials where a drug is being evaluated for its effectiveness (efficacy) in relieving the symptoms of a particular disorder the use of a placebo may be unethical or impractical. For example, if a drug is being evaluated for its antidepressant properties, it may be unethical to give depressed patients a placebo when there are drugs currently in use that have a 70–80% effectiveness rate. If these patients do not show symptom remission and they attempt or commit suicide or feel even more hopeless than they did before the treatment, the researchers might be held morally, if not legally, responsible. It is also understandable why some patients are reluctant to participate in such a trial when they know they might be part of a control group that receives an inactive substance. Thus it may be necessary for those who are placed in a control group to receive a substance that has a medically accepted level of effectiveness. The effectiveness of the experimental drug would then be compared with that of the control drug. Unfortunately, this procedure makes it more difficult to establish the experimental drug's true level of effectiveness because it is often easier to obtain results indicating that there is no difference between two treatments when they are in fact different, than it is to demonstrate that they are different.

For illustrative purposes, Figure 2–1 shows several idealized dose-response functions for some of the effects of the drug *d*-amphetamine that have occurred in laboratory rats. In Figure 2–1(a), we can see that as the dose of amphetamine administered increases, the percentage of time that the rats exhibit stereotypy (a repetitive, ritualistic, or compulsive set of behaviors, such as moving the head back and forth repetitively or gnawing at nonexistent objects) also increases.

In Figure 2–1(b), which expresses the relationship between the dose of amphetamine and the generalized locomotor activity of rats, we see that activity tends to increase with increases in amphetamine dosage up to a point. With larger doses of amphetamine, activity appears to be less and less apparent, and with a sufficiently large dose of amphetamine,

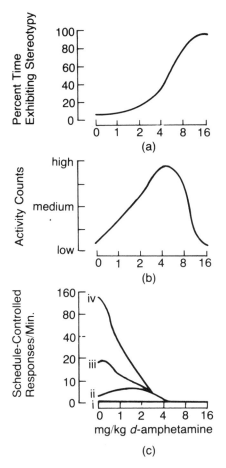

Figure 2–1

Various relationships between the dose of *d*-amphetamine and its behavioral effects in rats.

activity may actually occur at lower levels than with no drug at all (depicted as 0 mg/kg). Such functions are often called biphasic or curvilinear. For example, it has been suggested that a curvilinear relationship exists between clinical improvement and the blood plasma level (which may be directly related to dose) of some drugs used in the treatment of depression and psychosis. In this case, the optimal therapeutic results in schizophrenics and depressed patients can be obtained when the plasma levels are in a certain range, known as the **therapeutic window**; levels below and above the window are associated with poorer outcomes (Preskorn et al., 1988; Van Putten et al., 1988).

For the many drugs with a therapeutic threshold or range of effective drug levels, knowledge of these drugs' **plasma half-lives**—that is, the time it takes to eliminate half the drug from the bloodstream—can help to predict desirable drug doses and intervals between administrations (Swartz, 1991). For example, the antidepressant drug Prozac has a long plasma half-life of 1 to 3 days. Thus it may only need to be taken once a day to maintain plasma levels within the therapeutic window. If administered more frequently or in too large a dose, the plasma levels may progressively increase and exceed the therapeutic window; then it may induce toxic effects or side effects that decrease the overall well-being of the patient.

In Figure 2–1(c), we see that the effect of amphetamine on schedule-controlled behavior (that is, operant responses whose rate of occurrence is determined by the schedule of reinforcement) is quite complex. The effect depends on the dose of amphetamine and the normal rate of response without the drug (Seiden & Dykstra, 1977). That is, responses that occur at a fairly high rate to begin with become relatively less frequent with increasingly larger doses of amphetamine, whereas responses that occur somewhat infrequently become relatively more frequent with low to moderate doses of amphetamine, and then decrease with high doses of amphetamine. In the figure, condition *i* might occur if there were no reinforcement provided; condition *ii* might occur if responses were only reinforced if the animal spaced its responses with some minimum interval (such as 10 seconds) between them; condition *iii* might occur if responses were reinforced after variable periods of time had elapsed; and condition *iv* might occur if responses were reinforced after a specified number of responses had occurred. In each of these cases, the direction of amphetamine's effect at each dose—that is, whether there is a relative increase or decrease in the response frequency—depends on the normal rate of responding that occurs without the drug.

In summary, several observations may be made regarding dose-response relationships:

1. One cannot say what effect a drug will have unless one specifies what the dose of the drug is (and in what species).
2. There may be many different dose-response functions for any particular drug, depending upon the type of response monitored.
3. There is no "typical" dose-response function.
4. Larger doses of a drug do not necessarily mean a greater magnitude of response.

It should also be mentioned that there are two general types of dose-response functions, one describing the degree or magnitude of a specified response and another describing the percentage of organisms displaying a specified response.

Despite these difficulties in characterizing dose-response functions, let us look at some "typical" dose-response functions, shown in Figure

2–2, and discuss their various attributes. First, note that there are some doses that do not induce any noticeable effects. The arrow at point *a* indicates the **threshold dose** (or minimally effective dose), which is the dose just large enough to produce a detectable change in the response. The arrow at point *b* indicates the **maximum (or maximal) response**, which is the greatest degree of a given response that can be achieved with that drug. The maximal response is not necessarily produced by the largest effective dose of a drug, because at higher doses some agents (such as nicotine) antagonize the response brought about at lower doses, and some agents (such as amphetamine) induce effects that may compete with, interfere with, or suppress the behavior noted at lower doses. The arrow at point *c* depicts the **median effective dose**, which is the dose of the drug that produces a desired, and generally therapeutic, effect in 50% of the individuals tested. It is abbreviated **ED50**. If you draw a perpendicular line up from the ED50 to where it intersects the dose-response function, and then horizontally over to the response axis, it intersects with the 50th percentile—that is, the point at which 50% of the population is affected. Other EDs can be specified for a drug, but in practice such levels are rarely specified. For example, the ED5 would indicate the dose effective in 5% of the population. At this point it should be mentioned that because drugs are often used in different therapeutic contexts, a drug may have several ED50s. For instance, a barbiturate may have one ED50 for its sedative effects,

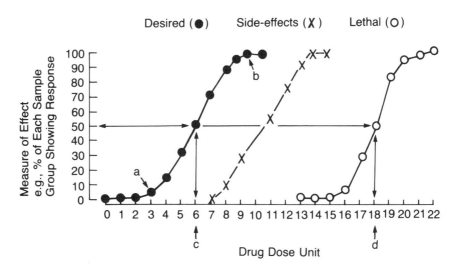

Figure 2–2

Stylized dose-response functions depicting (*a*) the threshold dose, (*b*) maximal (desired) response, (*c*) the ED50 of the drug, and (*d*) the LD50 of the drug.

another for its sleep-inducing effects, and another for its anesthetic actions.

All drugs can have lethal consequences, and clearly there is a relationship between the dose of a drug and lethality. Just as the ED50 for a drug can be specified, so can the **median lethal dose** or **LD50** (indicated by the arrow at point d in the figure). The LD50 is the dose that causes death in 50% of the population. Therapeutically speaking, one hopes that the LD50 for a drug is considerably larger than its ED50. In fact, a drug's relative margin of safety, called the **therapeutic index**, is often specified in terms of the drug's LD50 relative to its ED50. It is determined by simply dividing the LD50 by the ED50. For the hypothetical drug in Figure 2–2, the ED50 is 6 units and the LD50 is 18 units, so the drug's therapeutic index is 3. A drug with a therapeutic index of around 100—that is, where the LD50 is 100 times larger than the ED50—is generally considered safe, whereas a drug with a therapeutic index under 10 is generally considered quite hazardous. Unfortunately, though, the therapeutic index is a very gross measure of a drug's potential hazards, because many drugs have side effects, some of which may be very disabling, which can occur at doses much lower than the LD50. Also, one drug may have a considerably higher therapeutic index than another drug, but may have certain properties that increase the likelihood of the individual self-administering lethal amounts. For example, a person taking a drug that induces euphoria or mental confusion could accidentally take too large a dose.

By its very definition, the ED100 of a therapeutic drug would be most likely to exhibit positive effects in the greatest number of patients. However, the **maximum efficacy** of a drug is sometimes determined by other factors, such as side effects, which limit the largest amount of the drug that can be given to a patient. For example, in Figure 2–2, note that the ED100, which is about 9 units, produces side effects in about 30% of the subjects. With some drugs, variability in response from one patient to another is small, while in others it is very large, requiring each patient to be individually "titrated." (Most commonly, the variability is large when the slope of the dose-response function is steep.) Those individuals who overrespond to the ED50 of a drug are called **hyperreactors**; those who underrespond are called **hyporeactors**. The term **idiosyncrasy** is used to describe an unexpected response or unusual effect of a drug, such as drowsiness induced by amphetamine. The response may be independent of dose, and it implies more than just a hyper- or hyporesponsiveness.

The dose-response function can be used to illustrate a number of other concepts in pharmacology. Figure 2–3 depicts the dose-response functions for several analgesic drugs. Note that the doses of heroin needed to achieve analgesia are smaller than the doses of morphine needed to induce equivalent degrees of analgesia, which, in turn, are smaller than the doses of aspirin needed. The term **potency** refers to the

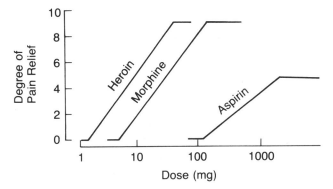

Figure 2–3

Dose-response relationships for aspirin, morphine, and heroin with respect to their relative potencies in reducing moderately severe pain, with 0 indicating no pain relief and 10 indicating complete absence of pain.

ability of a drug, relative to other drugs, to induce a given effect. It is not synonymous with a drug's potential lethality or toxicity, unless these are the specific effects in which one is interested. The smaller the dose needed to produce a given effect, the more potent the drug. Therefore, heroin is considered to be the most potent of the three drugs in inducing analgesia.

In the past much has been made of potency, but it is really of little clinical importance unless an increase in potency is associated with a decrease in undesirable side effects or with an increase in the maximal response achieved. Although heroin is more potent than morphine in inducing analgesia, morphine is capable of achieving the same maximal degree of pain relief as heroin. In fact, the clinical profiles of the two drugs are so similar that there is little reason to recommend one over the other. On the other hand, heroin and morphine are not only more potent than aspirin; they are also capable of achieving a higher maximal effect. Thus, they are said to have a greater **efficacy** or to be more **efficacious**—terms that refer to the degree to which a drug is able to induce a given desirable effect.

When discussing the dose-response function for any drug, one must take into consideration the route of administration, the time since the drug was administered, and the number and spacing of drug exposures. As we will see in Chapter 3, a given amount of a drug can have very different effects, in terms of intensity and duration, when administered orally versus intravenously. Once a drug has been administered, the type of effect and the magnitude of a given effect will vary across time because the concentration of a drug is rarely sufficient to exert much of an effect if the time period is too short or too long. Thus time-response curves are often graphed in much the same way that dose-response functions are graphed.

Finally, if a drug is administered on more than one occasion, a number of changes in the response to the drug may occur. The drug may accumulate in the body and produce greater and greater effects. In many cases, particularly with drugs used to treat mental and emotional disturbances, it may take several days or weeks of continued exposure before the beneficial effects of the drug are evidenced. In some cases, an enhanced response to a drug may occur because of previous exposure, but the drug is given at intervals far enough apart that the response cannot be attributed to drug accumulation. This effect, found with a variety of drugs, including amphetamine, cocaine, marijuana, antipsychotics, antidepressants, and antianxiety drugs, is known as **sensitization** (Antelman et al., 1987). However, in most cases, effects noted with initial drug exposures are no longer evidenced or are greatly reduced after chronic use—a phenomenon referred to as **tolerance**, which will be discussed in Chapter 6.

Drug Interactions

Sometimes the potency of a drug is reduced in the presence of another drug, and sometimes it is enhanced. The situation in which the response to one drug is decreased in the presence of another drug is referred to as **antagonism**. The opposite situation is referred to as **synergism**, whereby two drugs together produce a greater effect than either drug produces alone.

Various forms of antagonism and synergism for several hypothetical drugs are depicted in Figure 2–4. In the figure, note that while drugs *A*, *B*, and *D* are all effective in inducing sleep, drug *A* is most potent, whereas drugs *C* and *E* are incapable of inducing sleep at any dose. The *A* + *B*, *A* + *D*, *A* + *E*, *A* + *C*, and *B* + *C* dose-response functions show what may happen to the dose-response functions for drugs *A* and *B* when various doses of these drugs are combined with a given dose of the other drugs.

There are two basic types of antagonism: **pharmacological** and **physiological**. A **pharmacological antagonist** is a drug that has a definite affinity for a receptor but has little or no intrinsic activity after being bound to it. In the case of **pharmacological antagonism**—that is, when a pharmacological antagonist is in combination with a receptor—an agonist cannot bind to and activate that receptor. If the antagonist is capable of dissociating from the receptor, so that there is "competition" between the antagonist and agonist for the receptor, it is referred to as **competitive antagonism**. In Figure 2–4 the shift to the right (without change in

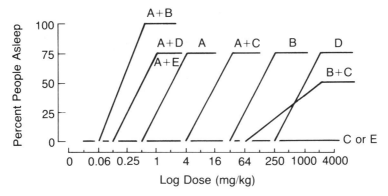

Figure 2–4

Dose-response functions for drugs *A, B, C, D,* and *E* when administered alone and in various combinations.

the slope or maximal response) in the dose-response function for *A* in the presence of 500 mg/kg of *C* (*A* + *C* function) would indicate that *C* is a competitive antagonist of *A*. If the antagonist is incapable of being dissociated or displaced from the receptor, the relationship is referred to as **noncompetitive antagonism**. In Figure 2–4 the shift to the right in the dose-response function of *B*, and the lower maximal response achieved in the presence of 500 mg/kg of *C* (*B* + *C* function), would indicate that *C* is a noncompetitive antagonist of B.

In both cases, in the presence of a given dose of the antagonist, the agonist's potency is reduced, as reflected in the agonist's dose-response function being shifted to the right. However, in competitive antagonism, since the number of receptors available does not change, the agonist's original maximal effect can still be achieved, assuming a large enough dose of the agonist is administered. In noncompetitive antagonism, the number of available receptors declines. Thus the maximal effect achievable decreases, and the slope of the agonist's dose-response function is likely to be shallower.

Physiological antagonism is a form of drug interaction in which two drugs (they may be either pharmacological agonists or pharmacological antagonists) act at two different kinds of receptors—that is, receptors whose biological actions oppose each other. For example, a drug may activate receptors that cause the heart to beat faster. Another drug may activate receptors that cause the heart to beat more slowly. Upon exposure to the first drug, the heart would speed up. Upon exposure to the second drug, the heart rate would return to normal levels; that is, the effects of the first drug would be counteracted (antagonized) by the second. Functionally, an inverse agonist is the same as a physiological antagonist, except that with the inverse agonist the receptor involved appears to be the same type that is activated by an agonist.

There are also several kinds of synergism, two of which are **addition** and **potentiation**. In the case of addition, two drugs produce the same overt effect, and the effect of the two drugs taken together is the sum of their individual effects. In Figure 2–4 the dose-response function for A in the presence of 500 mg/kg of D ($A + D$ function) would suggest that addition is involved, since D by itself is capable of inducing the same degree of effect as A and the maximal response to A was unchanged in the presence of D. For instance, two beers and two glasses of wine lead to greater intoxication than do two beers alone or two glasses of wine alone. Alcohol and barbiturates—two drugs that have similar sedative-hypnotic properties—also have an additive effect when used together.

Potentiation occurs when two drugs, only one of which generally produces a given effect, in combination induce effects greater than the sum of their individual effects. In Figure 2–4 the greater maximal response and shift to the left of the dose-response function for A in the presence of 64 mg/kg of B ($A + B$ function) would indicate that B potentiates the effects of A. However, the shift to the left in the dose response function for A in the presence of 500 mg/kg of E ($A + E$ function) would also indicate that E potentiates the effects of A, since E was incapable of inducing any effect by itself.

If two drugs are each capable of inducing the same overt effect (as is the case with drugs A and B in Figure 2–4), it is often difficult to distinguish whether addition or potentiation is occurring when the drugs are combined. For this reason, one often hears on the one hand that alcohol potentiates the effects of antianxiety agents, and on the other that their effects are additive. In general, however, potentiation is indicated if the maximal effect of two drugs together is greater than the maximal effect achieved with either drug alone or if the slope of the dose-response function for one drug is steeper when that drug is combined with the other drug.

Although some readers may find the concepts of potentiation and addition fairly easy to grasp, others have trouble with them—particularly with respect to drugs having a similar spectrum of effects. Perhaps an illustration will clarify matters. If 100 people drink 200 ml of ethanol in an hour, probably none of them will die, unless, of course, they go out and try to drive a vehicle under the influence of this amount of alcohol. However, if they drink an additional 100 ml of ethanol, for a total of 300 ml (about a fifth of 80 proof whiskey) in an hour, 10 of those people may die. If those 100 people drink 600 ml of ethanol in an hour—double the 300 ml—the number of people who die will not be 20, or double the deaths, but will be closer to 90. In other words, doubling the dose of alcohol that produces a given effect does not necessarily double the magnitude of the effect.

Now let's assume that, although drinking 200 ml of ethanol does not kill anybody, drinking 350 ml of ethanol is capable of killing 40% of the people in the sample. Furthermore, assume that 50 mg of Valium produces the same effects as 150 ml of ethanol. If 100 people were to take 50 mg of Valium along with 200 ml of ethanol, and 40 people died, it would be an illustration of addition. That is, the effects of 150 ml of ethanol plus the effects of 200 ml of ethanol equal the effects of 350 ml of ethanol, or 40 deaths; the effects of 150 ml of ethanol equal the effects of 50 mg of Valium; therefore, the effects of 50 mg of Valium plus the effects of 200 ml of ethanol equal the effects of 350 ml of ethanol, or 40 deaths, if the effects are additive. It would only be a case of potentiation if more than 40 people died. However, because neither 50 mg of Valium nor 200 ml of ethanol are lethal by themselves, and because their combination results in a sizable number of deaths, many people might assume that they potentiate each other.

Thus, to summarize, in order to determine whether the combination of two drugs that are capable of inducing the same effects involves addition or potentiation, one must

1. establish what the dose-response functions for the drugs are separately;
2. establish what the minimally effective doses of the two drugs are; and
3. determine whether the combination of these two doses results in an effect greater than that achieved by simply doubling the minimally effective dose of one of the drugs.

If the effect with the drug combination exceeds the effect of simply doubling the minimally effective dose of one of the drugs, it would indicate potentiation. If the effect of the drug combination and the effect created by doubling the minimally effective dose of one of the drugs are comparable, then you have addition. Since this three-step procedure is rarely followed, there generally are confusing differences in terminology used by different sources in distinguishing whether drugs like alcohol, "minor" and "major" tranquilizers, sleeping aids, and antidepressants induce additive or potentiating effects.

Antagonistic and synergistic effects are only some of the potential results of combining drugs. Drugs typically interact in inexplicable ways, and the more drugs given the more complex the situation becomes. Therefore, generally speaking, the fewer the drugs given the better. Nevertheless, it is not uncommon to see a schizophrenic treated with two or more antipsychotic drugs, despite the admonitions of most experts. The patient may also be prescribed an antidepressant (also contraindicated in most cases), drugs to counteract the motor disturbances induced by the antipsychotic, and a muscle relaxant. With such chemical "salads," it is almost impossible to predict what the outcome will be.

Unfortunately, people who see different physicians for different problems sometimes do not inform their physicians of this fact, or their physicians may not be aware of certain drug interactions, and the patients end up taking combinations in which the drugs negate or amplify each other or induce idiosyncratic reactions. Similarly, recreational drugs with very different biochemical properties—for example, alcohol and cocaine, alcohol and nicotine, or cocaine and heroin—are commonly combined to produce complex mixtures of synergistic and antagonistic actions and effects. Few empirical studies specifically concerned with these drug combinations have been published (Dial, 1992; Kerr et al., 1991).

Bibliography

Abel, E. L. (1974). *Drugs and behavior.* New York: John Wiley & Sons.

Antelman, S. M., Kocan, D., Edwards, D. J., & Knopf, S. (1987). A single injection of diazepam induces long-lasting sensitization. *Psychopharmacology Bulletin, 23,* 430–434.

Cooper, J. R., Bloom, F. E., & Roth, R. H. (1991). *The biochemical basis of neuropharmacology,* 6th ed. New York: Oxford University Press.

Dial, J. (1992). The interaction of alcohol and cocaine: A review. *Psychobiology, 20,* 179–184.

Kenakin, T. (1987). Agonists, partial agonists, antagonists, inverse agonists and agonist/antagonists? *Trends in the Pharmacological Sciences, 8,* 423–426.

Kerr, J. S., Sherwood, N., & Hindmarch, I. (1991). Separate and combined effects of the social drugs on psychomotor performance. *Psychopharmacology, 104,* 113–119.

Leavitt, F. (1982). *Drugs and behavior.* New York: John Wiley & Sons.

Preskorn, S. H., Weller, E., Jerkovich, G., Hughes, C. W., & Weller, R. (1988). Depression in children: Concentration-dependent CNS toxicity of tricyclic antidepressants. *Psychopharmacology Bulletin, 24,* 140–142.

Ross, E. M. (1990). Pharmacodynamics: Mechanisms of drug action and the relationship between drug concentration and effect. In A. G. Gilman, T. W. Rall, A. S. Nies, & P. Taylor (Eds.), *The pharmacological basis of therapeutics* (pp. 33–48). New York: Pergamon Press.

Seiden, L. S., & Dykstra, L. A. (1977). *Psychopharmacology: A biochemical and behavioral approach.* New York: Van Nostrand Reinhold.

Swartz, C. M. (1991). Drug dose prediction with flexible test doses. *Journal of Clinical Pharmacology, 31,* 662–667.

Van Putten, T., Marder, S. R., Mintz, J., & Poland, R. E. (1988). Haloperidol plasma levels and clinical response: A therapeutic window relationship. *Psychopharmacology Bulletin, 24,* 172–175.

Chapter Three

Pharmacokinetics

The effects of a particular drug on an organism depend heavily on the rate of accumulation and the concentration of the drug at its sites of action and the duration of contact at those sites (Shibanoki et al., 1987). These are a function not only of the amount of drug administered but of its **pharmacokinetics**. This term refers to the dynamic processes involved in the movement of drugs within biological systems with respect to the drug's absorption, distribution, binding or localization in tissues, metabolic alterations, and excretion from the body (see Benet et al. 1990, for a complete discussion of this area). Differences among organisms in their pharmacokinetics, due to genetic differences, the presence of other drugs, disease, and physiological and psychological status, can result in 5- to 20-fold differences (these are ballpark figures) in their reactions to a given amount of drug within species, and 20- to 100-fold differences in their reactions across species (Gillette et al., 1985). In some cases, a drug may not have the effect, at any dose, in one organism that it may have in another organism.

Drug Absorption

In order for drugs to reach their sites of action, they must first pass through several biological membranes, as diagrammed in Figure 3–1. The type and number of these membranes depend upon the drug's site(s) of action (in the case of psychotropic drugs this would be the nervous system) and the route of administration. For example, for an orally administered drug to exert an action on the brain, it must pass through a variety of biological membranes before it can reach the cells of the brain that are responsible for the drug's psychoactive properties. Several factors, such as the salt form of the drug, the particle size of the dosage

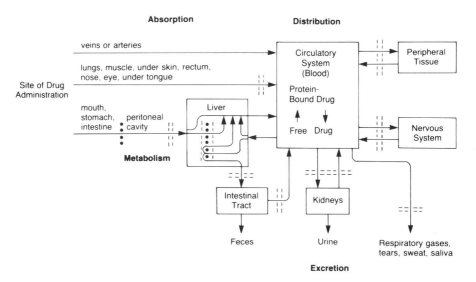

Figure 3–1

Summary diagram illustrating the major pharmacokinetic factors that influence the onset, duration, and intensity of psychoactive drug effects. Lipid membranes that must be crossed are indicated by ⫶. Enzymes that are capable of metabolizing drugs are indicated by ⫶ . From the site of administration, drugs must cross one or more lipid membranes in order to be absorbed into the circulatory system (unless injected directly into the blood supply). In addition, drugs taken orally or injected into the peritoneal cavity initially pass through the liver, where they may be structurally altered (metabolism) prior to entering the blood. Once in the blood supply, the free, unbound drug molecules—those not bound to plasma proteins—will be distributed to various organs (including the brain, liver, kidney, and adipose tissue) and then redistributed to other organs and tissues by the blood. At some point, an equilibrium is often established whereby the relative concentration of drug in tissue and blood is maintained at a constant level (the blood-to-tissue ratio varies depending on the tissue and whether there are specific binding sites for the drug). Metabolism of drugs may occur in many tissues, but most metabolism occurs in the liver. From the liver, drugs or their metabolites may then reenter the blood supply or may be absorbed into the bile, which eventually ends up in the intestinal tract. From the intestinal tract, drugs or their metabolites may be eliminated in feces or reabsorbed into the circulatory system. Water-soluble drugs or metabolites enter the kidneys and are excreted in urine. If they are still lipid-soluble, they will be reabsorbed into the circulatory system. A small (generally negligible) amount of drugs may be eliminated via the lungs, sweat, tears, saliva, or mother's milk. (See text for further details.)

form, and the suspending agent used, can affect the degree of absorption. Differences in these factors may account for why generic drugs, which are chemically identical to brand-name drugs, may occasionally not act like their brand-name counterparts; however, this appears to be a very rare situation.

One of the most fundamental factors affecting the passage of molecules from one side of a membrane to the other is the relative concentration of the molecule on the two sides. The greater the differential concentration of the molecules on the two sides, the more readily the molecules will diffuse from the site of higher concentration to the site of lower concentration. However, the most important factor in a drug's ability to pass through these biological membranes is its **lipid-solubility**—that is, its capability of being dissolved in fat (lipid material). These membranes, in general, are lipid in nature. Lipid-solubility is particularly important if a drug is to be psychoactive, for reasons that will be explained shortly. Although it is the case that very small water-soluble molecules and *ions* (positively or negatively charged particles) can diffuse through small aqueous channels located in the membranes, most drug molecules are too large to cross membranes in this manner and must diffuse through the substance of the membrane.

In order to dissolve in plasma and be effectively transported by the bloodstream, drugs must also be somewhat soluble in water. For these reasons, most drugs which are effective psychoactive agents are soluble to some extent in both oil and water. However, the relative solubility in each medium is a major factor in a drug's ability to get into the brain. To determine this relative affinity, a drug is often added to a mixture of water and refined olive oil. The mixture is shaken violently for a few seconds and then spun around to separate the oil and water. The drug concentration in the oil is divided by its concentration in the water. This figure is referred to as the drug's **oil/water partition coefficient**. The greater the drug's oil/water partition coefficient, the more easily the drug molecule can passively penetrate a lipoidal membrane, if other factors are held constant (Oldendorf & Dewhurst, 1978). For example, the differences in onset, intensity, and duration of the three analgesics morphine, meperidine (Demerol), and fentanyl (Innovar) are largely due to differences in their partition coefficients (van den Hoogen & Colpaert, 1987); that is, morphine's lower partition coefficient results in a slower onset of analgesia and less intensity, but a longer duration of action than fentanyl. A lower partition coefficient also increases the difference between a drug's ED50 when the drug is administered systemically—that is, into the general circulatory system—and its ED50 when it is administered directly into the brain. (See the next section for discussion of routes of administration.)

As stated earlier, two of the most important factors in a drug's effects are its concentration and its rate of accumulation at the site(s) of action. These, in turn, are heavily dependent on its concentration in the blood plasma (unless it is directly introduced into those sites), which is dependent on the drug's access to the blood, which is heavily influenced by the route of administration.

Routes of Administration

The most common route of drug administration is through the mouth (**per os** or P.O.) so that it is absorbed in various parts of the gastrointestinal (G.I.) tract. Rectal administration (through the rectal mucosa) may serve as an alternative *enteral* (within the intestine) route for drugs destroyed in the stomach or small intestine. The P.O. route is generally the safest, cheapest, and most convenient way of administering drugs. However, several factors can influence absorption of drugs from the G.I. tract, which can greatly alter the rate of drug accumulation, its concentration, and its duration at the site(s) of action.

Most drugs are thought to penetrate the G.I. mucosa by a process of passive diffusion, which in turn is limited mostly by the drug's lipid-solubility. Many drugs are weak bases (alkaloids) or weak acids, and this alkalinity or acidity often results in their being ionized. Such *ionization* reduces their solubility in cellular membranes because proteins embedded in these membranes have a mixture of positive and negative charges that tend to repel charged particles. Therefore, to facilitate their absorption, such drugs are commonly administered in the form of a *salt*, a compound formed by the combination of a *base* (often a negatively charged ion or *anion*) and an *acid* (often a positively charged ion or *cation*). However, because the components of a salt dissociate in a solution, the drug may exist as both the nonionized and ionized species. Since the nonionized form is more lipid-soluble than the ionized form, the proportion of nonionized to ionized drug molecules present in a given area is important for drug absorption.

The pH of the local area determines the ratio of ionized to nonionized drug in that area. Solutions with a pH of 7.0 are neutral; those with a pH of less than 7.0 are acid; and those with a pH of greater than 7.0 are basic. Weak acids, like aspirin, are less ionized in an acid medium and are therefore more lipid-soluble through the stomach, with a pH of less than 3. Alkaloids like heroin, morphine, and cocaine are poorly absorbed from the stomach. On the other hand, further down the G.I. tract, in the small intestine, where the contents are nearly neutral or slightly alkaline, the environment favors the absorption of weak bases.

However, local pH is only one factor influencing drug absorption. This explains why the greater surface area of the small intestine, combined with a longer duration of drug contact, favors drug absorption there. This is the reason why people get intoxicated faster with carbonated alcoholic drinks; the carbonation forces the alcohol quickly out of the stomach and into the small intestine, where it is absorbed more rapidly. Some drugs are poorly absorbed from any part of the G.I. tract because even in their nonionized state they have low lipid solubility. Neutral drugs, like alcohol, are readily absorbed all along the G.I. tract.

Other major factors in the absorption of drugs in the G.I. tract include the concentration of the drug, the rate of movement of the contents through the tract, G.I. blood flow, digestive secretions, and G.I. contents. The higher the concentration of the drug the easier it is for the drug to diffuse passively across the intestinal cell membranes. The effect of the movement of the contents through the G.I. tract would depend on where the drug is best absorbed; for example, rapid emptying of the stomach would decrease the rate of absorption of weak acids, like aspirin. Rapid movement through the intestine could decrease the amount of drug absorbed because of a shorter duration of contact (or because the drug is a weak acid) or increase it because of better contact with the absorbing cells lining the intestine. Slow movement through the intestines would generally favor drug absorption. Because intestinal blood carries drugs away from the intestine and maintains a concentration gradient conducive to drug absorption, increasing or decreasing blood flow would increase or decrease, respectively, drug absorption. Digestive secretions can inactivate some drugs or alter intestinal pH and drug ionization. Finally, the contents of the G.I. tract (that is, food) can bind to the drug or dilute it so that it is slowly absorbed.

From this discussion we see that although the oral route is the safest way to administer drugs, it also has several disadvantages:

1. Drugs taken orally are absorbed more slowly than drugs taken by most other routes, so the oral route is usually not good in emergencies.

2. Patients need to be conscious, because otherwise they might choke to death if the drug is given orally.

3. Because of the slow rate of absorption, concentrations of drugs given orally may not even reach levels sufficient to induce noticeable effects.

4. Drug absorption is much more variable with the oral route because of the constantly changing conditions of the G.I. tract.

5. Some substances are very irritating and may produce nausea and vomiting if given orally, unless they are given with food.

Conversely, the introduction of a drug directly into the blood, most commonly done through **intravenous (I.V.) injection**, results in very rapid onset of drug action and relatively intense effects. For example, the time it takes a drug to circulate between the vein of the forearm and the brain is less than 15 seconds. An amount of drug (such as heroin) that may exert minimal effects when administered P.O. may be extremely toxic when administered intravenously. Although fine adjustments in drug dosage are possible with the intravenous route (important in barbiturate anesthesia), if overdosage does occur, little can be done about it, unless a specific antagonist for the drug is readily available. Drugs injected I.V. must also be in solution or microsuspension and must have an aqueous vehicle. Repeated injections can lead to clot formation, vessel irritation, or vessel collapse. Finally, there is a high incidence of allergic reaction, pronounced cardiovascular action, and side effects with this route.

In addition to the P.O. and I.V. routes, there are several alternative ways of determining and controlling the intensity and duration of drug action. Because of the relatively good blood supply surrounding muscles, **intramuscular (I.M.) injection** generally results in a more rapid absorption than does the P.O. route. Drugs dissolved in an aqueous vehicle are more rapidly absorbed through the I.M. route than when dissolved or suspended in oil.

Because the lining of the inside of the lungs provides a large surface area in close proximity to many blood vessels, **drug inhalation** leads to fairly rapid onset of drug action and intense effects. However, irritants or oils can cause pneumonia, and long-term consequences, such as cancer associated with cigarette smoking, often occur with this route.

The injection of a drug underneath the skin into the tissue between the skin and muscle (that is, into the body fat) is referred to as **subcutaneous (S.C.) drug injection**. Because of the relatively poor blood supply in fatty tissue, this method can be used with nonirritating substances to produce fairly slow and even absorption. The rate of absorption can be controlled through the form of the drug. For instance, it can be in aqueous solution, promoting fast absorption; in suspension, promoting somewhat slower absorption; or in solid form, such as a pellet, allowing for very slow absorption.

Sublingual or **buccal administration** (through the oral mucosa under the tongue or between the cheek and gum) may be used with drugs that are destroyed in the stomach or intestines, such as nitroglycerin and nicotine. Other, but rarely used, routes of administration are **intraarterial administration** (generally very hazardous because the drug is so concentrated); bone marrow administration (used, for example, in an infant, or when the veins are collapsed); rubbing drugs over a large surface area of the skin (although normal skin is an effective barrier to drug absorption); application of drugs to the mucous membranes of the nose (**intranasal administration**), vagina, or urethra; and administration through the eye. **Intrathecal administration**, or injection of the drug into the subdural spaces of the spinal cord (for example, spinal anesthesia), and **intracerebroventricular injection,** or injection into the ventricular spaces of the brain, may be used to bypass the blood-brain barrier, which will be discussed shortly. Although rarely used in humans, injection of drugs into the abdominal cavity (peritoneum), called **intraperitoneal injection**, is commonly used with small animals such as mice and rats. Absorption by this route is somewhat faster and more uniform than with oral administration, and the drug is not affected by enzymes in the stomach or intestines.

The increasing awareness that drug-release patterns (continuous versus pulsatile) significantly affect therapeutic responses has led to research aimed at creating new drug delivery systems (Langer, 1990). For example, several experimental approaches have been developed that facilitate a drug's ability to cross the blood-brain barrier—for example, by rendering it more lipid-soluble or coupling it to a molecule that has a specific transport mechanism. Controlled-release systems have been developed that are even better than older "sustained-release" or "slow-release" preparations in maintaining drug plasma levels in the desired therapeutic range. Although the skin is often considered a barrier to all agents, including drugs, several transdermal delivery systems have been developed to allow clinically relevant doses of drugs to penetrate the skin—for example, scopolamine-containing patches to prevent nausea associated with motion sickness and nicotine-containing patches to alleviate nicotine withdrawal. Several approaches (e.g., subdermal, slow-release capsules) that will allow a wider variety of drugs to be administered transdermally are now being explored.

Drug Distribution

After a drug enters the bloodstream, it passes through various body compartments and is distributed throughout the body. Because of binding or dissolving in fat, most drugs accumulate in various tissues, often not at their sites of action. These sites of accumulation are often where the drug causes toxicity—for example, the liver and kidneys. These sites may also serve as storage depots within the body where the drug is in dynamic equilibrium with the free drug. The same factors that are involved in drug absorption determine whether and how a drug is accumulated or stored once it is in the body.

Drugs may bind to plasma proteins, which may be important drug storage depots. Drugs that are bound strongly to blood plasma proteins can compete for the same binding sites, such that the use of a competing drug can displace another from them. For example, several drugs used to treat mental illness can displace the anticoagulant warfarin (used in the treatment of some cardiovascular problems) from its plasma binding sites. The high concentration of free warfarin can, in turn, prevent the normal blood clotting process and produce unexpected internal bleeding.

One type of tissue in which there is a great deal of drug accumulation is adipose tissue (fat), which makes up approximately 18–28% of the body. Most psychotropic drugs are particularly prone to accumulating in adipose tissue because of their relatively high lipid solubility. Most drugs stored in human fat cause no overt symptoms unless the subject undergoes a rapid period of fat utilization, due to starvation or extreme dieting. The short duration of the action of some drugs, or the prolonged duration of others, can be explained on the basis of fat storage. For example, the drug thiopental (an ultrashort-acting drug used in anesthesia) is very lipid-soluble. When injected I.V., it rapidly enters the brain, leaving a relatively small concentration in the plasma. Thus the onset of its effects is very rapid, occurring within approximately 10–15 seconds. However, the drug is then taken up into skeletal muscle tissue and begins to leave the brain. The drug then enters fat tissue and remains there for some time. As a result, the intensity of the drug's effects is reduced fairly rapidly, but some small, residual effect of the drug may be experienced for many hours.

Because men and women generally differ in the proportion and distribution of their muscle and fat, the intensity and duration of drug action may differ between the sexes. For example, because women's bodies average a lower total water content (54% for females versus 60% for males) and a higher total fat content (28% versus 18%), peak plasma levels of alcohol (a water-soluble drug) tend to be higher in women. This difference occurs even if alcohol consumption is comparable with respect to total body weight (Schenker & Speeg, 1990). As a result, women may be more susceptible than men to the adverse effects of alcohol, particularly liver damage (discussed in Chapter 8).

The importance of fat in the effects of psychotropic drugs is also illustrated when patients who receive narcotic analgesics to relieve their pain do not achieve adequate plasma levels because the needles used to inject the drugs are often too short to get past the large padding of fat in the gluteus maximus (the buttocks).

To summarize, the dynamics involved in the distribution of a drug in the body depend on the lipid solubility of the drug, how lipoidal the tissue is, the blood flow through the tissue, the mass of the tissue, and the concentration gradient of the drug between the plasma and the tissue. A drug's pharmacokinetics may also depend on the species, sex, or, as we shall see, the age of the organism.

Some drugs can exert indirect influence on psychological processes. For example, a drug that paralyzes the muscles may induce emotional discomfort. However, in order to exert direct psychological effects, a drug must penetrate into the central nervous system (CNS). The entrance of drug molecules into the CNS and the cerebrospinal fluid (CSF) is a special aspect of cellular penetration.

Considering the fact that the brain comprises only about 2% of the body's entire mass but receives approximately 20% of the blood flow from the heart, we would expect a relatively large amount of a drug to enter the brain. However, the brain has evolved a way of preventing most nonnutritive substances from entering it and affecting nervous tissue. This is generally referred to as the **blood-brain barrier (BBB)** (Goldstein & Betz, 1986) and is a vital source of stability, as well as a defense. For example, after a meal, blood concentrations of numerous chemicals can rise sharply and could be very disruptive of brain functions if it were not for the BBB, which protects the brain against such fluctuations.

The BBB is actually a feature of the physical structure of the capillaries supplying blood to brain tissue. Figure 3–2(a) shows the structural relationship between brain capillaries, astrocytes, and neurons. *Astrocytes* are cells whose long processes (extensions) make contact with several other types of brain cells. The astrocyte processes touch neurons and the ependymal cells that line the ventricles, which are spaces at the center of the brain. In addition, each brain capillary is typically in contact with several astrocytes. Astrocytes are members of the largest class of brain cells, the glial cells. Although their function is not yet fully understood, they may influence capillary permeability. Unlike the cells of the capillaries elsewhere in the body, brain capillaries are made up of cells that are packed tightly together. Furthermore, ordinary capillaries have apertures, like small pores, through which drug molecules can pass. Brain capillaries have very few of these. Finally, there is a very lipid sheath that surrounds the brain capillaries and that is made up of extensions of "glial feet" from nearby astrocyte cells. As shown in Figure 3–2(b), astrocyte foot processes almost completely surround the brain capillary. Because of this relation, it was once thought that the astrocytes formed the blood-brain barrier. It is now known that the capillary endothelial cells constitute the barrier. Endothelial cells selectively transport nutrients into the brain, and their many mitochondria probably provide energy for transport. The endothelial cells of the brain have few pinocytotic vesicles. In other organs, such vesicles may provide relatively unselective transport across the capillary wall.

Thus, in order for a drug to get to CNS nerve cells (neurons), it must be (a) very small (this is unusual for psychotropic drugs), (b) lipid-soluble, or (c) compatible with one of the several *carrier-mediated* or *active transport systems* developed in the capillary and astrocyte cells. Active transport systems are systems in which ions or molecules are able to attach themselves to proteins embedded in the cell membrane. The proteins then transport the ions or molecules across the membrane through an energy-consuming process—a process that occurs at the expense of metabolic breakdown processes occurring within the cell. Apparently, these active transport systems have evolved in such a way that nutritive but nonlipid substances, such as glucose, vitamins, and minerals, can get into the brain (Pardridge, 1988). There are also carrier-mediated transport systems, which do not involve energy utilization, that can facilitate the diffusion of compounds across biological membranes. For example,

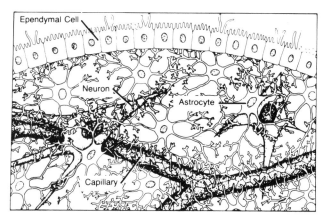

(a) Structural relationship between brain capillaries, astrocytes, and neurons.

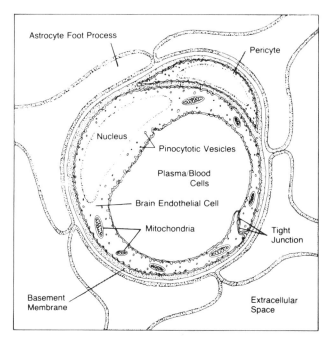

(b) Cross section of a brain capillary.

Figure 3–2

Schematic of the structural basis of the blood-brain barrier. (From "The blood-brain barrier" by G. W. Goldstein and A. L. Betz, *Scientific American*, 255, 74–83. Copyright © 1986 by Scientific American, Inc. All rights reserved.)

minute invaginations may form in the surface of cell membranes and close to form fluid-filled vesicles, known as *pinocytotic vesicles*, which then migrate across the membrane and spill their contents on the other side. Although rare, there are some drugs that penetrate the BBB by way of these two types of transport systems.

The BBB is not completely impermeable to chemicals that do not possess the characteristics just described. The capillaries atop the brain stem where the vomiting center is located are permeable to chemicals because the neurons there must monitor the blood for deadly poisons, detection of which induces vomiting. Also, the BBB may temporarily break down as a result of injury (e.g., a blow to the head or a stroke) or illness (e.g., meningitis), thus allowing chemicals to penetrate it. Such penetrability could be beneficial or detrimental to the person depending on whether a specific chemical is wanted in the brain or not.

Other factors limiting drug penetration in the CNS involve protein binding and degree of ionization. Drugs that are highly bound to plasma proteins are less likely to penetrate the BBB, because only free drug molecules can pass through. Drugs that are weak acids—that is, are highly ionized at the pH of blood plasma, which is approximately 7.4— are less likely to enter the CNS, because their lipid solubility is low.

Metabolism

Once a drug has been introduced into the body, it generally undergoes several chemical changes before it is eliminated from the body. The term **metabolism** (also known as **biotransformation**) refers to any process resulting in any chemical change in the drug in the body. This chemical change may result in the drug molecule becoming more active, less active, or unchanged in terms of its activity at its binding sites, so metabolism does not mean inactivation (Hoyumpa & Schenker, 1982). When complex chemical compounds are metabolized, or broken down, into simpler ones, the term *catabolism* is sometimes used; the reverse process is *anabolism*. It should be noted that drugs may be affected by all three types of metabolization. For example, codeine is transformed into the inactive codeine glucuronide, the more active molecule morphine, and the equally active compound norcodeine. The duration of action, or the drug's qualitative effects, may depend on which of these types of transformations is most rapid. Since the termination of a drug's action also is dependent to some extent on its being excreted from the body, metabolization of the drug into a more water-soluble compound generally must take place.

The fact that a drug may have several active metabolites is one reason why there are so many drugs of the same type and action on the market. That is, once a drug has been patented, the pharmaceutical company maintains the sole right to manufacture that drug for many years. However, if another company can determine that one of the drug's metabolites is also active, it can patent and market it. Pharmaceutical companies are also attempting to modify drugs into "prodrugs," inert substances converted by the body's own chemistry into active compounds, whenever the parent compound is hard to take or absorb or is slow to accumulate in target tissues (Hiller, 1991).

Many types of metabolic processes affect drugs in the body, and many drugs go through several metabolic changes before they are eliminated from the body. The major metabolic processes are *cleavage* reactions (the splitting of the molecule into two or more simpler molecules), *oxidation* (combining the molecule with oxygen or increasing the electropositive charge of the molecule through the loss of hydrogen or of one or more electrons), *conjugation* (the combining of the molecule with glucuronic or sulfuric acid), and *reduction* (the opposite of oxidation, where the molecule becomes more negatively charged by gaining one or more electrons). Nearly all tissues of the body are capable of carrying out some type of drug metabolic activity. The most active tissues are generally those involved in the excretion of drugs, particularly the liver, kidneys, and intestines. Within the cells of these tissues, the different subcellular parts carry out different metabolic activities.

It should be pointed out that some drugs are excreted intact, with only minimal metabolic transformation. This appears to be the case with the active ingredients of *Amanita muscaria,* a mushroom that is toxic and lethal in large enough quantities, but hallucinogenic in smaller quantities, which are passed into the urine and excreted. Siberian tribespeople, for whom the mushroom is quite a treat, take advantage of this fact by recycling the drug. (The recycling process they use and how they discovered it will be left to your imagination!)

As stated earlier, psychotropic drugs are generally lipid-soluble. Before there is any significant elimination of them from the body, they must become more water-soluble, because the excretion of drugs and their metabolites by way of the kidneys into the urine is, by far, the most important in terms of volume. Also, with the exception of the removal of volatile substances through the lungs, other excreta, like feces and perspiration, are aqueous in nature.

Drugs administered orally must initially pass through portions of the G.I. tract where various enzymes may metabolize them. After the drug molecules cross the membranes of the cells in the G.I. tract, they move into a blood circulation system that goes directly to the liver before getting into the blood that supplies the body and brain. Thus the molecules can be further metabolized in the liver—that is, the hepatic system (see Figure 3–1). It is for this reason that plasma or brain concentrations of drugs administered in this fashion are generally lower than those of drugs administered through other routes—a phenomenon known as

first-pass metabolism. For example, blood ethanol levels are approximately 60% lower following oral administration than following I.V. administration if ethanol is given after a meal, and approximately 20% lower if given after overnight fasting (DiPadova et al., 1987). For most drugs, first-pass metabolism is primarily hepatic, although for some drugs, notably ethanol, it occurs predominantly at an upper G.I. site (Frezza et al., 1990).

By far, the organ most responsible for metabolizing drugs is the liver. Within the membranes of the primary liver cells exists a large complex of *enzymes*. Enzymes are proteins secreted by cells that act as a catalyst to induce chemical changes in other substances, but which themselves are unchanged in the process. These particular enzymes—technically the *hepatic microsomal enzyme system*—have apparently been developed through evolution in order to deal with toxic substances that animals may ingest in their food. Because the actions of these enzymes are nonspecific in nature—that is, they may act on many different types of substances—they also metabolize drugs. To differentiate between these enzymes and a multitude of others in the body, I will refer to these as **drug-metabolizing enzymes**.

As blood passes through the liver, drugs diffuse into the liver cells and are acted on by drug-metabolizing enzymes. The metabolites (or, in some cases, the unchanged drugs) then diffuse back into the plasma or are secreted into the bile. Metabolites that are in the plasma and are sufficiently water-soluble are excreted primarily in the urine. If they are not sufficiently water-soluble, they may undergo further metabolization in the liver. Metabolites in the bile are delivered into the intestines. If they are water-soluble, they are excreted in the feces. However, if they are still lipid-soluble, they may be reabsorbed from the intestines to undergo further metabolization.

In most cases, the rate of drug metabolization is proportional to the plasma concentration of the drug (in log units), a relationship which is referred to as **first-order kinetics**. Some drugs exhibit **zero-order kinetics**; that is, they are metabolized at a fairly constant rate regardless of the amount taken—for example, ethanol (the alcohol we drink) (Ritchie, 1985) and certain antidepressants taken in very large doses (Jarvis, 1991). The rate is also dependent upon the number of drug-metabolizing enzymes in the liver. This level can be elevated several times over with continuous exposure to certain drugs, although the process generally takes several days or weeks (Shoaf & Linnoila, 1991). This is an important factor in many cases of drug tolerance, where the effects of a given amount of drug are decreased because of previous exposure to the drug. For example, long-term exposure to alcohol can induce a 30% elevation in the amount of drug-metabolizing enzymes of the liver, and barbiturates can elevate these levels to five times that of the normal level. Since all psychotropic medications (except lithium) are metabolized by these enzymes, their plasma levels can be considerably reduced due to this factor (Shoaf & Linnoila, 1991).

In fact, most drugs that depress brain functions (such as sedatives) tend to induce higher levels of the drug-metabolizing enzymes. Such effects are not restricted to sedative-type drugs. Tobacco smoking, for example, can enhance the metabolism and elimination from the body of many psychotropics (e.g., antipsychotics, antidepressants, and caffeine) because of its ability to enhance the hepatic microsomal enzyme system (Shoaf & Linnoila, 1991).

Drugs can also inhibit the metabolization of other drugs through various mechanisms. Some drugs, including estrogens (female hormones) in oral contraceptives, have been suggested to reduce the level of enzymes (Benet et al., 1990). Other drugs, including Antabuse, a drug used in the treatment of alcoholism, may combine with the active sites of the enzyme complex and prevent them from being available for metabolizing other drugs. Alcohol normally undergoes several metabolic changes. It first changes into acetaldehyde, which is fairly toxic. Normally, acetaldehyde is metabolized into nontoxic acetic acid. However, Antabuse competes for the enzyme that changes acetaldehyde into acetic acid. Thus, if the person who is taking Antabuse drinks alcohol, acetaldehyde levels build up and cause the person to become nauseated and to throw up. Supposedly the alcoholics' knowledge of these consequences prevents them from drinking alcohol. Finally, one drug may reduce the metabolization of another because the two drugs share a common metabolic pathway. For example, higher-than-normal brain levels of barbiturates and other sedative-hypnotics may occur if accompanied by alcohol intake because the enzymes are busy metabolizing the alcohol (Hoyumpa & Schenker, 1982).

Not only can a drug influence the rate of metabolizing other drugs, but also the presence of one drug may alter the types of metabolites formed from another drug. A notable example occurs when the liver enzymes, in the presence of alcohol, convert cocaine into cocaethylene, a metabolite that appears to be more potent than cocaine in terms of its reward properties as well as its toxicity (Barinaga, 1990).

Because there are vast differences in the ways in which different species metabolize drugs, it is very difficult to predict the response of humans to drugs on the basis of the response of other animals. In humans it is now recognized that there are marked between- and within-race variations in the level of drug-metabolizing enzymes and the rates of metabolizing drugs, and perhaps as much as 50% of this variation is due to genetics (Reed & Hanna, 1986). Age may also be a factor in drug metabolization, because older people tend to lose their ability to produce many of these enzymes, making them particularly susceptible to the toxic effects of drugs. In the developing fetus and in newborn infants, where drugs are metabolized chiefly in the liver, the activity and concentration of many metabolizing enzymes is less than in adults, prolonging and exaggerating drug effects (Ramirez, 1989). Children do not have a full complement of these enzymes until they are a year or two old.

Other important factors in drug metabolization are nutrition and disease (Hoyumpa & Schenker, 1982). For example, in animals, blood alcohol concentration has been found to be lowered and alcohol clearance from the body accelerated with high-carbohydrate (such as simple sugar) diets, whereas alcohol concentration is increased and clearance is reduced with low-carbohydrate diets (Rao et al., 1986). In the initial stages of starvation, drug metabolization may be enhanced, whereas in later stages it will be reduced. Severe liver diseases, such as cirrhosis, obstructive jaundice, and hepatitis, can significantly reduce the ability of the organism to metabolize drugs. The ability of skid-row alcoholics to get drunk on as little as a half pint of wine—what some people might refer to as **reverse tolerance**—is probably due to both nutritional deficiencies and disease (Wilson et al., 1986).

Very little work has been done on human sex differences in metabolizing drugs. Although some studies have concluded that gender differences are not very significant for most drugs (Dawkins & Potter, 1991), recent studies have indicated that there may be notable differences in the ways in which men and women metabolize some drugs. One study indicated that the blood levels of alcohol in women were significantly higher than in men who had been given the same amount of alcohol (relative to their body weights), because women exhibit lower gastric first-pass metabolism of alcohol (Frezza et al., 1990). Other studies have indicated that women tend to metabolize some antianxiety drugs slower than men do (Wilson, 1984). Therefore, women are prone to accumulate higher, and potentially more dangerous, levels of these drugs with repeated administrations.

Drug Excretion

The liver excretes drugs into the bile by a secretory process. Highly water-soluble metabolites are not reabsorbed and are removed from the body by way of the feces. However, renal (kidney) excretion of drugs—primarily their metabolites—is the primary way in which they are removed from the body. Because of their lipid-solubility, psychotropic drugs are always excreted slowly in their active forms. To a great extent, the metabolites' rate of excretion depends on their lipid-solubility, on whether they are actively secreted (as opposed to passively diffused) into the urine by the kidney cells, and on their pH and the pH of the urine. For example, an increase in the urinary pH (that is, a decrease in acidity) enhances the excretion of a weak organic acid, like aspirin, but reduces the rate of excretion of a weak base, like morphine. Therefore,

the rate of excretion of certain acidic drugs can be enhanced by al-
kalinization of the urine—for example, with bicarbonate of soda (Alka-
Seltzer)—while the excretion of alkaline drugs can be enhanced by
acidification—for example, with vitamin C. It should be noted that urine
is usually acid, although it may not be if a person's drinking water is
highly alkaline.

Like metabolism, renal function and, therefore, ability to excrete
drugs, varies considerably with age. Fetal excretion of most drugs, via
the placenta and fetal urine, is delayed. Excretion through urine increases to maximal levels in humans between the ages of 5 and 10. Renal
functioning then declines somewhat, tends to stabilize between the ages
of 10 and 40, and then begins to decline thereafter. Thus the plasma half-
life of most drugs progressively increases from childhood to old age
(Geller, 1991). (See Chapter 14 for further discussion of pharmacokinetics of the elderly.)

Implications of Pharmacokinetics in the Fetus and Neonate

One can make an argument that adults who take drugs are doing so by
choice and that they are responsible for whatever consequences a drug
may have on their body. Unfortunately, the developing fetus or newborn
of a woman who takes psychotropic drugs does not have that choice. As
many as 80% of all pregnant women take prescribed drugs, and up to 35%
take psychotropic drugs, none of which have been proven safe for use
during pregnancy (Kerns, 1986). The tissue through which most psychotropic drugs can easily pass, and which expectant parents should be
fully aware of, is the *placenta*. This tissue is specialized to allow transport
of oxygen, nutrients, and waste between the woman and the fetus, but it
is no different from other cell membranes in its general permeability to
drugs. In fact, drugs can cross the placenta, nearly always through passive diffusion, even more easily than they can penetrate the BBB in the
adult brain. Therefore, any psychoactive drug, when taken orally, passes
through the placenta and accumulates in the developing fetus in significant quantities. Passive diffusion through the placenta is dependent upon
characteristics of the drug (such as molecular size, lipid-solubility, and so
on), drug concentration, and duration of exposure.

In a fetus, a greater proportion of blood flow is distributed to its
brain than is the case in adults. Combined with the less-developed BBB
of the fetus and fewer plasma proteins for drug binding, this greater
flow leads to more rapid and complete drug exposure of the fetal brain.
Furthermore, with greater cerebral blood flow, a less-developed BBB,
fewer protein-binding molecules, a lower level of hepatic metabolizing
enzymes, and slower drug excretion, the fetus and newborn are much
more susceptible to the potential toxic effects of drugs than adults are

(Kerns, 1986; Guyon, 1989). This lesson was most agonizingly learned more than 30 years ago when a large number of women who had been taking a mild sedative called thalidomide during their pregnancy gave birth to infants with missing or malformed limbs.

The risks to the fetus include **teratogenic effects** (abnormal development), long-term behavioral effects, and direct toxic effects. Teratogenic effects may be apparent immediately and result in spontaneous abortion, malformation, or altered fetal growth, or they may be delayed and not measurable or manifested for years after birth. The majority of drugs of abuse, including alcohol, nicotine, marijuana, cocaine, and opiates, have been found to impair fetal growth, resulting in lower birth weights and shorter gestational periods (Kaye et al., 1989; Zuckerman et al., 1989).

In addition to obvious physical abnormalities, psychotropic drugs can disturb nerve cell proliferation, differentiation, and neurotransmitter concentrations. Disruptions in psychomotor activity, behavioral development, and performance may occur. For example, in humans, alcohol, opiates, and some anticonvulsants are well-established behavioral teratogens, producing disturbances of arousal and motor coordination, specific learning disabilities, and mental retardation.

Whether subtle or transient, behavioral effects may still cause problems. Subtle ones may only be evidenced if the infant is exposed to certain environments, such as an impoverished one. Transient ones, like neonatal withdrawal symptoms when drug exposure ceases at birth, can disrupt early mother-infant interactions and bonding, which can lead to long-term consequences for the child's psychological development.

Unfortunately, some emotional or mental disorders require that the pregnant female be maintained on medication in order to protect the fetus. For example, an actively psychotic, manic, or severely depressed female may engage in activities that would endanger the fetus. An epileptic fit, with the likelihood of experiencing seizures, has a significant potential for fetal damage. Fortunately, most studies indicate that the majority of psychotropic drugs used to treat these disorders have minimal teratogenic potential (Hawkins, 1989). Problems with medications that have some teratogenic potential (e.g., lithium and anticonvulsants) can be minimized by reducing dosage or eliminating drug treatment during the first trimester or by taking other precautions. (See Elia et al., 1987, and Hawkins, 1989, for a more complete description of potential teratogenic effects of specific psychotherapeutic drugs.)

Bibliography

Barinaga, M. (1990). Miami vice metabolite. *Science, 250,* 758.

Benet, L. Z., Mitchell, J. R., & Sheiner, L. B. (1990). Pharmacokinetics: The dynamics of drug absorption, distribution, and elimination. In A. G. Gilman, T. W. Rall, A. S. Nies, & P. Taylor, *The pharmacological basis of therapeutics* (pp. 3–32). New York: Pergamon Press.

Dawkins, K., & Potter, W. Z. (1991). Gender differences in pharmacokinetics and pharmacodynamics of psychotropics: Focus on women. *Psychopharmacology Bulletin, 27,* 417–426.

DiPadova, D., Worner, T. M., Julkunen, R.J.K., & Lieber, C. S. (1987). Effects of fasting and chronic alcohol consumption on the first-pass metabolism of ethanol. *Gastroenterology, 92,* 1169–1173.

Elia, J., Katz, I. R., & Simpson, G. (1987). Teratogenicity of psychotherapeutic medications. *Psychopharmacology Bulletin, 23,* 531–586.

Frezza, M., Di Padova, C., Pozzato, G., Terpin, M., Baraona, E., & Lieber, C. S. (1990). High blood alcohol levels in women. *New England Journal of Medicine, 322,* 95–99.

Geller, B. (1991). Psychopharmacology of children and adolescents: Pharmacokinetics and relationships of plasma/serum levels to response. *Psychopharmacology Bulletin, 27,* 401–410.

Gillette, J., Weisburger, E. K., Kraybill, H., & Kelsey, M. (1985). Strategies for determining the mechanisms of toxicity. *Clinical Toxicology, 23,* 1–78.

Goldstein, G. W., & Betz, A. L. (1986). The blood-brain barrier. *Scientific American, 255,* 74–83.

Guyon, G. (1989). Pharmacokinetic considerations in neonatal drug therapy. *Neonatal Network, 7,* 9–12.

Hawkins, D. F. (1989). Drugs used to treat medical disorders in pregnancy and fetal abnormalities. In E. M. Scarpelli & E. V. Cosmi (Eds.), *Reviews in perinatal medicine* (pp. 91–131). New York: Alan R. Liss.

Hiller, S. (1991). A better way to make the medicine go down. *Science, 253,* 1095–1096.

Hoyumpa, A. M., & Schenker, S. (1982). Major drug interactions: Effect of liver disease, alcohol, and malnutrition. *Annual Review of Medicine, 33,* 113–149.

Jarvis, M. R. (1991). Clinical pharmacokinetics of tricyclic antidepressant overdose. *Psychopharmacology Bulletin, 27,* 541–550.

Kaye, K., Elkind, L., Goldberg, D., & Tytun, A. (1989). Birth outcomes for infants of drug abusing mothers. *New York State Journal of Medicine, 89,* 256–261.

Kerns, L. L. (1986). Treatment of mental disorders in pregnancy. *Journal of Nervous and Mental Disease, 174,* 652–659.

Langer, R. (1990). New methods of drug delivery. *Science, 249,* 1527–1533.

Oldendorf, W. H., & Dewhurst, W. G. (1978). The blood-brain barrier and psychotropic drugs. In W. G. Clark & J. D. Giudice (Eds.), *Principles of psychopharmacology* (pp. 183–192). New York: Academic Press.

Pardridge, W. M. (1988). Recent advances in blood-brain barrier transport. *Annual Review of Pharmacology and Toxicology, 28,* 25–39.

Ramirez, A. (1989). The neonate's unique response to drugs: Unraveling the causes of drug iatrogenesis. *Neonatal Network, 7,* 45–49.

Rao, G. A., Larkin, E. C., & Derr, R. F. (1986). Biologic effects of chronic ethanol consumption related to a deficient intake of carbohydrates. *Alcohol and Alcoholism, 21,* 369–373.

Reed, T. E., & Hanna, J. M. (1986). Between- and within-race variation in acute cardiovascular responses to alcohol: Evidence for genetic determination in normal males in three races. *Behavioral Genetics, 16,* 585–598.

Ritchie, J. M. (1985). The aliphatic alcohols. In A. G. Gilman, L. S. Goodman, T. W. Rall, & F. Murad (Eds.), *The pharmacological basis of therapeutics* (pp. 372–386). New York: Macmillan.

Schenker, S., & Speeg, K. V. (1990). The risk of alcohol intake in men and women. *New England Journal of Medicine, 322,* 127–129.

Shibanoki, S., Kubo, T., & Ishikawa, K. (1987). Comparative study of phenothiazine derivatives on monoamine metabolism—Direct correlation between the concentrations of drugs and monoamine metabolites in the brain. *Journal of Pharmacology and Experimental Therapeutics, 240,* 959–965.

Shoaf, S. E., & Linnoila, M. (1991). Interaction of ethanol and smoking on the pharmacokinetics and pharmacodynamics of psychotropic medications. *Psychopharmacology Bulletin, 27,* 577–609.

van den Hoogen, R.H.W.M., & Colpaert, F. C. (1987). Epidural and subcutaneous morphine, meperidine (pethidine), fentanyl and sufentanil in the rat: Analgesia and other in vivo pharmacologic effects. *Anesthesiology, 66,* 186–194.

Wilson, J. S., Korsten, M. A., & Lieber, C. S. (1986). The combined effects of protein deficiency and chronic ethanol administration on rat ethanol metabolism. *Hepatology, 6,* 823–829.

Wilson, K. (1984). Sex-related differences in drug disposition in man. *Clinical Pharmacokinetics, 9,* 189–202.

Zuckerman, B., Frank, D. A., Hingson, R., Amaro, H., Levenson, S. M., Kayne, H., Parker, S., Vinci, R., Aboagye, K., Fried, L. E., Cabral, H., Timperi, R., & Bauchner, H. (1989). Effects of maternal marijuana and cocaine use on fetal growth. *New England Journal of Medicine, 320,* 762–768.

Chapter Four

Conduction and Neurotransmission

All thoughts, emotions, and behaviors come about because of biochemical and electrochemical processes that take place in specialized cells in the nervous system called *neurons*. Drugs that affect these psychological variables do so because they alter these biochemical and electrochemical processes. Therefore, in order for the student to appreciate how psychotropic drugs work and what their short- and long-term consequences are, he or she should be familiar with these basic processes. The purpose of this chapter is to describe the biochemical and electrochemical activities that neuroscientists believe take place in the nervous system, and how they are related to psychotropic drug action.

Many of the descriptions that follow are theoretical in nature, rather than factual, because they deal with what goes on in the *central nervous system* (comprised of the brain and the spinal cord) or CNS. The neurons of the CNS are packed together so tightly and their functions are so interrelated that it is extremely difficult to say precisely what happens in the CNS, whether it is with respect to the normal activities taking place there or with respect to drug action. Neurons are also mixed in with numerous other nonneuronal cellular elements called *neuroglia* or *glia*, which serve important metabolic and supportive functions. Therefore, much of the evidence for the activities of these cells is based on what has been demonstrated to occur in neurons of the *peripheral nervous system* or PNS (made up of all neurons outside the brain and spinal cord), which are much easier to isolate and manipulate. However, most evidence suggests that the neurons and the interactions among them in the two systems are very similar, so in most cases information about one should provide us with a reasonably good idea of what goes on in the other.

It has been estimated that the human nervous system contains approximately 85 billion neurons (Williams & Herrup, 1988). To illustrate how enormous this number is, if you were to lose 100,000 neurons a day for 70 years, you would still have around 82 billion left. (Since CNS neurons are not replaced, the ones you die with are the ones you were born with minus the ones you lose.) So, just in terms of sheer numbers, the CNS is a very complex system. Neurons comprise a communication network in which the information is analogous to codes made up of on and off signals, which correspond to the two drastically different states between which neurons are capable of rapidly alternating. Neurons are specialized to perform different functions. For example, some communicate between the senses and the nervous system, some communicate between neurons within the nervous system, and some communicate between the nervous system and the organs of the body, such as the heart, blood vessels, and muscles. However, they all appear to work in basically the same fashion (Stevens, 1979).

Two basic processes are involved in the communication network: *conduction*, which refers to changes within a neuron that allow the information to be transmitted from one part of the neuron to another part; and *neurotransmission*, which refers to changes that take place within one neuron because of the release of biologically active chemicals from adjacent neurons (Stevens, 1979). Conduction is basically an electrochemical process that is "all or none." Neurotransmission is basically a chemical process and may be "graded." Psychotropic drugs are simply chemicals that alter the normal processes of conduction, neurotransmission, or both. However, before we get into a description of these processes, the primary parts of the neuron that are instrumental in the processes must be identified.

The Neuron

Figure 4–1 depicts a stylized neuron and parts of other neurons that interact with it. Note that each neuron in the figure has numerous excitatory (E) and inhibitory (I) inputs or synapses, which regulate the frequency of action potentials (discussed in the next section) produced by them. The large arrows indicate the direction of information flow.

The main body of the neuron is called its *soma*, parts of which serve integrative functions in the communication of information. Extensions from the soma are termed *dendrites* and *axons*. Normally, there are many dendrites extending from the soma, which serve as receivers of information from other neurons, and one axon, which serves as the pathway over which signals pass from the soma to other neurons. Thus, in a sense, information flows from dendrite to soma to axon. Dendrites tend to be relatively short, but axons can be quite long. For

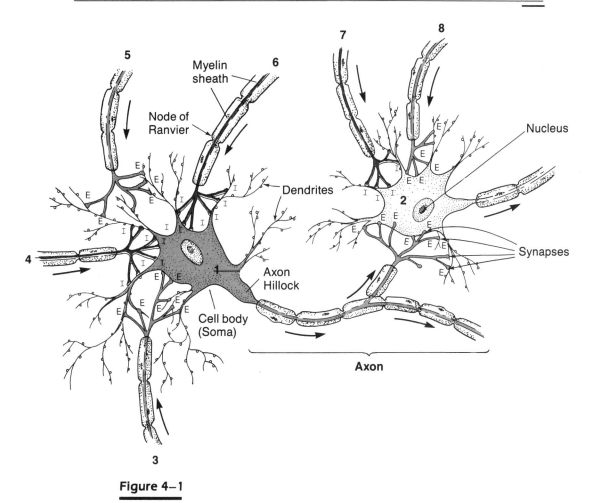

Figure 4–1

Schematic of the major parts of two CNS interneurons (1 and 2) depicting the relationship between them and the axons and terminals of other neurons (3–8). (Adapted from Carlson, 1988.)

instance, a spinal motor neuron may have an axon several feet long, although they too may be quite short in CNS neurons. The enlarged region where the axon emerges from the soma is called the *axon hillock*. A short distance from their origin, many axons have a coating called the *myelin sheath*, which is analogous to the insulation on a wire. Gaps in the myelin sheath, where the axon comes into direct contact with the extracellular fluid, are called the *nodes of Ranvier*. The presence of these gaps allows for an increase in the rate of conduction down the axon. Conduction in nonmyelinated axons tends to be rather slow. Near its end, the axon branches, and at the tip of each branch is an enlargement called a *terminal button,* which will be referred to hereafter as an *axon terminal.* Chemicals found within the axon terminal can be released into an exceedingly small gap between the neurons, called a *synaptic cleft,* allowing the neuron to affect the excitability of adjacent neurons. The region itself is called a *synapse,* and it consists of the presynaptic membrane of the axon terminal, the cleft, and the postsynaptic membrane of the "target" neuron.

Conduction

As with all body cells, neurons consist of a cell membrane filled with fluid, within which are subcellular structures that sustain the cell and help carry out its particular function. There is also fluid surrounding neurons (extracellular fluid), from which the cells take up oxygen, various nutrients, and, if present, drugs. Waste products and drug metabolites are discharged in this fluid. In the intra- and extracellular fluids are different concentrations of negatively and positively charged ions. The four primary ions important for conduction are sodium (designated as Na^+ where the Na is the abbreviation for the sodium atom and the $+$ stands for the positive charge the atom possesses), potassium (K^+), chloride (Cl^-), and large negatively charged protein molecules (which will be designated as A^- because the general term for a negatively charged particle is *anion*). A fifth ion (Ca^{++}, a calcium ion with two positive charges) is also involved, as it appears to be involved in the permeability of Na^+ ions through *sodium channels* in the neuronal membrane. As you might guess, the extracellular fluid is quite similar to the environment in which organisms originally evolved—that is, seawater made up of Na^+ and Cl^- ions and water.

There are two primary forces that influence the concentrations of these ions across neuronal membranes. A *concentration gradient* force refers to the fact that when there are different concentrations of molecules on the two sides of the membrane, they travel from the high-concentration region to the low-concentration region. *Electrostatic pressure* refers to the force exerted by the attraction of oppositely charged ions or by the repulsion of similarly charged ions. As was mentioned earlier, neurons can be in one of two states. One state is called the resting state, although the term "resting" is not really appropriate because the cell is actually expending a considerable amount of energy maintaining this state. In this state, there is a much higher concentration of negatively charged ions on the inside of the cell membrane than on the outside of the membrane, as shown in Figure 4–2. In the figure, the size of the symbol for the various ions indicates their relative abilities to cross the cell membrane by way of the channels located in the membrane. Also shown are examples of two of

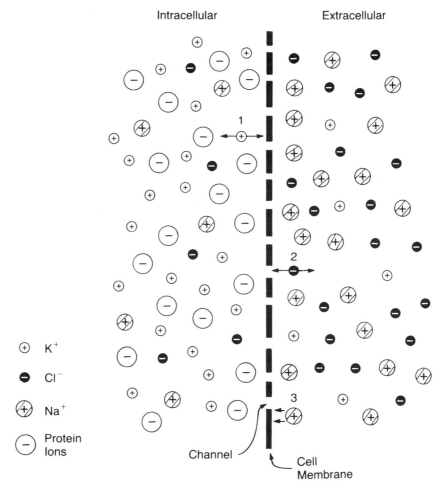

Figure 4–2

Relative distribution of the major ions in the intracellular (inside) and extracellular (outside) fluids of a neuron under resting conditions.

the primary forces maintaining these ion distributions: 1 shows a potassium ion (K+) being "pulled" out of the cell because of concentration gradient pressure and "pulled" in because of electrostatic pressure; 2 shows a chloride ion (Cl−) being "pulled" into the cell because of concentration gradient pressure and "pushed" out because of electrostatic pressure; 3 shows a sodium ion (Na+) being "pulled" into the cell by both electrostatic and concentration gradient pressure. Not shown is the sodium/potassium pump, which is another major factor in maintaining these ion concentrations. Note that the large negatively charged protein ions are clustered close to the inside membrane, and the positively charged sodium ions are clustered close to the outside of the membrane. The close proximity of these two ions on the two sides of the cell membrane and their attraction for each other produces a considerable amount of pressure (voltage potential) at the membrane.

In the resting state, the cell is referred to as being *polarized*. In the other state, in which there is a rapid exchange of ions across the neuron membrane, the cell is referred to as being *depolarized*, a process resulting in what will be called an *action potential*. (The term "depolarized," which might suggest a loss of potential, is a misnomer; as we shall see, the depolarized state is actually a reversal in polarity.)

The neuron is analogous to a tiny biological battery with positive poles outside the cell and negative poles inside the cell. At rest, the neuron normally maintains an *electrical potential* (electrical pressure measured in volts) of approximately 70 millivolts (mV). Since the inside of the cell membrane is negative relative to the outside of the cell membrane, it is conventional to refer to this voltage potential as -70 mV. (The resting potential of individual neurons varies between -60 and -90 mV, but -70 mV will be used here as a ballpark figure for purposes of discussion.) The cell membrane is a protein and lipid barrier that contains small pores or channels. The differential concentration of ions is believed to be due to the different capabilities of the ions to pass freely through these pores of the cell membrane, where K^+ and Cl^- diffuse freely through them, Na^+ diffuses through with difficulty, and the protein ions essentially do not diffuse through them at all. This phenomenon is referred to as *selective permeability*. The differential permeability of the cell membrane to these ions is believed to be due to their relative sizes: Na^+ ions are approximately 50% larger in diameter (in water) than K^+ and Cl^- ions.

In addition to concentration gradient and electrostatic forces, the concentration of the different ions under resting conditions is determined by what is referred to as *sodium-potassium pumps* embedded in neuronal membranes. These are energy-dependent pumps responsible for the active transport of both Na^+ out of the cell and K^+ into the cell. (They are termed energy-dependent because they derive their energy from metabolic processes in the interior of the cell.) The concentration gradient would normally result in equal concentrations of the ions on both sides of the neuron membrane. However, because of the A^- ions retained inside, the Cl^- ions are repelled through the membrane (remember, like charges repel, opposite charges attract), so the net effect is a greater concentration of Cl^- ions outside the neuron. Conversely, the K^+ and Na^+ ions are "pulled" inside because of the A^- ions. However, there is a greater concentration of K^+ inside and a greater concentration of Na^+ outside because of the sodium-potassium pumps. The sodium-potassium pump is more effective in transporting Na^+ than K^+; for every three Na^+ ions pumped out, two K^+ ions are pumped in. This is another process allowing the inside of the cell membrane to be negative relative to the outside.

As long as the cell membrane of the neuron remains undisturbed, the resting potential remains at approximately −70 mV. However, all of this changes if for some reason the voltage potential shifts approximately 10 mV toward 0—that is, goes to −60 mV. This point is referred to as the *threshold potential.* As soon as this threshold potential is reached, it triggers a rapid sequence of events lasting about 4 milliseconds (ms), which is referred to as an *action potential.* It is also common to say that the neuron "fires" when this happens. During this sequence, the electrical potential is reversed, going from −70 mV to approximately +30 mV, and then returns to the original electrical potential, with an actual overshoot of the −70 mV level (approximately −80 mV) before the final resting potential is reachieved. This sequence of events and the resulting changes in electrical potential are summarized graphically in Figure 4–3.

In most excitable cells, the action potential consists of three phases, each resulting from shifts in voltage that selectively open ion channels and allow ions to flow across the cell membrane (Catterall, 1988). Because these channels open and close as a result of shifts in membrane voltage potential, they are referred to as *voltage-sensitive* or *voltage-gated channels.* During the first phase, there is a rapid flow of Na^+ into the neuron mediated by voltage-sensitive Na^+ channels that cause depolarization (point *a* in Figure 4–3). In the second phase, the neuron remains depolarized because of inward movement of Ca^{++} ions through voltage-sensitive Ca^{++} channels. The Ca^{++} entering the neuron serves a variety of biochemical functions—for example, activating release of neurotransmitters from the neuron. The action potential is terminated by activation of voltage-sensitive K^+ channels that mediate outward movement of K^+ ions, which *repolarize* the neuron (point *b* in the figure). The K^+ ions (repelled by the Na^+ ions) flow so rapidly outside the cell (point *c* in the figure) that there is an overshoot of K^+ ions, and the electrical potential at that part of the cell becomes even more negative than the normal resting potential (point *d* in the figure). This event is referred to as *hyperpolarization.* Finally, the −70 mV resting potential is reachieved as the sodium-potassium pump works to pump Na^+ ions out of and K^+ ions back into the cell (point *e* in the figure).

The point of origin of what has just been described generally is the region where the axon emerges from the cell body, called the axon hillock. The axon hillock may be viewed as a decision-maker regarding the production of action potentials, since it is the region where the integration of all the inputs to the cell occurs (some of which are inhibitory and some of which are excitatory). With all of this activity, depolarization of adjacent regions (at the nodes of Ranvier in myelinated axons)

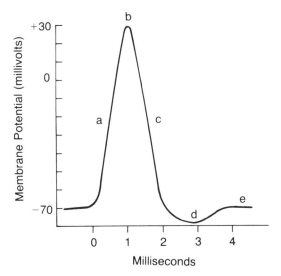

Figure 4–3

The action potential depicted here is the result of the rapid exchange of sodium (Na^+) and potassium (K^+) ions across the neuron cell membrane. (See text for explanation of the dynamics occurring at points *a–e.*)

occurs, and the same sequence that was just described occurs, resulting in what is termed *propagation* of the impulse down the axon, eventually reaching the axon terminals. Once the action potential reaches the axon terminals, it initiates a whole different sequence of events, which will be described in detail shortly. The propagation of the action potential down the axon takes place without a change in the action potential's magnitude; that is, the changes in ionic exchange are the same from beginning to end. However, the rate of propagation depends directly upon the size of the axon and the thickness of the myelin sheath: the larger the fiber and the thicker the sheath, the faster the propagation. It should be added that only a small amount of the available ions are exchanged during a single action potential, so thousands of action potentials in succession do not radically alter the relative concentrations of ions inside and outside the cell.

The excitability of a neuron—that is, its ability to initiate an action potential as a result of an outside stimulus—is dependent upon the degree of polarization when stimulation is applied. If the cell is hyperpolarized (the resting potential moves further from the threshold), it is less excitable; if it is slightly depolarized (between −70 and −60 mV), it is more excitable. Its excitability is also dependent upon whether an action potential has already occurred. Immediately following the action potential, there is a *refractory period* of a millisecond or two, during which no new action potential is generated. During the last part of the refractory period, an action potential can be triggered, but only if the stimulus is much stronger than normal. The cell is also less excitable during phase *d*, a form of hyperpolarization.

To summarize, information transmitted through neurons begins at the dendrites and soma, through processes that will be described shortly. It then travels to the axon hillock, where an action potential may be generated and propagated down the axon to its many terminals. (Normally this action potential goes from cell body to axon terminal, but under abnormal conditions, such as epilepsy, it can backfire—that is, originate in the axon terminals and get propagated to the cell body.) The information is actually in the form of shifts in the electrical potential in the different parts of the cell due to the opening and then closing of Na^+ channels. The regulation of the density of Na^+ channels in the neuronal membranes of the dendrites, soma, axon, and terminals may be an important determinant of their different functional roles in the process.

How do drugs fit into this picture? First of all, they can affect the properties of the membrane itself. For example, phenytoin (Dilantan), one of the most common drugs used in the treatment of epilepsy (see Chapter 14), has a variety of neuronal membrane-stabilizing properties (Pincus & Kiss, 1986). These properties decrease the Na^+ flow during the resting and action potentials, thus reducing the cell's excitability, and decrease the outward flow of K^+ during the action potential, thus increasing the duration of the refractory period. In addition, phenytoin decreases the flow of Ca^{++} ions into the axon terminals, thus decreasing the depolarization-linked release of several types of neurotransmitters (see the next section).

Alcohol and **general anesthetics**—including volatile solvents found in glue, industrial solvents, and aerosol sprays (such as toluene, acetone, benzene, hexane, and ether)—expand cell membranes and make them more "fluid" (Chin & Goldstein, 1977). The likely result is a disturbance in the sodium and potassium channels and improper exchange of Na^+ and K^+. The net result is a less excitable cell that is less able to propagate an action potential (see Chapter 8 for a further discussion of alcohol's neuropharmacological properties). This process in turn is also going to disrupt neurotransmission because of the decrease in the amount of chemicals released from the axon terminal. The psychological effects of these drugs are not very specific because they affect all neurons in the same way. However, certain effects may be noted at some doses and not at others because of differential sensitivity of different types of neurons that regulate psychological processes.

The second way in which drugs can affect conduction is by altering the structure or function of sodium channels located in the axonal membranes. As an example, one of cocaine's pharmacological properties in the PNS makes it useful as a **local anesthetic** (it induces a lack of sensation from a specific part of the body). Its local anesthetic properties are believed to be due to its ability to occupy sodium channels, preventing the influx of Na^+, and thereby preventing the triggering and conduction of an action potential (VanDyke & Byck, 1982). This action prevents any sensory information from reaching the CNS. There has been considerable debate over whether these properties are involved in cocaine's effects on mood and mental functions—that is, its CNS effects. Most of the evidence points to cocaine having an entirely different mechanism of action in the CNS.

Third, drugs can alter the balance of ions on the two sides of the membrane. For example, lithium is a small, positively charged ion (Li^+). Studies have indicated that when Na^+ and K^+ are deficient outside neurons, Li^+ substitutes for K^+ and is pumped inside. When Na^+ and K^+ are deficient inside the cell, Li^+ substitutes for Na^+ and is pumped outside the cell (Tosteson, 1981). The ramifications of these actions are still not understood, but they may have something to do with the ability of lithium salts to stabilize mood.

Neurotransmission

This chapter began with a discussion of the process of conduction where the action potential first begins—in the region of the axon hillock. Yet how does the neuron "know" when to generate an action potential? The process actually begins at the dendrites and the soma of the cell in areas that come into very close contact with parts (predominantly axon terminals) of other neurons. It is at these sites that chemicals released at these junctions, referred to earlier as synapses, cause very small, localized fluctuations in the electrical potential of the neuron. It is this process to which we now turn. (More extensive details of this process can be found in Bloom, 1985, and Weiner & Taylor, 1985.)

Getting information across the synapse was once believed to be due to an electrochemical process like conduction, similar to a spark crossing the gap between two electrical wires. While some neurons in the human brain may be electrically coupled in this way, the extent of such coupling appears to be quite limited. We now believe that the vast majority of neurons are coupled through a chemical process (actually a multitude of chemical processes) referred to as *neurotransmission*, which is perhaps even more complicated than the process of conduction. Although drugs do affect conduction, as I just discussed, most psychotropic drugs appear to induce their effects by altering the neurotransmission process. Therefore, I will discuss the events that theoretically take place in this process in some detail. The word "theoretically" was used because we are dealing with an immensely large and complicated system, the CNS, whose workings are largely inferred from what is known about the PNS.

Figure 4–4 displays in highly simplified form the basic steps in neurotransmission. On one side of the synapse is an axon terminal, containing enzymes used to synthesize the active neurotransmitter molecules, the neurotransmitter substance, and small granular spheres called *vesicles*, which store and release the neurotransmitters. (Because a number of dilated regions of an axon may make functional contact with parts of other neurons before the ultimate termination, the term "axon terminal" connotes a functional transmitting site rather than the end of the axon.) Terminals also contain small specialized subcellular parts, called *organelles*, serving individual functions. One type of organelles are the *mitochondria*, some of which have an important function in the regulation of the overall amount in the terminal of certain neurotransmitters we will call monoamines. The membrane of the axon terminal at the synaptic cleft is referred to as the *presynaptic membrane.*

On the other side of the cleft is the *postsynaptic membrane.* This membrane may be part of a dendrite, soma, or axon terminal of another neuron, or it may be part of a nonnervous system cell under neuronal control, such as a contractile (muscle) cell. The synapses of these four different junctions are called, respectively, axodendritic, axosomatic, axoaxonal, and neuromuscular synapses. It is not clear how these synapses differ in terms of the processes involved in neurotransmission, so for our purposes, unless stated otherwise, we will assume that the functions are basically the same in all of them, at least with respect to presynaptic activity. Synapses between dendrites of neurons (dendro-dendritic synapses) have been identified in the CNS, but the neurotransmission processes involved at these synapses are still very speculative. In most instances, synaptic transmission involves the passage of chemicals called *neurotransmitters* (or simply *transmitters* for short) from the endings of one neuron to an adjacent neuron. Somehow recognition of the transmitter by *postsynaptic receptors* in the membrane surface of the receiving (target) cell alters ion permeability in that area of the target neurons, and this alteration in turn influences their excitability. In some cases it increases the excitability, and in others it decreases it.

Before neurotransmission can take place, the synthesis of the active neurotransmitter substances must occur. In many cases this requires a series of enzymatically induced changes in chemicals obtained in our food that take place in our body. Because these chemicals come before the neurotransmitter, they are referred to as *precursors*. Neurotransmitter synthesis generally takes place in various parts of the neuron, such as the cell body and the axon terminal, where precursor molecules called *amino acids* (organic acids with a nitrogen atom combined with one or more hydrogen atoms, such as NH_2) are transported

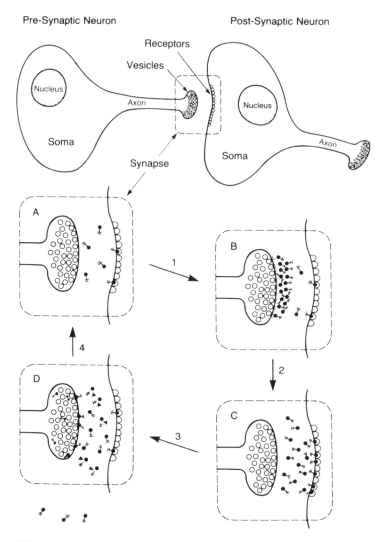

Figure 4–4

The general sequence of events believed to be involved in neurotransmission. (*A*) Between impulses only small amounts of transmitter (symbolized by ↦) leak through the presynaptic membrane, and very few postsynaptic receptors are activated. (*B*) An action potential arrives and causes release of transmitters into the cleft. (*C*) Transmitters diffuse through aqueous material of cleft and bind to postsynaptic receptors. At excitatory synapses, postsynaptic membrane potential is reduced (that is, goes toward threshold potential); at inhibitory synapses, it is increased (that is, becomes more negative). (*D*) Transmitters dissociate from receptors and then diffuse throughout extracellular fluid, undergo reuptake, or are inactivated by enzymes (symbolized by ▲).

across the BBB and then taken up from the extracellular fluid. If synthesized in a part of the neuron other than the axon terminal, the neurotransmitter is transported down the axon until it reaches the terminal. Transmitter synthesis takes place continuously, and the rate of synthesis is often inversely related to intracellular concentrations of the transmitter (i.e., the more transmitter used, the lower the concentration inside the neuron, and the higher the rate of synthesis), as well as by the amount of synthesis enzymes and precursor molecules. The speed with which a neurotransmitter is used and replenished is sometimes referred to as *turnover rate.*

Transmitters are found in heavy concentrations in the axon terminals. The heaviest concentrations are found in the synaptic vesicles, which appear to serve several functions. First, they serve as storage depots for future use in neurotransmission. Second, they serve to protect the transmitters from further enzymatic changes by enzymes in the terminal that can make them chemically inactive (that is, no longer able to induce biological changes at the postsynaptic membrane). Third, it has long been thought that vesicles that are in direct contact with the presynaptic membrane serve an active role in neurotransmission by fusing with the neuronal membrane and releasing their contents into the synaptic cleft when an action potential arrives at the terminal. More recent evidence suggests, however, that at least with one type of neuron (neurons releasing acetylcholine), the neurotransmitter molecules are more readily released from the cytoplasm of the terminal rather than from the vesicles (Dunant & Israel, 1985). Whether this occurs with other types of neurons or not remains to be determined.

For many years it was believed that each neuron released only one type of neurotransmitter, but recent evidence indicates that many neurons simultaneously release more than one chemical that can serve as a transmitter or play a modulating role in the activity of postsynaptic cells (Bartfai et al., 1988). In many cases the different neurotransmitters—that is, *cotransmitters*—in an axon terminal are stored in different types of vesicles, which in turn may release their contents at different frequencies of stimulation. Thus there is the possibility of pharmacologically manipulating one type of vesicle population without affecting the other.

Present theory has it that when an action potential arrives it allows calcium ions (Ca^{++}) to enter the axonal cytoplasm and promote the fusion of vesicles with the presynaptic membrane (Zucker & Lando, 1986). Only those vesicles close to the membrane fuse with it, while other vesicles seem to be held in reserve some distance away. The contents of the fused vesicles, including the transmitter(s), enzymes, and other proteins, are then discharged into the cleft. (As mentioned previously, an alternative is for cytoplasmic transmitter substances to be released.) Once released into the synaptic cleft, the transmitters passively diffuse through the aqueous material to the postsynaptic membrane, are briefly bound to receptors, and alter cellular functions of the receiving cell. (Neurotransmitters are sometimes referred to as ligands, since this is a general term for a natural body substance that acts on specific receptors.) Transmitters are then inactivated rapidly by diffusion into the extracellular fluid, by enzymatic degradation, or by *reuptake*. In the case of reuptake, the transmitters are actively taken back up into the neurons that released them or into other neurons or glia (the nonneuronal supportive cells of the nervous system) through an energy-dependent "pump" mechanism. The neuron is then ready to start the process all over again. With some transmitters, all three processes take place, but in others, the metabolites of the degradation process go through reuptake for later resynthesis into active transmitters. Transmitters that have undergone reuptake by the neuron may be rebound to vesicles for use again at a later time.

Once a neurotransmitter molecule binds to a receptor on the postsynaptic cell, the receptor briefly initiates a chain of events that allow ion channels to open up (Sakmann, 1992). This allows ions to flow across the postsynaptic membrane, generating a change in postsynaptic membrane potential. The size, duration, and direction of this ion flow, as well as the nature of the ions traversing the postsynaptic membrane, determine whether this response will either activate voltage-sensitive ion channels and initiate action potentials or instead reduce the cell's electrical activity.

At the present time it appears that there are two general classes of receptors, "fast" and "slow" (Cooper et al., 1991). *Fast receptors* are directly linked to an ion channel and are responsible for responses that last, at most, tens of milliseconds (see Figure 4–5). In contrast, *slow receptors* (see Figure 4–6) are responsible for slower and longer-lasting responses, lasting hundreds of milliseconds to tens of seconds, that are generally modulatory; that is, they either dampen or enhance the signal that acts on fast receptors. Slow receptors are coupled to a class of proteins, called G proteins, which in turn are directly coupled to ion channels or linked to what are termed *second messenger systems*. That is, receptor-ligand binding appears to activate specific enzymes in the target cell membrane that convert energy-carrier molecules into small molecules called nucleotides inside the target cell (Enna & Karbon, 1987). The nucleotides then serve as *secondary messengers*, which trigger the cell's internal machinery, leading to a momentary opening up of ion channels in the neuronal membrane. Two well-researched enzymes involved in this process are adenylate cyclase, which converts adenosine triphosphate (ATP) into cyclic adenosine monophosphate (cAMP), and guanylate cyclase, which converts guanosine triphosphate (GTP) into cyclic guanosine monophosphate (cGMP); cAMP and cGMP then serve as the secondary messengers.

It is unknown to what extent receptor activation leads to the formation of secondary messengers in CNS neurons or how many of these

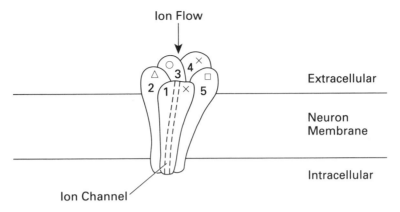

Figure 4–5

Model of a fast-receptor-ion-channel complex. It is made up of a protein with five different subunits (labeled 1–5) that form an ion channel in the middle. Each subunit is shown to have different receptor
binding sites (indicated by x, ○, △, and □) for different ligands
(neurotransmitters). Depending on which site or sites are occupied,
ligand or drug binding may result in ion channel opening directly,
thus allowing selected ions to flow into the cell, may facilitate channel opening by another ligand, may inhibit channel opening, or may
close the channel after it opens. (Note: other combinations are possible, and ion flow may be in the opposite direction.)

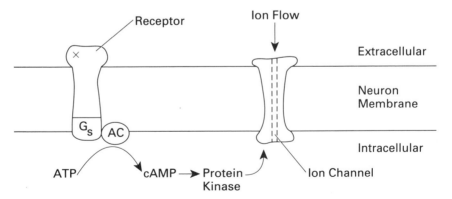

Figure 4–6

Model of one type of slow receptor. A ligand (the primary messenger) binds to the receptor site (x), which activates adenylate cyclase
(AC) via the stimulatory G protein (G_s), which forms cAMP, which
activates protein kinase (both of which can be viewed as secondary
messengers), which opens the ion channel and allows ions to flow
into the cell (or out of the cell).

messengers exist. Also, some receptors may be involved in the inhibition of the enzymes responsible for secondary messenger formation (Cooper et al., 1991). Unfortunately, this lack of knowledge complicates our attempt to understand what is going on in the nervous system, since some neurotransmitters may inhibit a secondary messenger system via one type of receptor and activate it via another type of receptor. (For example, see the discussion in Chapter 12 regarding the two major types of receptors for dopamine.) However, this apparent contradiction does explain how the same neurotransmitter may have excitatory actions in one area and inhibitory actions in another.

In many cases, the actions of a neurotransmitter or its cotransmitters at different receptors on the same cell are synergistic (Bartfai et al., 1988). For example, one cotransmitter may block or slow down the enzymatic degradation of a more active cotransmitter or may change the affinity for or the number of functional receptors available for another cotransmitter. In some cases coexisting and coreleased neurotransmitters may induce apparently opposite signals; for example, one may activate a secondary messenger system and the other may subsequently inhibit it, producing a sharp, well-defined signal.

In any case, receptor activation allows for negatively or positively charged ions on the two sides of the membrane to pass through the membrane (Nicoll, 1988). Since these channels open as a function of a chain of biochemical events triggered by receptor activation, they are often referred to as *chemically sensitive* or *chemically gated channels*. (This terminology distinguishes these channels from the voltage-sensitive channels referred to earlier in the discussion of the conduction process.)

Chemically gated channels that allow Na^+ or Ca^{++} to enter the cell cause a small momentary decrease in polarization. This shifts the electrical potential more toward threshold and thus makes the receiving cell more excitable. When this shift occurs, the voltage change is referred to as an *excitatory postsynaptic potential* or EPSP. Conversely, channels that allow Cl^- to enter the cell or K^+ to leave the cell cause a small momentary increase in polarization, called *hyperpolarization*. This shifts the electrical potential away from the threshold, making the receiving cell less excitable, and the voltage change is referred to as an *inhibitory postsynaptic potential* or IPSP.

Each CNS neuron generally has thousands of synapses, some of them excitatory and some of them inhibitory. A neuron's excitability is determined by the algebraic sum of IPSPs and EPSPs which, as mentioned earlier, can last from several milliseconds to several seconds (Sakmann, 1992).

The influences of EPSPs and IPSPs on neuronal activity are shown graphically in Figure 4–7. Sites 1 and 2 are at the postsynaptic membrane of an excitatory (B) synapse and an inhibitory (C) synapse, respectively. (Of the typical CNS interneuron's several thousand such synapses, only

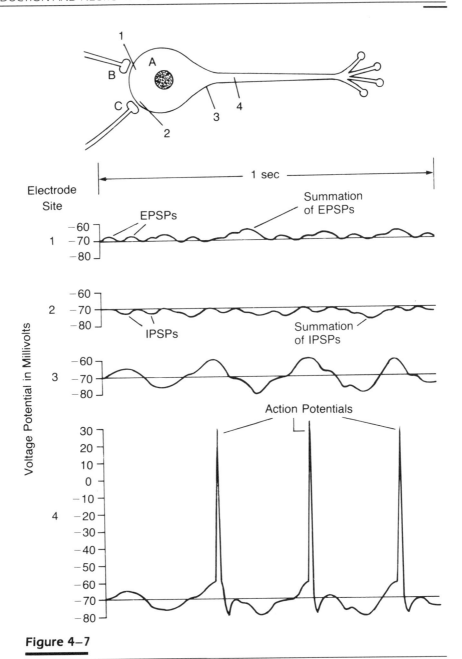

Figure 4–7

Variations in electrical potential at the cell membrane of a neuron (*A*) as a function of where the recording electrode is located.

two are shown here.) Site 3 is located in the region where the axon emerges from neuron A's cell body. Site 4 is located in the axon of neuron A. Variations in electrical potential at sites 1 (EPSPs) and 2 (IPSPs) are quite small, are unidirectional, and occur a millisecond or two after the arrival of action potentials at the presynaptic axon terminals at B and C. Variations at site 3 are somewhat larger and are bidirectional. (Fluctuations at site 3 do not necessarily coincide with fluctuations at sites 1 and 2, since the voltage potential at site 3 is a summation of fluctuations at hundreds of such sites.) Variations at site 4 are relatively large, with the largest shifts (the action potentials created in A) coinciding with the shifts at site 3 that reach the -60 mV threshold potential.

In addition to there being many putative neurotransmitters, virtually all neurotransmitters have at least two distinct receptor subtypes coupled to different ion channels on different cells or even the same cell, and each may have several functions. For example, a neurotransmitter may activate fast receptors at low concentrations and slow receptors at higher concentrations (Nicoll, 1988).

The fact that there are different receptors for the same transmitter may explain why a particular transmitter may be inhibitory in one part of the nervous system (that is, its release causes the receiving neuron to become hyperpolarized) and excitatory (causing depolarization) in another part (Cooper et al., 1991). As more and more receptor subtypes become identified, the selectivity of drug action can be greatly enhanced. Future drugs can be designed to fit only a single receptor subtype, which could then reduce or eliminate the side effects that limit the usefulness of currently employed drugs.

Autoreceptors and Presynaptic Receptors

In addition to the several types of postsynaptic receptors, there is considerable evidence that there are receptors on neurons that are activated by the very neurotransmitters they release (Carlsson, 1987). Thus they are sometimes called *autoreceptors.* These receptors appear to be located in regions of the neuron outside of synapses. Thus these receptors most likely are activated under conditions where there is a relatively high concentration of extracellular neurotransmitter. They appear to perform an "inhibitory feedback" function; that is, when activated, they decrease the neuron's physiological activity or decrease the synthesis or release of its neurotransmitters, which then reduces the influence of the neuron on its target cells' activity. Some neurons have autoreceptors located on their cell bodies or dendrites (see Figure 4–8). These appear to play a role in the modulation of the physiological activity of these neurons, such as their rate of firing. Autoreceptors

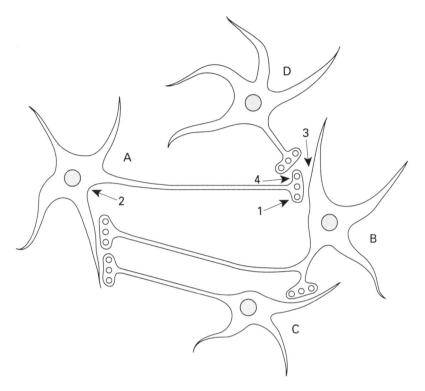

Figure 4–8

Schematic of several potential "negative feedback systems" through
which a neuron's activity may be modulated. Depicted are three different receptor sites for the transmitter released from neuron *A*.
Autoreceptor activation at site 1 (on *A*'s axon terminals) reduces neuron *A*'s transmitter synthesis or release, whereas autoreceptor activation at site 2 (on *A*'s cell body or dendrites) reduces neuron *A*'s physiological activity, for example, by hyperpolarizing the cell.
Postsynaptic receptor activation at site 3 alters neuron *B*'s activity. In
turn, axons from neurons *B* or *C* may form a "collateral negative feedback loop," which modulates neuron *A*'s physiological activity. Finally, neuron *D* may modulate neuron *A*'s ability to release its
neurotransmitters by releasing its own neurotransmitters and activating presynaptic receptors on *A*'s axon terminals at site 4 (an example
of an axoaxonal synapse).

may also be localized on the axon terminals of some neurons. These
appear to modulate the rate of both transmitter biosynthesis and action
potential–induced transmitter release, although these two functions
may be mediated via different autoreceptor subtypes. In general, it
appears that autoreceptors localized on different parts of the neuron act
synergistically. Their stimulation reduces the overall influence of the

neuron on its target postsynaptic cells, while their blockade enhances its influence on the postsynaptic cells.

Several drugs alter neurotransmission because of their high affinity for these autoreceptors. For example, clonidine is a drug that works by activating (thus, it is an agonist) specific autoreceptors for noradrenaline, thus reducing the amount of noradrenaline released into the synapse. This property makes clonidine a potentially useful drug in a variety of clinical and research settings. For example, it can reduce blood pressure and alleviate some narcotic and alcohol withdrawal symptoms (Svensson, 1986).

The presence or absence of autoreceptors on neurons containing the same neurotransmitter may be an important factor in their differential sensitivity to certain types of drugs and to the development of drug tolerance with chronic drug exposure (discussed in Chapter 6). For instance, it has been suggested that this may be responsible for the differential tolerance to the effects of antipsychotics (dopamine receptor blockers) (Cooper et al., 1991). That is, following chronic administration, the influence of many antipsychotic drugs decreases with respect to the dopaminergic neurons possessing autoreceptors (the neurons presumed to be responsible for many of the motor disturbances induced by these drugs; see Chapter 12), but is maintained with respect to those dopaminergic neurons lacking autoreceptors (presumably those neurons responsible for the symptoms of schizophrenia).

A neuron's activity may also be modulated by *collateral feedback mechanisms* via other neurons. In such cases, the activity of one neuron on another is modulated via collateral axons, which form a kind of negative feedback loop (see Figure 4–8).

As was just discussed, autoreceptors may play a role in neurotransmitter release. Unlike the all-or-none process of conduction, the process of releasing transmitters from the terminal appears to be graded, in that the amount of transmitter released is dependent on the ability of Ca^{++} ions to enter the terminal when the action potential arrives (Cooper et al., 1991). The greater the flow of Ca^{++} into the terminal, the greater the quantity of neurotransmitter released. The flow of Ca^{++} may be affected because of activation of the neuron's autoreceptors or because receptors on the terminal have been activated by transmitters released from another axon terminal (that is, activity at an axoaxonal synapse such as depicted in Figures 4–8 and 4–9). The latter receptors are often referred to as *presynaptic receptors* because they are located on the axon terminals and affect the amount of neurotransmitter released from those terminals. (It should be noted that, from the perspective of the neurotransmitter activating these receptors, they are postsynaptic receptors.) It is likely that both autoreceptors and presynaptic receptors are of the slow type. In both cases, the presumed activity decreases Ca^{++} flow into the axon terminal, thereby decreasing the amount of transmitter re-

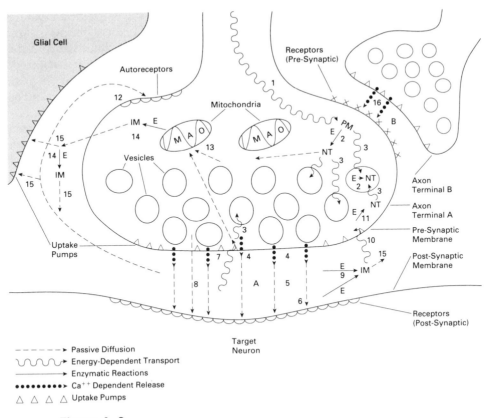

Figure 4–9

Major steps (numbered 1 through 16 in the figure) involved in neurotransmission that are often altered by psychotropic drugs. See text for a discussion of each of these steps.

leased from the terminal when an action potential arrives (Duckles & Budai, 1990). However, in some cases activity at axoaxonal synapses (shown in Figure 4–8 in which axon terminal *D* might synapse with axon terminal *A*, which synapses with dendrite *B*) may enhance transmitter release (from axon terminal *A*) by prolonging depolarization when an action potential arrives.

To summarize, very small electrical potential changes in the dendrites, caused by activity at the synapses, are graded and represent the sum of the contributions of multiple synaptic inputs, some of them inhibitory and some of them excitatory. The summed potentials reach the soma and are modulated by additional synaptic inputs directly to the soma, where there may be enough sodium channels in the soma for action potentials to be initiated there. However, in many neurons, a high density of sodium channels at the axon hillock reduces the threshold for the generation of action potentials, so this initial segment acts as a summation point for the graded potentials from both the dendrites and the soma. In any case, once the threshold potential of the neuron is reached, an action potential is created and propagated down the axon to the axon terminals, which then release the neurotransmitters stored there, and so on and so on and so on.

Figure 4–9 combines all the processes discussed in this chapter that are involved in neurotransmission and that are often altered by psychotropic drugs. Synapse *A* depicts an axodendritic synapse consisting of axon terminal *A* and a postsynaptic membrane of a target neuron's dendrite. Synapse *B* depicts an axoaxonal synapse consisting of axon terminal *B* and a portion of axon terminal *A*'s membrane.

In step 1, precursors (PM) to neurotransmitters (NT) obtained from one's diet must cross the blood-brain barrier, be taken into the neuron, and be transported to the axon terminal. Drugs that are precursors to neurotransmitters found to be deficient in some neurological diseases— for example, Parkinson's disease and Alzheimer's disease—have been used to lessen the symptoms of these diseases.

In step 2, the active neurotransmitter is synthesized from the precursors by way of enzymes (E) located in the axon terminal. Often the synthesis process involves several stages and enzymes and is modulated by step 12. A variety of drugs are available that enhance or reduce these metabolic activities and thus increase or decrease the level of neurotransmitter available for use.

Step 3 depicts the uptake of neurotransmitter molecules or precursors into the synaptic vesicles. Reserpine, a drug originally used to treat extremely agitated patients, prevents several kinds of neurotransmitters from binding to vesicles. This action leaves these neurotransmitters "unprotected" so that they are metabolically inactivated at a higher than normal rate (via step 13). This discovery led to early hypotheses on the biochemical basis of some mood disorders.

Step 4 depicts the entry of Ca^{++} into the axon terminal when an action potential arrives. This results in neurotransmitter release from the vesicles into the synaptic cleft. A variety of drugs affect this process either directly, by blocking Ca^{++} ion channels, or indirectly by activating autoreceptors (step 12) or presynaptic receptors (step 16) that affect Ca^{++} ion channel opening.

Step 5 depicts the passive diffusion of neurotransmitters across the synaptic cleft—a step that drugs rarely alter directly.

Step 6 depicts the binding to and activation of receptors on the postsynaptic membrane of a target neuron, which then results in ion channel opening and a shift in the target neuron membrane's voltage potential. Many drugs discussed in upcoming chapters alter this step because of their agonist or antagonist properties.

Step 7 depicts the reuptake of neurotransmitter back into the axon terminal—a primary mechanism for terminating many neurotransmitters' actions. Cocaine, amphetamine, and some antidepressant drugs inhibit the reuptake of several kinds of neurotransmitters and thus indirectly enhance the amount of neurotransmitter molecules available for receptor binding.

Step 8 indicates that between action potentials some spontaneous leakage of unbound neurotransmitter through the presynaptic membrane can occur. This is one of several processes altered by psychostimulants like amphetamine.

Step 9 indicates the extraneuronal enzymatic alteration of neurotransmitter into inactive metabolites (IM)—another common mechanism for terminating neurotransmitter activity. Some drugs that may potentially reduce the symptoms of Alzheimer's disease alter this step.

Step 10 indicates that some neurotransmitter metabolites may also undergo reuptake so that they can be resynthesized into the active neurotransmitter molecules again (step 11).

Step 12 indicates that neurotransmitters may diffuse through the extracellular fluid and bind to autoreceptors on the axon terminal or other parts of the neuron (not shown), which, when activated, inhibit synthesis or release of neurotransmitters. Most of the drugs that affect step 6 also affect this step.

Step 13 indicates that enzymatic alteration of neurotransmitters into inactive metabolites may also occur intraneuronally when the neurotransmitter is not bound to vesicles. Inhibition of one type of these intraneuronal enzymes, MAO, is believed to be the primary mechanism of action of some types of antidepressant drugs, because this allows neurotransmitter levels to build up in neurons that are deficient in the neurotransmitter.

Step 14 indicates that neurotransmitters may undergo several metabolic alterations, either intraneuronally or extraneuronally. Step 15 indicates that neurotransmitters or their metabolites may also undergo uptake into nonneuronal glial cells or may diffuse through the cerebrospinal fluid to possibly act at sites far removed from their release site. Drugs affecting other steps are also likely to alter steps 14 and 15.

Step 16 depicts the modulating influence of one neurotransmitter on another's activity via an axoaxonal synapse. In this situation the amount of neurotransmitter released from axon terminal *A* can be reduced or enhanced (by altering step 4) through the activity of neurotransmitters released from axon terminal *B* that bind to receptors on axon terminal *A*. (From the perspective of axon terminal *A*, these are presynaptic receptors, but from the perspective of axon terminal *B*, they are postsynaptic receptors.) A variety of drugs, most notably opiates like morphine, are believed to act at this step.

As one might expect, each of these steps interacts in an extremely complicated fashion, so that it is very difficult to determine what the overall consequences of a particular drug's actions might be. Thus, for example, a drug that simply reduces a particular neurotransmitter's reuptake can have far-reaching consequences. This action could increase the number of neurotransmitter molecules available for acting at postsynaptic receptors. On the other hand, it could also increase the number of neurotransmitter molecules acting at autoreceptors. If this results in the decrease in the synthesis or release of the neurotransmitter, it could actually decrease the number of neurotransmitter molecules available for acting at postsynaptic receptors.

This picture will likely be further muddied when you get to subsequent chapters and find out that the number or the sensitivity of various kinds of receptors can change with chronic drug exposure. To reiterate, any drug action, no matter how simple, initiates a cascade of events— some of which eventually are reflected in behavioral effects. Which of these processes are most relevant for the behavioral effects is as yet largely a matter of speculation.

The process of neurotransmission is exceedingly complex—considerably more complicated than it was thought to be just five or 10 years ago. We now recognize the fact that each axon terminal may release one, two, three, or even four different neuroactive chemicals, depending on how frequently the neuron fires. We now know that each of these chemicals generally has more than one type of postsynaptic receptor, presynaptic receptor, or autoreceptor to act on. Some of these receptors induce rapid but short-lived actions on cells, whereas others induce slower-onset and longer actions. Thus the nervous system is capable of considerably more complex signals than we ever imagined. This makes our understanding of how our nervous system works even more difficult than ever. But these new findings do suggest that we will be able to pharmacologically manipulate mood, cognitive functions, and behavior in much more selective ways than ever before—to the point of being able to enhance psychological processes or alleviate dysfunctional ones without inducing the often uncomfortable and sometimes debilitating side effects that present psychotropic drugs induce. We certainly look forward to these advances.

Bibliography

Bartfai, T., Iverfeldt, K., & Fisone, G. (1988). Regulation of the release of coexisting neurotransmitters. *Annual Review of Pharmacology and Toxicology, 28*, 285–310.

Bloom, F. E. (1985). Neurohumoral transmission and the central nervous system. In A. G. Gilman, L. S. Goodman, T. W. Rall, & F. Murad (Eds.), *The pharmacological basis of therapeutics* (pp. 236–259). New York: Macmillan.

Carlson, N. R. (1988). *Foundations of physiological psychology*. Boston: Allyn & Bacon.

Carlsson, A. (1987). Perspectives on the discovery of central monoaminergic neurotransmission. *Annual Review of Neuroscience, 10*, 19–40.

Catterall, W. A. (1988). Structure and function of voltage-sensitive ion channels. *Science, 242*, 50–61.

Chin, J. H., & Goldstein, D. B. (1977). Drug tolerance in biomembranes: A spin label study of the effects of ethanol. *Science, 196*, 684–685.

Cooper, J. R., Bloom, F. E., & Roth, R. H. (1991). *The biochemical basis of neuropharmacology* (6th ed.). New York: Oxford University Press.

Duckles, S. P., & Budai, D. (1990). Stimulation intensity as critical determinant of presynaptic receptor effectiveness. *Trends in the Pharmacological Sciences, 11*, 440–443.

Dunant, Y., & Israel, M. (1985). The release of acetylcholine. *Scientific American, 252*, 58–66.

Enna, S. J., & Karbon, E. W. (1987). Receptor regulation: Evidence for a relationship between phospholipid metabolism and neurotransmitter receptor-mediated cAMP formation in the brain. *Trends in the Pharmacological Sciences Reviews, 8*, 21–24.

Nicoll, R. A. (1988). The coupling of neurotransmitter receptors to ion channels in the brain. *Science, 241*, 545–551.

Pincus, J. H., & Kiss, A. (1986). Phenytoin reduces early acetylcholine release after depolarization. *Brain Research, 397*, 103–107.

Sakmann, B. (1992). Elementary steps in synaptic transmission revealed by currents through single ion channels. *Science, 256*, 503–512.

Stevens, C. F. (1979). The neuron. *Scientific American, 241*, 54–65.

Svensson, T. H. (1986). Clonidine in abstinence reactions: Basic mechanisms. *Acta Psychiatrica Scandinavica, 73*, 19–42.

Tosteson, D. C. (1981). Lithium and mania. *Scientific American, 244*, 164–174.

VanDyke, C. & Byck, R. (1982). Cocaine. *Scientific American, 246*, 128–141.

Weiner, N., & Taylor, P. (1985). Neurohumoral transmission: The autonomic and somatic motor nervous systems. In A. G. Gilman, L. S. Goodman, T. W. Rall, & F. Murad (Eds.), *The pharmacological basis of therapeutics* (pp. 66–99). New York: Macmillan.

Williams, R. W., & Herrup, K. (1988). The control of neuron number. *Annual Review of Neuroscience, 11*, 423–453.

Zucker, R. S., & Lando, L. (1986). Mechanism of transmitter release: Voltage hypothesis and calcium hypothesis. *Science, 231*, 574–578.

Chapter Five

Neuroactive Ligands and the Nervous System

There are literally hundreds of neuroactive chemicals found in and among the billions of cells making up the brain. Some of them appear to exert actions of very short duration (for example, a few milliseconds), while others appear to exert actions of relatively long duration (for example, several seconds or minutes). Some travel very short distances from the cells in which they originate, and others travel relatively long distances. Some exert an action by themselves, while others appear to exert an action only in the presence of other endogenous chemicals. Specific neuroactive ligands are highly localized in some areas of the brain, while others are distributed widely throughout the nervous system.

The nervous system itself has a variety of highly interrelated subsystems, all of which allow us to engage in extremely complex psychological activities such as thinking, planning, learning, speaking, experiencing emotions, preparing the body for action, and so on. By interacting with the natural neuroactive ligands in various areas of the brain, drugs can shift normal psychological activities carried out by the brain into abnormal ones and, in some cases, can serve to normalize abnormal psychological activities. The purpose of this chapter is to familiarize you with some of the more important ligands found in the nervous system and to review briefly some of the major subsystems of the nervous system, so that you can get a better understanding of how psychotropic drugs act and why they induce the effects they do.

Neurotransmitters, Neuromodulators, and Neurohormones

Neurotransmitters are commonly viewed as chemicals that are located in specific regions of neurons, are released under specific stimulation, act on a specific set of receptors, and induce short-duration changes in membrane potentials. Closely related to neurotransmitters are *neuro-hormones*. These are chemicals that are synthesized in one area of the nervous system, are released into circulation, travel to some site that is distant from the release site, and then produce some effect on the brain or body. It is not clear just how far apart the release and receptor sites must be before the status of a chemical changes from that of a neurotransmitter to that of a neurohormone. Furthermore, there are chemicals which have some of the characteristics of neurotransmitters or neurohormones, but by themselves have no intrinsic activity except in the presence of other synaptic activity. These are referred to as *neuromodulators* because they modify responses to other transmitters presynaptically or postsynaptically while not showing any direct shifts in membrane potential or conductance when tested for actions on their own. For example, a neuromodulator may induce a change in the binding of a neurotransmitter to its receptor, or it can act through secondary messengers to modulate neural responses to a neurotransmitter (Kow & Pfaff, 1988).

To further confuse matters, a chemical that appears to play the role of a neurotransmitter in one area of the nervous system may play the role of a neuromodulator or neurohormone somewhere else in the body (Cooper et al., 1991). Because of this potential confusion and because, in a way, neurotransmitters, neurohormones, and neuromodulators are all involved in chemical communication among neurons, throughout this text we will simply refer to them all collectively as neurotransmitters. On occasion, when it is important to distinguish a more specific role for a neuroactive ligand, we will apply the more specific term.

Finally, there are numerous chemicals that play an indirect role in these processes. Some of these are precursors, while others are enzymes involved in the synthesis or breakdown of neuroactive chemicals. Others may be the remnants of the active chemicals that have been inactivated through metabolic processes, but which may still influence neurotransmission because their presence reduces the access of the active chemicals to their receptors.

Hundreds of chemicals in the nervous system have been identified as either being or having the potential to be neurotransmitters (or neuromodulators). They range in structural complexity from molecules of two atoms—for example, simple gases such as nitric oxide (NO) and carbon monoxide (CO)—to molecules comprising hundreds of atoms. The major chemical classes of transmitters are *amines* (molecules with a group consisting of one nitrogen atom in combination with one or more hydrogen atoms), amino acids, and *peptides* (molecules made up of two or more amino acids). With respect to the CNS, most of these chemicals have yet to meet several criteria that would definitely indicate their roles as neurotransmitters. In order for a chemical to be designated as a neurotransmitter,

1. it should be found in presynaptic neurons;
2. enzymes necessary for its synthesis must also be present in the neuron;
3. there should be a mechanism for terminating its action;
4. its direct application to the postsynaptic neuron should be equivalent to stimulation of the presynaptic neuron;
5. when the presynaptic neuron is stimulated, the synaptic cleft should contain the neurotransmitter;
6. drugs interfering with the synthesis or reaction at the postsynaptic membrane should block the effects of presynaptic neuronal stimulation; and
7. drugs blocking the actions of the inactivating enzyme should prolong the transmitter's actions (Cooper et al., 1991).

Though most of the chemicals to be discussed here satisfy one or more of these criteria, only acetylcholine and norepinephrine in the peripheral nervous system satisfy all of them.

Virtually every drug that alters psychological function does so by interacting with one or more neurotransmitter systems in the brain. Drugs have been shown to alter the synthesis, storage, release, enzymatic inactivation, and reuptake of the neurotransmitters. Many drugs either mimic (that is, they are agonists) or block (that is, they are antagonists) specific neurotransmitters at their receptors, both presynaptic and postsynaptic.

The fact that a drug can act on both presynaptic and postsynaptic receptors can cause considerable confusion as to what behavioral effects the drug will have. If, for example, the drug mimics the neurotransmitter at its postsynaptic receptors, it will enhance the neurotransmitter's ability to alter activity of the postsynaptic, or receiving, cell. If the drug mimics the action of the neurotransmitter at its autoreceptors and inhibits the release of the neurotransmitter, it will reduce the neurotransmitter's ability to alter the activity of the postsynaptic cell. (It may help to refer back to Figures 4–8 and 4–9.)

The situation is even more complicated if a drug mimics a neurotransmitter at both its autoreceptors and its postsynaptic receptors, but has a greater affinity for its autoreceptors—a situation that is not uncommon. In such cases, the drug may reduce the neurotransmitter's action at postsynaptic receptors when administered in low doses (because activation of the autoreceptors decreases the amount of endogenous neurotransmitter available for activating the postsynaptic receptors), but it may activate the transmitter's postsynaptic receptors when administered in higher doses. In such cases, even though there is less endogenous transmitter available for the receptors, the drug takes its place so that there is more postsynaptic receptor activation than might occur normally with the transmitter alone (Skirboll et al., 1979).

Although the preceding scenario is indeed confusing, it does give promise for the development of more specific-acting therapeutic drugs in the near future. One of the primary problems we currently have with respect to drugs is their relative lack of specificity, which can result in dependence and side effects that may, in the long run, be worse for patients than the condition they took the drug to counteract.

To summarize, a psychoactive drug can alter any number of the processes involved in the communication system I have just described. It can

1. increase or decrease the rate of synthesizing one or more neurotransmitters;
2. increase or decrease the amount of neurotransmitter released;
3. enhance or prevent the storage of neurotransmitter;
4. increase or decrease a neurotransmitter's rate of metabolic breakdown;
5. bind to the presynaptic or postsynaptic receptors for the neurotransmitter (depending on whether or not the drug activates the receptor), it can accentuate or blunt the neurotransmitter's effects;
6. reduce or enhance the neurotransmitter's reuptake; and
7. serve as a **neurotoxin** or **neurotoxic agent**, a substance that causes the destruction of neural tissue.

Specific Neurotransmitters

There are many putative neurotransmitters. As we see in Figure 5–1, GABA, aspartate, and glutamate are amino acids believed to serve a neurotransmitter role. Serotonin is shown to be composed of an indole nucleus and an amine; norepinephrine is shown to be composed of a catechol nucleus and an amine. Leu-enkephalin is shown to be composed of a string of amino acids; that is, it is a peptide. Histamine is generally found in non-CNS cells made up of connective tissue (mast cells). It is also found in the brain. Although it shares a molecular similarity to the monoamines (norepinephrine, dopamine, serotonin), and blocking its action with antihistamines produces substantial CNS actions such as drowsiness and hunger, the role of histamine in brain function is still very speculative. However, these are only a few that we know much about with respect to drug action, and even in these cases there is a great deal of speculation. Some of these will be described briefly here in terms of some of their properties, and they will be discussed with respect to drug actions later in this book. During this discussion, you should keep in mind that each neuron releases a specific type (or types) of neurotransmitter. In some cases, two or more substances may be released, each substance playing a different role in synaptic transmission (Bartfai, Iverfeldt, & Fisone, 1988). However, neurons are generally referred to by the neurotransmitter that is released that plays the most predominant

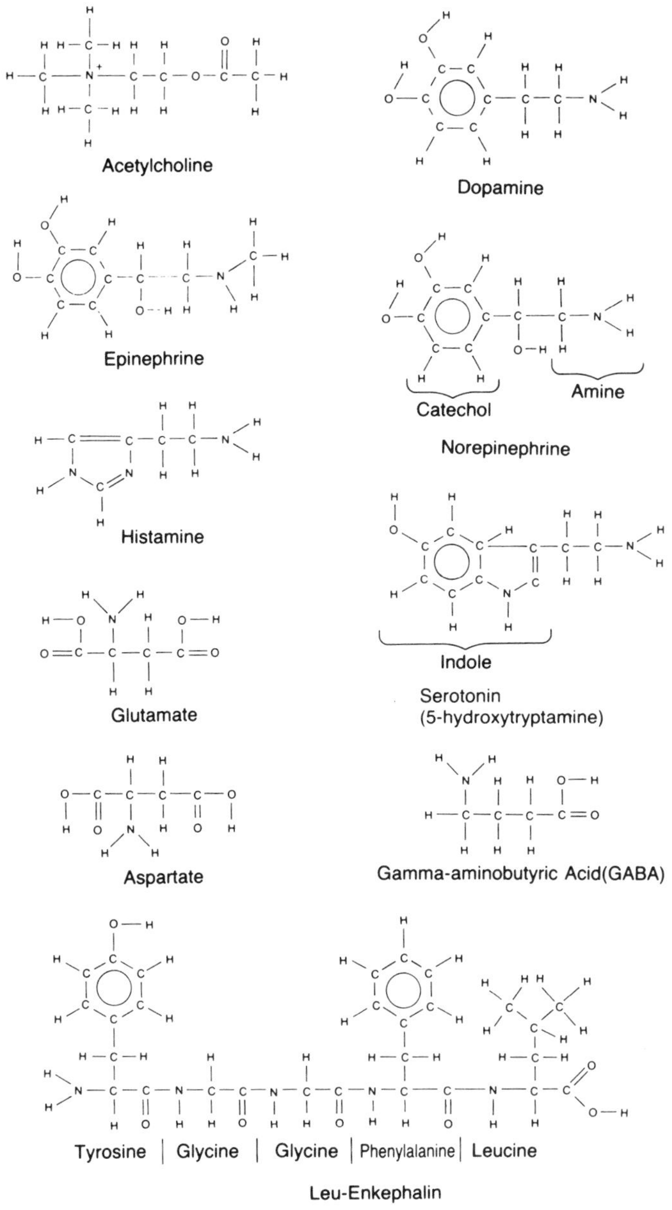

Acetylcholine

Dopamine

Epinephrine

Catechol   Amine

Norepinephrine

Histamine

Indole

Serotonin
(5-hydroxytryptamine)

Glutamate

Aspartate

Gamma-aminobutyric Acid(GABA)

Tyrosine | Glycine | Glycine | Phenylalanine | Leucine

Leu-Enkephalin

Figure 5–1

Molecular structures of chemicals found in the mammalian nervous
system that are believed to serve either a neurotransmitter or
neuromodulatory role. The symbols stand for atoms: C, carbon; H,
hydrogen; O, oxygen; and N, nitrogen. A single bond between atoms is indicated by −, and a double bond by =.

role in the process. Such terms are commonly formed by adding the suffix "ergic" to a root designating the neurotransmitter. For example, adrenergic neurons are those that release adrenaline or noradrenaline, noradrenergic neurons release noradrenaline, dopaminergic neurons release dopamine, cholinergic neurons release acetylcholine, and so forth.

Acetylcholine (Ach) was the first transmitter to meet all of the criteria listed at the beginning of the preceding section (Taylor, 1985). It is found in various parts of the PNS and numerous areas of the CNS. It has excitatory properties in the PNS (it depolarizes the membrane of target cells), whereas in the CNS it can have either excitatory or inhibitory influences on neurons, depending on the area being monitored. It is one of the transmitters that undergo inactivation in the cleft by way of an enzyme. In this case the enzyme is acetylcholinesterase. (Whenever a chemical name ends with "ase," it is an enzyme.) Reuptake then occurs with one of the metabolites (choline).

Cholinergic neurons are found in many different areas of the nervous system, and it is likely that they play a role in a multitude of psychological activities. In the CNS, Ach is particularly important in memory functions. Alzheimer's disease, which results in severe memory loss, is due to the destruction of a relatively small portion of acetylcholine-containing neurons. Drugs that block Ach in the brain (anticholinergics) profoundly reduce the ability to form new memories. On the other hand, drugs that enhance Ach activity may be useful in alleviating some types of memory dysfunctions. Ach is probably involved in certain forms of aggression and grand mal seizures, since both have been noted to occur when there is excessive Ach activity. Excessive Ach activity, when coupled with low norepinephrine activity (discussed below), has been suggested to be a factor in certain kinds of depression as well. Cholinergic mechanisms play an important role in the initiation and maintenance of REM sleep (see Chapter 8). Since abnormalities in REM sleep are found in clinical disorders such as major depression, narcolepsy, obsessive-compulsive disorder, and some forms of schizophrenia (all discussed in later chapters), it is possible that abnormal activation of central cholinergic mechanisms may be involved in these disorders (Shiromani et al., 1987).

Ach also plays numerous roles in the PNS. It is released from the preganglionic nerve endings of both the parasympathetic and the sympathetic nervous systems (these will be briefly discussed a little later on), the postganglionic nerve endings of the parasympathetic nervous system, and the nerve endings at neuromuscular synapses. Many of the peripheral side effects of drugs used for the treatment of mental illness are attributed to the reduction of Ach activity at some of these synapses.

Ach has two primary types of receptors, referred to as *muscarinic* and *nicotinic* because the former are easily activated by the drug muscarine (that is, like Ach, it is an agonist at these receptors) and the latter by nicotine. These drugs exert only minimal influence on the opposite receptors. Recent evidence suggests that there are four or five subtypes of these receptors, differing in terms of where they are found, what types of drugs are agonists and antagonists for them, and their functions. For example, at least one of the nicotinic Ach receptors is a "fast" receptor, whereas all the muscarinic Ach receptors are "slow" receptors (Cooper et al., 1991).

In addition to nicotine and muscarine, some other drugs known to alter cholinergic functioning are curare, which blocks Ach at neuromuscular synapses; atropine, which blocks Ach at muscarinic receptors; and physostigmine, which enhances cholinergic activity at both nicotinic and muscarinic sites by inhibiting acetylcholinesterase.

Norepinephrine (NE, also known as *noradrenaline*) was the second neurotransmitter to be identified as such by neuroscientists (Weiner, 1985). It has a major influence on both the PNS and the CNS. On peripheral cells it has a depolarizing action; that is, it is excitatory. In the CNS, it appears to be predominantly inhibitory with respect to its target neurons, although this may be the case only when the organism is in a quiet environment. With sudden changes in environment, such as a noise, NE activity at its target neurons may enhance their physiological activity (Olpe et al., 1983). Approximately 95% of released NE undergoes reuptake, and the remaining 5% undergoes enzymatic inactivation through the action of the extraneuronal enzyme COMT, which stands for catechol-O-methyl-transferase. NE that is not bound to vesicles can also be changed into an inactive metabolite intraneuronally by MAO (*monoamine oxidase*).

The NE metabolites produced through COMT and MAO activity are different. The former are referred to as *O-methylated metabolites* (because a methyl group, CH_3, is attached to an oxygen atom of the molecule), and the latter are referred to as *deaminated metabolites* (because the amine group, NH_2, is removed). This topic needs to be mentioned here because researchers have attempted to measure their relative amounts in the CNS to provide clues to disorders, such as manic-depression, and drug effects that may be mediated by NE activity. However, as one gets away from the actual sites of NE activity, the metabolites are further metabolized into a common metabolite. That is, O-methylated metabolites get deaminated when they come into contact with MAO, and deaminated metabolites get O-methylated when they come into contact with COMT. Therefore, measuring urinary metabolites of NE, or any other neurotransmitter, is not particularly useful in determining CNS NE activity.

While the brain content of NE is exceedingly small relative to other putative transmitters, it appears to play a crucial role in arousal and mood, where decreased NE activity is associated with low arousal and depression, and high levels are associated with mania and increased motor activity (Stein, 1978). In conjunction with these CNS properties, during acute stress or excitement, NE is released by the postganglionic nerve endings of the sympathetic nervous system.

NE also has two primary types of receptors, with at least two sub-types for each. These are designated as *alpha$_1$*, *alpha$_2$*, *beta$_1$*, and *beta$_2$* receptors, and all are slow receptors (Cooper et al., 1991). Stimulation of alpha$_1$ receptors, which are postsynaptic receptors, generally produces an excitatory effect on the target organ, whereas stimulation of beta receptors depresses ongoing functions (except at the heart). Receptors of the alpha$_2$ type are predominantly autoreceptors on presynaptic axon terminals (although they may also have postsynaptic functions), such that their activation produces effects opposite to those induced by alpha$_1$ receptor activation.

Epinephrine (Epi, also known as *adrenaline*), is closely related to NE, in both structure and function in the PNS. The structural similarity comes about because NE is the immediate precursor to Epi. Their functional similarity comes about because during times of acute stress, when the organism is frightened or must be ready to fight or flee (the *fight-flight-fright* syndrome), Epi is released from the adrenal gland into the bloodstream and is taken to NE sites of action in the sympathetic nervous system, where it is an agonist. In this context, Epi may be viewed more as a neurohormone than as a neurotransmitter. Because Epi is found in very small amounts in the brain, our understanding of Epi's role in CNS functions is very limited. It may be a factor in the control of neuroendocrine function and blood pressure (Cooper et al., 1991).

Closely related to NE and Epi is the transmitter *dopamine* (DA). It is one of the neurotransmitters whose primary role appears to be inhibitory on its target neurons in the CNS. While it appears to serve its own transmitter role in some neurons, it is also the immediate precursor to NE in those neurons where NE is the transmitter. (Because NE, epinephrine, and DA molecules have two common parts—a "catechol" nucleus and an amine group [NH$_2$]—they are often referred to as *catecholamines*.) Dopamine's and NE's actions are terminated in the same way; most DA undergoes reuptake, and some undergoes COMT transformation. Intra-neuronal metabolization by way of MAO may also occur with DA.

At least two classes of DA receptors have been distinguished (designated D$_1$ and D$_2$), and both classes appear to consist of slow receptors (Cooper et al., 1991). Recent cloning studies have subsequently identified four subtypes of D$_2$ receptors and two subtypes of D$_1$ receptors. Postsynaptic D$_2$ receptors appear to be primarily responsible for the antipsychotic activity of many drugs, as well as the motor disturbances induced by them. There is considerable evidence that both DA synthesis and DA release in CNS neurons are regulated via D$_2$ autoreceptors, and there is evidence that both processes are independent of each other (Zetterstrom, Sharp, & Ungerstedt, 1986).

Like NE, DA comprises a relatively small proportion of putative neurotransmitters in the brain, but it appears to exert profound influence on many emotional, mental, and motor functions, as well as drug-induced effects (Stein, 1978). In many cases, DA appears to play a modulatory role in behavior, with its effects dependent on slow, sustained DA secretion—referred to as *tonic* release—which is relatively independent of nerve impulse patterns (McGinty & Szymusiak, 1988). In other dopaminergic tracts, DA release is very much dependent on nerve impulse pattern and frequency—referred to as *phasic* release.

Brain DA systems are believed to mediate the euphoric effects of drugs like cocaine. An overactive DA system, because of overly sensitive receptors, too many receptors, too much DA release, or too little DA reuptake, has been suggested to be the cause of many symptoms of most cases of schizophrenia, whereas the destruction of a small subset of DA-containing neurons in the brain is responsible for Parkinson's disease. DA neurons have also been suggested to be involved in tic and movement disorders, such as Huntington's chorea and Gilles de la Tourette's syndrome; affective disorders; sexual activity and drive; hyperactivity in children and adults; and long-lasting motor disturbances associated with prolonged use of antipsychotics. Each of these will be discussed later on.

Structured somewhat along the lines of the catecholamines just described is a neurotransmitter called *serotonin*. Its more technical name is *5-hydroxytryptamine* or 5-HT. (It would be nice if all neuroscientists could agree on one term for these chemicals so we would not have to learn so many names for the same thing, but unfortunately that is not the case.) It also consists of one amine group attached to what is referred to as an indole nucleus. (Because their structures contain one amine group, 5-HT and the catecholamines are often referred to as *monoamines*.) Termination of 5-HT action appears to be entirely through reuptake. Several distinct subtypes of 5-HT receptors have been identified (designated in a variety of ways, e.g., 5-HT_{1A}, 5-HT_{1B}, 5-HT_{1C}, 5-HT_{1D}, 5-HT_2, 5-HT_3, 5-HT_{1P}) (Cooper et al., 1991), but as yet little is known about their different functions. At least two of these appear to be slow receptors.

Although 5-HT has some PNS activity (for example, it regulates contractions of various blood vessels), it plays a profound role in many CNS activities, where at the cellular level it is predominantly an inhibitory neurotransmitter. Serotonergic systems have been implicated in the modulation of a variety of psychological processes—for example, sexual activity, mood, degree of pain sensitivity, aggression, sleep, and some psychotic symptoms (Cooper et al., 1991). Several depression-relieving drugs, such as amitriptyline (Elavil), as well as hallucination-inducing drugs, like LSD and mescaline, appear to act by altering serotonergic functioning.

In addition to its role as a neurotransmitter, serotonin may play a vital role in learning because it has been shown to strengthen the synapses formed between neurons (of mollusks) that have been grown in cultures (i.e., two or three neurons that have been removed from the animal and grown in a medium of molluscan fluids and factors), much as it does between neurons in the intact animal after a learning session (Barinaga, 1990).

Though amino acids are often intermediary substances in the metabolic synthesis of the types of neurotransmitters just described, many also fulfill several of the criteria for being neurotransmitters themselves. In fact, in sheer quantity, amino acids are probably the major neurotransmitters in the mammalian CNS (Cooper et al., 1991). Some amino acids are excitatory; that is, they depolarize neurons. Others are inhibitory; that is, they hyperpolarize neurons. Perhaps the most widespread inhibitory neurons in the CNS utilize gamma-aminobutyric acid (GABA) as a neurotransmitter. Almost every major division of the brain and spinal cord includes some of them. Enhancing the activity of GABA at its receptor complex appears to be a major common pathway for a diversity of drugs with sedative and sleep-inducing properties—for example, alcohol, diazepam (Valium), and barbiturates (Gottlieb, 1987). There appear to be at least two functionally distinct types of GABA receptors. $GABA_A$ receptors are fast receptors directly associated with a Cl^- ion channel, whereas $GABA_B$ receptors are slow receptors coupled to secondary messenger systems that either enhance K^+ flow out of neurons or inhibit Ca^{++} flow into neurons (Cooper et al., 1991).

A great deal of interest has been generated recently over the excitatory amino acids glutamate and aspartate, because they act at a type of receptor termed the NMDA receptor. This receptor has been linked to a variety of processes ranging from learning and memory formation to neurotoxicity associated with low blood sugar or low oxygen levels, seizures, and other disturbances resulting from excess excitatory amino acid activity (Olney, 1990). Because the NMDA ion channel is selective for Ca^{++}, it may be possible to prevent many brain disorders—for example, epilepsy, Parkinson's disease, Alzheimer's disease, Huntington's chorea, AIDS dementia—through the use of calcium channel blockers. The ion channel regulated by NMDA receptors also appears to be one of the sites of action of phencyclidine, a psychosis-mimicking drug.

A variety of *peptides*, or strings of amino acids, have neuroactive properties (Krieger, 1983). Peptides may serve as neurotransmitters, in which they generally act slowly (e.g., actions that may last 2–3 minutes), or as neuromodulators, in which they generally act even more slowly (e.g., actions lasting 45 minutes or longer) (Kow & Pfaff, 1988). Several important peptides that have become prominent are called *endorphins*, which stands for *end*ogenous m*orphin*e-like substances. This class of peptides was first identified in the mid-1970s, and they appear to serve as prototype neuromodulators; that is, they may not serve as transmitters in the traditional sense but may modulate the activity of the transmitters. The term "endorphin" is used in two different contexts. In one it refers specifically to endogenous peptides with opiate-like properties found primarily in the pituitary, but also found throughout the various parts of the body. This usage contrasts with the term *enkephalin* (in the head), which refers to a number of endogenous peptides with opiate-like properties found in the CNS. In the other context, endorphin is a general term encompassing all endorphin and enkephalin molecules in the body (in most cases this is how they will be referred to throughout this text).

There has been considerable speculation recently that endorphins are involved in a wide variety of processes and activities, including pain perception, attention, primary reward, crying, laughing, thrills from music, acupuncture, placebos, stress reactions, depression, compulsive gambling, aerobics, masochism, massage, labor and delivery, appetite, immunity, near-death experiences, and playing with pets (Hopson, 1988). For example, studies on maternal calming of infants have shown that certain substances, milk and sucrose among them, cause the release of endorphins in infants, which, in turn, is manifested in increased pain tolerance, decreased vocalization, decreased activity, reduced heart rate, and bringing the hand to the mouth (Blass, 1992). The effects of narcotics such as morphine and heroin are due to their agonist activity at endorphin receptors. Several subtypes of endorphin receptors (most of them slow receptors) have been identified and will be discussed in Chapter 10.

The majority of this section has focused on the neurotransmitter systems that most likely mediate the psychological effects of psychotropic drugs, because these systems play such a generalized role in the way we process information, in our readiness to respond to the external environment, and in our emotions and motivational states (Panksepp, 1986). In very general terms, we can say that the cholinergic system is an action system in the brain (in both motor and sensory-processing terms) that helps elaborate the ability to focus on the environment and achieve a coherent behavioral response to it. Practically every type of motivated and emotional behavior is affected by alterations in serotonergic and noradrenergic activity. They exert a direct influence on attentional processes, and hence affect learning and memory formation. Dopaminergic systems mediate a generalized ability for response initiation, having perhaps a more specific role in triggering instinctual processes related to positive and negative incentives. Most motivated and emotive behaviors, ranging from feeding to aggression, are also affected by alterations in GABA activity. Finally, the global function of opioid systems appears to be one of counteracting any major perturbation of physiological homeostasis (i.e., stress). However, as the preceding account should indicate, virtually every psychobehavioral process is mediated by more than one brain area and more than one neurochemical system and affected by drugs with very different mechanisms of action (Panksepp, 1986).

Neurotransmitters and Diet

Neurotransmitters (and other neuroactive substances) and their precursors are chemical substances that are essentially nutrients obtained in the food we eat. In most cases, it is the precursors that are likely to be found in the diet, since most neurotransmitters are unable to cross the blood-brain barrier. One of the most common precursors to a variety of neuroactive ligands is glucose, which follows a number of metabolic pathways to form ligands such as aspartate, glutamate, GABA, and acetylcholine (Cooper et al., 1991). A variety of amino acids also serve as neurotransmitter precursors. For example, tryptophan, an amino acid found in protein-rich foods like dairy products, meat, fish, and poultry, is a precursor of the neurotransmitter serotonin. (Tryptophan is one of eight essential amino acids, so-called because our bodies cannot synthesize them; they must be obtained from our diet.) Tyrosine, a precursor of dopamine, norepinephrine, and epinephrine, is another amino acid found in proteins. Choline, the precursor of acetylcholine, is a component of the lecithin found in egg yolks, soy products, and liver. Therefore, it makes sense that altering one's diet can give rise to important changes in the chemical composition within the brain and can modify brain function and alter mood and behavior in specific ways (Wurtman, 1982).

For example, loading up on protein-rich foods might be expected to enhance the brain's production of serotonin, which is believed to promote relaxation and hasten the onset of sleep (Radulovacki, 1982). It has been suggested that people who have trouble sleeping should drink warm milk, which contains high levels of tryptophan, before bedtime. Protein-rich foods might also be expected to elevate levels of norepinephrine, believed necessary for positive mood states (Stein, 1978). Loading up on lecithin-containing foods may be beneficial in cognitive and memory disorders such as Alzheimer's disease, which have been associated with acetylcholine deficiencies.

Unfortunately, however, it is not that simple. Numerous biochemical processes must follow in sequence if the consumption of a meal rich in a particular nutrient is to increase the synthesis of a neurotransmitter in the brain (Wurtman, 1982). First, there must be a significant elevation of the plasma level of the nutrient; in some cases, the level of a nutrient in the plasma is regulated by inhibitory feedback mechanisms. Second, the nutrient's concentration in the brain must vary with the plasma concentration; that is, the nutrient must be able to penetrate the blood-brain barrier. Third, the transport system involved in the nutrient's movement between the plasma and the brain must not be easily saturated with the nutrient or other nutrients that compete for the same transport system. Fourth, the enzymes necessary for the conversion of the precursor into the neurotransmitter in the brain must not be easily saturable. Fifth, these enzymes must not be susceptible to negative feedback inhibition when the intracellular levels of the neurotransmitter rise.

In many cases, not all of these requirements can be fulfilled simultaneously. For example, in the case of tryptophan, you might think that a high-protein meal would make you drowsy. However, high-protein foods contain several amino acids, not just tryptophan, and they all compete for the same transporter molecules in the blood-brain barrier. Because tryptophan occurs in food in relatively small quantities, it does not have much of a chance of getting into the brain if all one eats is protein. If one eats food with carbohydrates (for example, sweets, bread, pasta, potatoes), which stimulate the production of insulin, all the other amino acids can get drawn out of the blood while having little effect on tryptophan blood levels. Therefore, the proper mixture of proteins and carbohydrates must be consumed in order to increase the chances of tryptophan making it into the brain. In fact, many of the behavioral effects that have been attributed to eating carbohydrates may be due to the ability of carbohydrates to enhance the influx of tryptophan into the brain (Spring et al., 1987).

Because various nutrients in food interact in such complicated ways, most of which are not well understood, it is very difficult to predict in advance what a particular nutrient or combination of foods will do with respect to mood and behavior. In most studies showing links between diet and behavior in human beings, the effects have been subtle, in comparison with a multitude of other factors influencing mood and behavior. Furthermore, the relationships may depend on the age of the individual, the time of day the nutrient or food is consumed, or individual genetic variations.

Structures and Subsystems of the Nervous System

Moods, thoughts, and behavior do not come about through the activity of single neurons, nor are the actions of drugs due to their actions at single neurons. Neurons make up a number of structures and subsystems of the nervous system, which have different functions and involve different neurotransmitters, which in turn are affected by drugs. Some of these will be briefly described here; they will be discussed with respect to drug action at later points in this book.

Peripheral Nervous System

The *peripheral nervous system* (PNS) is composed of all nervous tissue outside of the spinal cord and the brain. The PNS can be differentiated into nerves (bundles of axons outside the CNS) serving sensory functions (for example, allowing light, sound, and chemicals from the environment to impact on the CNS) and motor functions (such as allowing the CNS to induce changes in bodily functions). *Motor nerves* are further differentiated into the *somatic nervous system,* which controls skeletal muscles, and the *autonomic nervous system,* which controls smooth and cardiac muscle activity and several glands, including the adrenal glands, salivary glands, and sweat glands. Virtually all of these organs are innervated (connected to nerves) by two opposing systems within the autonomic nervous system. One is called the *parasympathetic nervous system,* which is responsible for controlling vegetative, restorative, and energy-saving processes. It is particularly active in calm situations. The other is called the *sympathetic nervous system,* which is responsible for preparing the body for dealing with situations requiring fighting or fleeing, or times when the organism is frightened (the *fight-flight-fright* system). It is particularly active during times of acute stress and excitement. Drugs whose actions mimic those associated with sympathetic activity are often referred to as **sympathomimetics**, and those whose actions mimic parasympathetic activity are referred to as **parasympathomimetics**. Table 5–1 indicates the major activities carried out by the sympathetic and parasympathetic nerve fibers comprising the autonomic nervous system.

The axons from both the parasympathetic and sympathetic systems that originate from neurons in the spinal cord and brain are referred to as preganglionic fibers, and they release the neurotransmitter acetylcholine. The target neurons for these fibers are clustered together in groups of cell bodies called *ganglia* (a *ganglion* is a grouping of neuron cell bodies outside the CNS). The receptors on the target neurons are those I referred to a little earlier as nicotinic receptors. The axons that originate from these ganglionic cells and connect with, or innervate, the organs are referred to as postganglionic fibers. Postganglionic axons of the sympathetic system release norepinephrine, which activates three different types of receptors (alpha$_1$, alpha$_2$, and beta$_2$) in the membranes of target organ cells. Postganglionic axons of the parasympathetic system release acetylcholine, which activates muscarinic receptors in the target organ cells. Because NE activates receptors in the sympathetic part of the PNS, and Ach activates receptors in the parasympathetic part of the PNS, the functions of these two neurotransmitters are generally in opposition in the PNS (Weiner & Taylor, 1985). An exception is the case where activation of Ach receptors in the adrenal gland results in the release of epinephrine, a neurohormone that enhances sympathetic activity.

The relatively high degree of localization of noradrenergic and

Table 5–1

Effect of Activity of Autonomic Nerve Fibers

Organ	Sympathetic	Parasympathetic
Adrenal medulla	Secretion of epinephrine and norepinephrine	
Bladder	Inhibition of contraction	Contraction
Blood vessels		
Abdomen	Constriction	
Muscles	Dilation	Constriction
Skin	Constriction or dilation	Dilation
Heart	Faster rate of contraction	Slower rate of contraction
Intestines	Decreased activity	Increased activity
Lacrimal glands	Secretion of tears	
Liver	Release of glucose	
Lungs	Dilation of bronchi	Constriction of bronchi
Penis	Ejaculation	Erection
Pupil of eye	Dilation	Constriction
Salivary glands	Secretion of thick, viscous saliva	Secretion of thin, enzyme-rich saliva
Sweat glands	Secretion of sweat	
Vagina	Orgasm	Secretion of lubricating fluid

cholinergic nerve fibers and several types of receptors for noradrenaline and acetylcholine in the PNS has allowed neuroscientists to assess neurotransmission processes and drug actions in a fairly specific manner. This has led them to develop models of what is happening with respect to these processes and actions in the brain, where neurons of various types are tightly packed together and are difficult to isolate. In fact, much of what is thought to go on in the synapses in the CNS is based on studies conducted on the PNS, on the assumption that the two operate in basically the same fashion.

Central Nervous System

The *central nervous system* or CNS, shown in Figure 5–2, is comprised of the brain and spinal cord. The top portion of the brain is actually comprised of two semisymmetrical halves called the *cerebral hemispheres*. The outer surface of these is called the *cerebral cortex,* and it is composed of several densely packed layers of neuron cell bodies. Certain parts of the cortex are called *sensory projection areas* because these are areas of the cortex where the information from the senses is processed. The *temporal lobes* contain the primary receiving area for auditory information and visual recognition. The *parietal lobes* are the primary receiving area for bodily sensations and are involved in spatial perception. The *occipital lobes* are the primary receiving area for visual information.

The cortex in the *frontal lobes* allows us to ascribe meaning to the incoming stimuli initially processed in the sensory projection areas. It is essential for higher-order thought processing, such as synthetic reasoning and abstract thought, and it allows us to organize events from independent places and times and to make plans. The cortex comprising the back part of the frontal lobe, called the *motor projection area,* allows us to act voluntarily on these higher level processes; that is, it is from this region that directives that ultimately go to the muscles are issued.

Finally, while the two hemispheres are viewed as specializing in processing different kinds of information—for example, language in the left and visual-spatial in the right—they are connected by some 200 million nerve axons collectively referred to as the *corpus callosum,* which allows them to communicate with one another.

Considering the variety of functions carried out by these portions of the brain, it should not be surprising that a vast mixture of neurotransmitters and other biologically active chemicals are found in these regions. It should also come as no surprise that we know relatively little about the complex drug interactions that take place in these regions. Any drug affecting these regions is going to have a multiplicity of effects on perceptual and cognitive functions.

Figure 5–3 shows the part of the brain below the cerebral hemispheres and some important subcortical structures comprising the limbic system. The *medulla* controls vital reflex functions such as respiration, heartbeat, and blood pressure. The *pons* connects higher brain centers with the cerebellum and, along with the medulla, contains most of the cell bodies of the reticular activating system (discussed later in this section). In these regions of the brain, relatively high concentrations of catecholamines, serotonin, and enkephalins have been noted. The *cerebellum* controls automatic skeletal motor activities and coordinates balance and the body's movements. Collectively, the medulla, pons, and cerebellum are often referred to as the *hindbrain.*

The *midbrain* contains primitive centers for auditory and visual processing. It is also important for the perception of pain, a function which is consistent with the high concentrations of enkephalins found there. The midbrain also contains dopaminergic neurons, whose axons project into areas in the frontal cortex and the basal ganglia (see the last paragraph of this section), which have been suggested to be involved in disorders such as schizophrenia and Parkinson's disease (discussed in

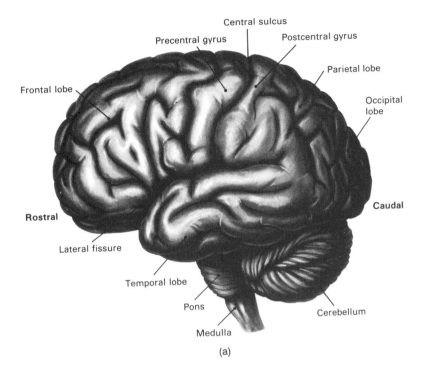

Central sulcus
Precentral gyrus
Postcentral gyrus
Parietal lobe
Frontal lobe
Occipital lobe
Caudal
Rostral
Lateral fissure
Temporal lobe
Pons
Cerebellum
Medulla

(a)

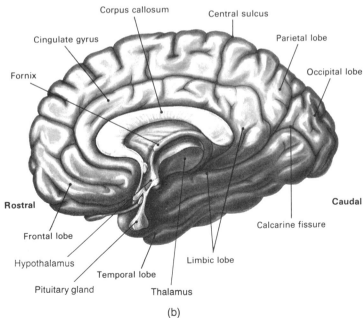

Corpus callosum
Central sulcus
Cingulate gyrus
Parietal lobe
Fornix
Occipital lobe
Rostral
Caudal
Frontal lobe
Calcarine fissure
Hypothalamus
Pituitary gland
Temporal lobe
Limbic lobe
Thalamus

(b)

Figure 5–2

The human brain: (*a*) lateral view of the left side; (*b*) midline section showing the inside part of the right hemisphere.

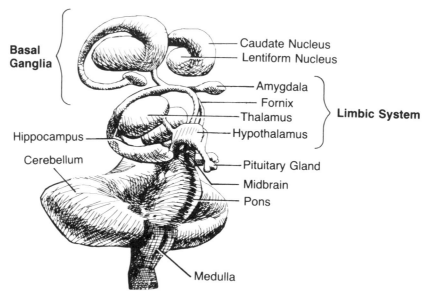

Figure 5–3

Some of the important internal structures of the brain, including the thalamus, basal ganglia, limbic system, hypothalamus, and lower brain structures.

Chapters 12 and 14). The *thalamus* is the great "relay" station in the brain in that it relays incoming sensory information to the appropriate areas of the cortex, as well as relaying information from higher regions of the brain to lower ones. It also appears to play a part in regulating the overall level of excitability of cortical neurons.

The *limbic system* is a conglomeration of diverse structures in the cerebral hemispheres where a large number of circuits relating to different functions come together. It is thought to play a key role in the cognitive arousal of emotion and the formation of memory (McGinty & Szymusiak, 1988). The primary reward and punishment centers are believed to exist in this diffuse system, since mild electrical stimulation applied to various limbic regions can serve as very effective reinforcement for instrumental responding in animals, whereas electrical stimulation in other regions appears to be highly aversive. Limbic structures may also be involved in many mood and thought disorders in humans, since electrical stimulation and lesions in various areas of the limbic system have been found to induce paranoid ideation (characterized by suspiciousness and beliefs that one is being plotted against and persecuted), depersonalization (feelings of strangeness and an unreality of experience), perceptual distortions or hallucinations (compelling perceptual experiences without the pres-

ence of a physical stimulus), catatonia (immobility), thought disturbances, and mood and emotional disturbances.

Some parts of the limbic system are critically important for certain
kinds of learning and memory formation—for example, the *hippocampus*.
Others are critically involved in mood, emotionality, and emotional
expressions—for example, the *amygdala* and *cingulate gyrus*. Relatively
heavy concentrations of catecholamines (primarily norepinephrine),
GABA, serotonin, and enkephalins have been found in the limbic system. However, to say that any of these are the major neurotransmitters
of this system would be misleading, as there are more than 20 different
neurotransmitters or modulators found in the hippocampus alone (Nicoll, 1988).

The *hypothalamus* regulates the expression of basic drive states—
such as hunger, thirst, sex, and aggression—and body temperature, and
it exerts major control over the autonomic nervous system. It is also the
nervous system's way of mediating control over the endocrine system
because it has numerous neuronal connections and hormones that can
influence the activity of the pituitary gland, whose hormones control
numerous functions of the other endocrine glands of the body. As is the
case with the limbic system, heavy concentrations of catecholamines and
enkephalins are found in the hypothalamus. Thus drugs that alter activity at catecholamine receptors (such as cocaine, amphetamine, and chlorpromazine) or enkephalin receptors (such as morphine and heroin) profoundly influence mood, emotion, emotional reaction, and primary
drive.

The *reticular activating system* or RAS, shown in Figure 5–4, is comprised of a diffuse network of neurons whose cell bodies originate in the
pons and medulla and send axons (ascending and descending) to most
regions of the brain and spinal cord. The RAS participates in a wide
variety of psychological processes ranging from perception to mood to
our ability to associate events (McGinty & Szymusiak, 1988). It may be
thought of as setting "brain tone," by regulating mood and the responsiveness of target neurons to incoming stimulation from the senses or to
internally produced stimuli (that is, mental activity). The ascending RAS
regulates the level of alertness and screening of information—that is,
attentional processes—by filtering out unimportant sensory information
and allowing important information to reach higher brain centers for
further processing. These functions also suggest that thought and perceptual disturbances may be the result of malfunctions in the reticular
activating system. Although several types of neurons play roles in this
system, serotonergic and noradrenergic neurons appear to be particularly important (McGinty & Szymusiak, 1988). Their influence is primarily inhibitory with respect to their target neurons if the organism is in a
vegetative state or if there is little environmental stimulation. However,
with sudden changes in environmental stimulation, the activity of the

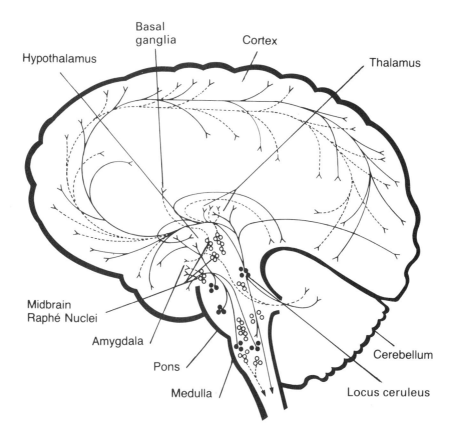

Basal
ganglia   Cortex

Hypothalamus   Thalamus

Midbrain
Raphé Nuclei

Amygdala

Pons   Cerebellum

Medulla

Locus ceruleus

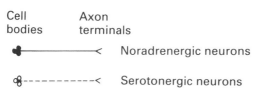

Cell   Axon
bodies   terminals

Noradrenergic neurons

Serotonergic neurons

Figure 5–4

Stylized schematic of the reticular activating system (RAS) comprised
predominantly of serotonergic and noradrenergic cells and axon fibers (although other neurons, such as adrenergic cells, play a role in
the RAS). Note that both types of fibers are very diffusely distributed
and greatly overlap. They differ, however, in the details of distribution and target cells they innervate.

target neurons may actually be enhanced with RAS noradrenergic input. During certain stages of sleep, these serotonergic and noradrenergic neurons cease firing almost completely, and this cessation of activity may account for some of the phenomena associated with dreaming, such as the vivid mixtures of strange images, sounds, and emotions.

Along with the descending RAS, numerous brain structures, including the motor cortex and cerebellum, are involved in regulating the activity of motor neurons that control the skeletal muscles. One group of these brain structures comprises the *basal ganglia* (actually this is a misnomer since ganglia are located *outside* the CNS). This group of structures, just above and to the side of the thalamus (see Figure 5–3), serves in the regulation of slow, voluntary, smooth movement of different speeds, which can be modified by sensory feedback while the movement is occurring. Loss of dopaminergic input (from a midbrain area called the *substantia nigra*) to the basal ganglia leads to progressive deterioration of walking, standing, and many other postures and movements involving the body as a whole. Excessive dopaminergic input may result in repetitive or stereotypic movements. The symptoms of Parkinson's disease and several side effects of drugs used to treat schizophrenia arise from disturbances in the basal ganglia.

Drugs, the Nervous System, and Behavior: A Perspective

This chapter has dealt very briefly with a number of complex processes through which drugs may act to bring about alterations in mood, emotions, cognitions, and behavior. In some cases, the processes involve molecular activities; in other cases, they involve cellular or multicellular activities and functions in the nervous system. Understanding drug action at these levels is important. However, one of the greatest challenges for neuroscientists is to be able to translate the actions of a drug at the subcellular, cellular, or multicellular level into an understanding of its actions at the psychological level. At present, it is a challenge with which we only vaguely know how to deal.

For example, what does it mean to become excited? Personally, when I sink a crucial 30-foot putt on the last hole of a golf match, I get excited. I yell and throw my fist into the air, my heart pounds, my blood pressure shoots up, and I breathe heavily. However, when a neuron gets excited, it means something entirely different. It means that the electrical gradient that is present between the inside and the outside of the cell has been reduced to the point at which it is no longer sufficient to keep the Na^+ channels closed, which then initiates a whole chain of biochemical events. Is this what we mean when we say the CNS is excited? Probably not. The CNS is a collection of around 85 billion cells, with perhaps 600 trillion connections among them. It is certainly not the case that most or all fire simultaneously or that all the synapses are filled with neurotransmitters. That would be chaos. (This issue will be discussed more fully in the context of drugs with stimulant or depressant properties in Chapter 7.)

In conclusion, we may be able to determine that a drug activates, or excites, a specific set of receptors, which in turn opens ion channels, which allows negatively charged ions to flow inward, which hyperpolarizes the cell, which decreases its rate of firing, and so on. As impressive as such knowledge might be, it would have little value in leading us to an understanding of how that drug brings about changes in mood, emotion, or cognitive functioning. That is, there is no reason to assume that such a drug action at the cellular level will depress mood or slow one's thought (Cooper et al., 1991). The fact is there are a multitude of intermediate steps between the cellular activities of the nervous system and the behavior, emotions, and thoughts evidenced in the intact organism. While we may discuss neurotransmitter effects as excitatory or inhibitory, it should be made clear that these effects are on neuron membrane potentials, not on behavior. Conversely, when we say an organism has become aroused or excited, we must not confuse this state with alterations in membrane potentials.

Bibliography

Barinaga, M. (1990). The high culture of neuroscience. *Science, 250,* 206–207.

Bartfai, T., Iverfeldt, K., & Fisone, G. (1988). Regulation of the release of coexisting neurotransmitters. *Annual Review of Pharmacology and Toxicology, 28,* 285–310.

Blass, E. M. (1992). The ontogeny of motivation: Opioid bases of energy conservation and lasting affective change in rat and human infants. *Current Directions in Psychological Science, 1,* 116–120.

Cooper, J. R., Bloom, F. E., & Roth, R. H. (1991). *The biochemical basis of neuropharmacology* (6th ed.). New York: Oxford University Press.

Gottlieb, D. I. (1987). GABAergic neurons. *Scientific American, 258,* 82–89.

Hopson, J. L. (1988, July/August). A pleasurable chemistry. *Psychology Today,* pp. 29–33.

Kow, L. M., & Pfaff, D. W. (1988). Neuromodulatory actions of peptides. *Annual Review of Pharmacology and Toxicology, 28,* 163–188.

Krieger, D. T. (1983). Brain peptides: What, where, and why? *Science, 222,* 975–985.

McGinty, D., & Szymusiak, R. (1988). Neuronal unit activity patterns in behaving animals: Brainstem and limbic system. *Annual Review of Psychology, 39,* 135–168.

Nicoll, R. A. (1988). The coupling of neurotransmitter receptors to ion channels in the brain. *Science, 241,* 545–551.

Olney, J. W. (1990). Excitotoxic amino acids and neuropsychiatric disorders. *Annual Review of Pharmacology and Toxicology, 30,* 47–71.

Olpe, H. R., Jones, R.S.G., & Steinmann, M. W. (1983). The locus coeruleus: Actions of psychoactive drugs. *Experientia, 39,* 242–249.

Panksepp, J. (1986). The neurochemistry of behavior. *Annual Review of Psychology, 37,* 77–107.

Radulovacki, M. (1982). L-tryptophan's effects on brain chemistry and sleep in cats and rats: A review. *Neuroscience and Biobehavioral Reviews, 6,* 421–428.

Shiromani, P. J., Gillin, J. C., & Henriksen, S. J. (1987). Acetylcholine and the regulation of REM sleep: Basic mechanisms and clinical implications for affective illness and narcolepsy. *Annual Review of Pharmacology and Toxicology, 27,* 137–156.

Skirboll, L. R., Grace, A. A., & Bunney, B. S. (1979). Dopamine auto- and postsynaptic receptors: Electrophysiological evidence for differential sensitivity to dopamine agonists. *Science, 206,* 80–82.

Spring, B., Chiodo, J., & Bowen, D. J. (1987). Carbohydrates, tryptophan, and behavior: A methodological review. *Psychological Bulletin, 102,* 234–256.

Stein, L. (1978). Reward transmitters: Catecholamines and opioid peptides. In M. A. Lipton, A. DiMascio, & K. F. Killam (Eds.), *Psychopharmacology* (pp. 569–582). New York: Raven Press.

Taylor, P. (1985). Cholinergic agonists. In A. G. Gilman, L. S. Goodman, T. W. Rall, & F. Murad (Eds.), *The pharmacological basis of therapeutics* (pp. 100–109). New York: Macmillan.

Weiner, N. (1985). Norepinephrine, epinephrine, and the sympathomimetic amines. In A. G. Gilman, L. S. Goodman, T. W. Rall, & F. Murad (Eds.), *The pharmacological basis of therapeutics* (pp. 145–180). New York: Macmillan.

Weiner, N., & Taylor, P. (1985). Neurohumoral transmission: The autonomic and somatic motor nervous systems. In A. G. Gilman, L. S. Goodman, T. W. Rall, & F. Murad (Eds.), *The pharmacological basis of therapeutics* (pp. 66–99). New York: Macmillan.

Wurtman, R. J. (1982). Nutrients that modify brain function. *Scientific American, 246,* 50–59.

Zetterstrom, T., Sharp, T., & Ungerstedt, U. (1986). Effect of dopamine D-1 and D-2 receptor selective drugs on dopamine release and metabolism in rat striatum in vivo. *Naunyn-Schmiedeberg's Archives of Pharmacology, 334,* 117–124.

Chapter Six

Tolerance and Dependence

Now that you are familiar with some of the basic principles behind drug action and the theoretical processes involved with conduction, neurotransmission, and brain function, two phenomena that can have a profound influence on drug action and drug abuse may be discussed. These are drug tolerance and drug dependence, which in some cases are related. These phenomena are important theoretically because they tell us something about the mechanism of drug action. Perhaps more important is the fact that, although the processes resulting in tolerance and dependence may not be directly detrimental to the organism, their occurrence may result in severe repercussions for the individual and society.

What Is Tolerance?

Drug tolerance (hereafter referred to as tolerance) occurs when there is decreased susceptibility (or diminished response) to the effects of a given amount of drug as a result of previous exposure, typically caused by repeated exposures to the drug. This implies that increasingly larger doses of the drug are required to induce the same behavioral effect, although in some cases tolerance can be so dramatic that no amount of drug is capable of inducing its original effects. Tolerance due to drug exposure is different from so-called genetic or dispositional tolerance, whereby an individual may not be affected by the drug as much as other individuals are because of genetic or dispositional factors. For example, recent evidence suggests that some individuals predisposed to alcoholism metabolize alcohol at a faster rate than those not predisposed to alcoholism, even if they have not been exposed to alcohol before. This characteristic would allow such persons to consume quantities of alcohol much larger than normal before becoming intoxicated.

Although tolerance generally requires several drug exposures before it is evidenced, there is a special case of tolerance in which a noticeable decrease in the organism's sensitivity to the drug occurs over a very short period of time—on the order of a few hours. This is referred to as **tachyphylaxis**. In this form of tolerance, the same amount of drug administered on two separate occasions a couple of hours apart may induce greater effects with the first dose than with the second dose. Tachyphylaxis is also evident when the behavioral or physiological effects of a given dose of a drug dissipate at a faster rate than the rate at which the drug is eliminated from the brain (through catabolization or excretion). For example, a person may experience much greater effects of alcohol as the alcohol is accumulating in the brain than an hour or so later when it is being eliminated from the brain, despite the fact that at the two points in time the brain has the same concentration of alcohol in it (see Figure 8–1).

Cross-tolerance refers to the phenomenon in which the development of tolerance to one type of drug results in decreased sensitivity to the effects of another type of drug. For example, a heavy drinker who has developed tolerance to alcohol's sleep-inducing properties may not even get sleepy when given a dose of a barbiturate that normally induces sleep in other individuals.

While tolerance per se is not a particularly large problem, it can have severe repercussions. First, most psychoactive drugs we take in our culture are not especially harmful in and of themselves when taken in reasonable quantities with sufficient time between administrations. However, once tolerance to a drug's effects develops, larger and more frequent doses that do become toxic are often administered. Second, tolerance to the effects of drugs does not develop uniformly; that is, some effects may show profound tolerance, whereas others may show little or no tolerance (Pohorecky et al., 1986; Seiden & Dykstra, 1977). This is a distinct problem with alcohol and many sedative-hypnotic drugs, where the beneficial or recreational effects of the drugs may show considerable tolerance, but little tolerance develops to the lethal effects of these drugs (Jaffe, 1985). In effect, with this type of tolerance, the therapeutic index for these drugs gets smaller and smaller. With other drugs, tolerance to the desirable effects of a drug may occur while the person actually becomes more sensitive to the side effects of the drug. For example, the ability of amphetamine to induce euphoria decreases with regular use, but the ability for amphetamine to induce psychotic-like effects may actually increase with regular use of large doses.

Tolerance Mechanisms

There are two distinct types of drug tolerance: **pharmacodynamic tolerance** (also called **functional** or **nonassociative tolerance**) and **context-**

specific tolerance (also called **behavioral**, **learned**, or **associative toler-ance**). Pharmacodynamic tolerance is produced by exposure to high doses of a drug and is not affected by environmental or behavioral ma-nipulations of the organism. Context-specific tolerance is very sensitive to behavioral and environmental manipulations and involves learning and memory. What follows is a description of the various processes that are involved in these two forms of drug tolerance.

Mechanisms of Pharmacodynamic Tolerance

One mechanism already discussed involves the ability of the liver to synthesize more drug-metabolizing enzymes than normal when ex-posed to a drug (Cochin, 1970). Generally, this process requires several exposures to the drug for some length of time. Once this repeated expo-sure has taken place, the liver can metabolize the drug at a faster rate than it could previously, thereby decreasing its duration of action. How-ever, the peak intensity of the drug's action may not be reduced very much through this mechanism, particularly if administered intrave-nously, because the drug must first pass through the liver before it can be metabolized. This mechanism is also responsible for some cross-tolerance between drugs, since the actions of the drug-metabolizing en-zymes are not specific to one particular drug. (This form of tolerance is sometimes referred to as metabolic, or dispositional, tolerance by other authors. However, at the beginning of this chapter, I used the term "dispositional tolerance" to refer to a type of genetically based tolerance that is unrelated to previous drug exposures. Therefore, if you run across this term in other sources, look at the context in which it is used to determine what the author means by it.)

Tolerance to a drug may also develop because of a depletion of neurotransmitters critical to the drug's effects (Cochin, 1970). That is, some drugs (such as amphetamine and cocaine) act by augmenting a specific type of neurotransmitter activity in the synapse; that is, the drug may enhance the transmitters' release or inhibit their reuptake and increase the transmitters' access to receptors. However, the drug's actions may lead to a depletion of the transmitters (Gold & Dackis, 1984), either because they are used faster than they can be replenished or because the actual synthesis of the transmitters is decreased (per-haps because of excessive activity at autoreceptors). Therefore, with fewer transmitter molecules available, a larger drug dose must be ad-ministered. If this cycle continues long enough, this form of tolerance can lead to the drug's becoming completely ineffective, regardless of the dose administered. A drug's ability to deplete neurotransmitters can also be a factor in some forms of cross-tolerance. For example, one drug may act by enhancing the transmitters' release, and another may act by reducing the transmitters' reuptake. With either drug, depletion of the transmitters will reduce the effects of the drug. Finally, depletion of neurotransmitters can lead to the person experiencing symptoms that are the opposite of those he or she experienced with the drug; that is, where the drug initially induced its effects by amplifying neurotransmitter levels in the cleft, absence of the drug results in a reduction in neurotransmitter levels in the cleft (Gold & Dackis, 1984).

Another possible tolerance mechanism involves the drug's occupation and saturation of receptor sites, whereby the drug molecules exert their action at the time of occupation of receptor sites (Cochin, 1970). However, once binding occurs, the drug no longer exerts an effect other than preventing the initiation of a new response by other drug molecules combining with the receptor. For example, nicotine is an agonist at nicotinic receptors for Ach, which results in membrane depolarization. However, because nicotine disassociates from the Ach receptor rather slowly, the cell remains depolarized, and a new action potential cannot be initiated until the nicotine is removed from the receptors. Thus large doses of nicotine may actually exert an antagonistic action at Ach receptors (after the initial agonistic action).

There appear to be several mechanisms for tolerance involving cellular adaptations related to *homeostasis* (the processes that maintain a state of equilibrium in the body with respect to various functions and to the chemical compositions of the fluids and tissues). One rather novel explanation for drug tolerance was that something akin to an immune reaction occurred (Cochin, 1970). The drug molecules would be the antigen to which the organism would develop antibodies. This explanation for tolerance was originally invoked to explain how rats, whose mothers were made physically dependent on narcotics and then withdrawn from the drug several weeks before becoming impregnated (so that no drug molecules were present), were more resistant to the effects of morphine than rats whose mothers had not been exposed to narcotics. Presumably, the antibodies formed in the mothers crossed over the placenta into the fetuses, so that when they were later grown and given morphine the antibodies reduced the drug's effectiveness. This mechanism would account for the persistence of some kinds of tolerance for long periods of time and would account for some forms of cross-tolerance. Recently, the involvement of the immune system in a variety of phenomena associated with chronic use of morphine has been extended to opiate withdrawal symptoms. Several studies have demonstrated that a variety of treatments that suppress the immune system also significantly reduce the severity of withdrawal signs in morphine-dependent animals (Pellis et al., 1987). Thus, at least with opiates, it appears that the immune system may play a role in both tolerance development and abstinence symptoms.

Lately, a great deal of consideration has been given to homeostatic adaptations taking place in the neuronal membranes or neuronal receptors. For example, as mentioned in Chapter 4, alcohol increases the fluidity of neuronal membranes, possibly leading to the neurons' decreased ability to generate and propagate action potentials. However, the membrane's rigid characteristics return rather quickly (within a few hours), in spite of the fact that brain levels of alcohol are maintained (Chin & Goldstein, 1977). This phenomenon, although clearly a potential factor in tachyphylaxis, is still being explored as a possible factor in long-term tolerance and physical dependence.

Drug-induced alterations in the sensitivity of receptors in neuronal membranes have also been identified by recent research, and it is likely that homeostatic processes are involved. The alterations may reflect either qualitative changes in the neurotransmitters' receptor configuration or changes in the actual number of receptors, which, in turn, affect the transmitters' binding or intrinsic activity (Lefkowitz et al., 1989). It has been suggested that the ability of agonists and antagonists to bind to neuronal receptors is altered when drug exposure exceeds several hours. In many cases, drugs that mimic or amplify the action of neurotransmitters at their receptors tend to decrease receptor activity through processes referred to as **down-regulation** and **desensitization** (Ross, 1990). Down-regulation refers to a decrease in the number of functional receptors available for activation, whereas desensitization refers to a decrease in the receptors' ability to elicit cellular changes upon activation but no change in receptor number. In contrast, drugs that act as antagonists or dampen the action of neurotransmitters at receptors tend to increase receptor activity, as if there were more receptors, which may involve **up-regulation** or **sensitization** of receptors—that is, processes that are just the reverse of down-regulation and desensitization.

According to this model of tolerance, with fewer receptors with which the drug molecules or transmitter can interact, higher doses of the agonist must be administered so that the original effect can be induced. This dosage increase, of course, may decrease the receptor population further, so that successively higher doses of the agonist are needed to activate the increasingly smaller population of receptors. With drug antagonists, the reverse process may occur; that is, with a greater population of receptors, higher doses of the antagonist are needed to block them. This model of drug tolerance has great appeal because it explains cross-tolerance between different classes of drugs and because it makes a direct connection between tolerance and physical dependence (Redmond & Krystal, 1984). Figure 6–1 graphically displays in a step-by-step fashion these theoretical processes for both drug antagonists, seen in Figure 6–1(a), and agonists, in Figure 6–1(b).

If, for example, the actions of drug A are due to its ability to block

Figure 6–1(a)

Model for drug tolerance involving alterations in neurotransmitter (NT) receptor population on postsynaptic membrane, how these might affect the magnitude (in mV) of an excitatory postsynaptic potential (PSP), and how the behavioral effect or effector organ activity, e.g., heart rate (HR), may be altered. (1) Normal NT release (with action potential), receptor activation (receptors activated indicated by +), PSP, and HR. (2) Drug antagonist blocks receptors, decreases PSP, and lowers HR. (3) Receptor population increases, so despite drug blockade of other receptors, normal PSP is created, and HR is normal. (4) Drug dose is increased so that more receptors are occupied and blocked; PSP is reduced and HR decreases. (5) Receptor population increases further; PSP and HR return to normal. (6) Drug not given; with greater number of receptors available, NT has increased probability of activating more of them, which results in greater PSP than normal and an exaggerated behavioral effect (i.e., HR elevation). (7) With no further drug exposure, receptor population, PSP, and effector organ activity eventually return to normal.

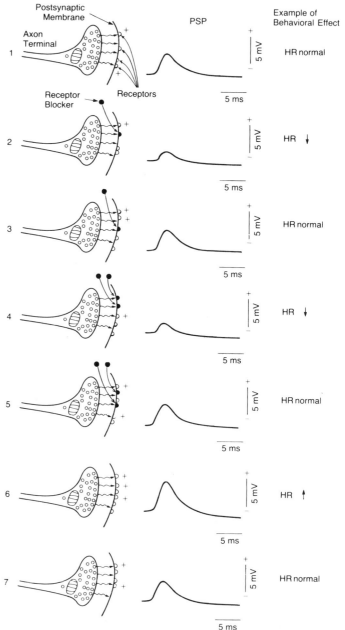

Figure 6–1(b)

The same model for drug tolerance depicted in Figure 6–1(a), except the drug is an agonist. (1) Normal NT release, receptor activation, PSP, and HR. (2) Drug agonist activates additional receptors, increases PSP, and increases HR. (3) Receptor population decreases, so despite subsequent exposure to the original concentration of the drug, normal PSP is created, and HR is normal. (4) Drug dose is increased so that more receptors are occupied and activated; PSP is enhanced and HR increases. (5) Receptor population decreases further, so that despite the presence of the drug molecules, the PSP and HR are maintained at normal levels. (6) Receptor population is at minimal levels, so that even though the concentration of the drug may be increased with larger doses, no further amplification of the PSP is possible, and HR stays at normal levels. (7) Drug is eliminated from the body; with smaller number of receptors now available, NT has decreased probability of activating those that remain, which results in smaller PSP than normal and reduced behavioral activity (i.e., HR declines). (8) With no further drug exposure, receptor population, PSP, and effector organ activity eventually return to normal.

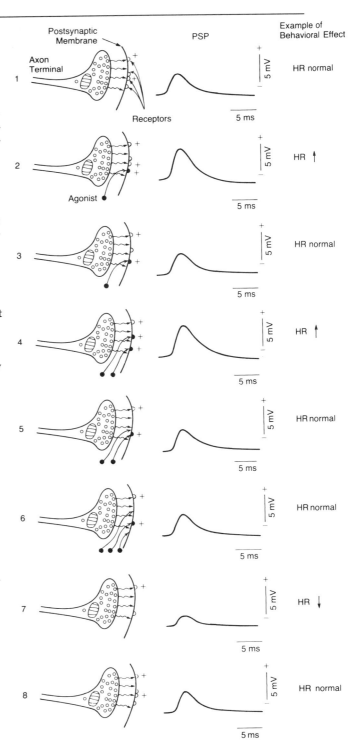

the postsynaptic receptors for neurotransmitter B, and this blockade is maintained for several hours, the population of postsynaptic receptors may increase. With more receptors available for activation by neurotransmitter B, a greater dose of drug A will be needed in order to block a sufficient number of receptors to bring about the original drug effects; that is, tolerance occurs. Now if the actions of drug C are due to its ability to block the release of neurotransmitter B, and drug C is substituted for drug A, drug C's effects will also be decreased. Conversely, if drug A is not given, there will be more than the normal population of receptors for neurotransmitter B to activate, and effects directly opposite to those induced by the drug—that is, withdrawal effects—will occur.

For how long must exposure to a drug occur for the receptor population to change? Studies with a variety of drugs suggest that several hours of continuous exposure to high drug concentrations may be sufficient to induce significant alterations in many hormone and neurotransmitter receptors (Nathanson, 1987). This time period may be linked to the approximate "lifetime" for a receptor. For example, the receptor for the hormone insulin has been estimated to have a half-life of between 7 and 12 hours in different cell types, which is shortened by exposure of the cell to the insulin ligand; that is, receptor down-regulation occurs (Rosen, 1987). Other receptors may have considerably longer half-lives. For example, adrenergic receptors have been shown to have half-lives greater than 20 hours (Mahan et al., 1987). Nevertheless, agonist exposure markedly shortens their half-life. Thus we can speculate that the lifetime of a receptor is reduced when extensively activated, and increased when activation is prevented. Furthermore, the number of receptors gradually returns to normal values, after the drug is removed, on a time course that depends on many factors. For example, when some muscarinic receptors are down-regulated with exposure to cholinergic agonists, it appears that they must first be newly synthesized from proteins and then slowly converted to physiologically functional forms before normal cholinergic activity returns (Nathanson, 1987).

This receptor phenomenon coincides with behavioral studies showing that a single dose of morphine, if large enough to maintain morphine concentrations in the rat for approximately 12 hours, can increase the perceived intensity of mild shock (indicative of a withdrawal-like increase in pain perception) 24 to 72 hours later (Grilly & Gowans, 1986). On a more personal level, if you have ever had an alcohol hangover (which may very likely constitute a mini-withdrawal syndrome), it is probably because you drank sufficient amounts of alcohol to maintain significant brain concentrations of alcohol for at least 12 hours. If you drink enough alcohol to become legally intoxicated in most states—0.10 percent blood alcohol content—it takes approximately 7 hours to eliminate it from your body. (A 0.10 percent blood alcohol content means that in every 1,000 ml of blood there is 1 ml of pure ethanol.) Therefore, if you experience a hangover after a night of drinking, it is likely that you were well over the legal limit by the time you finished drinking.

A somewhat similar mechanism for inducing tolerance might involve the reduced synthesis of a neurotransmitter as a result of the action of a drug that mimics it. In other words, if a drug is added to the normal pool of neurotransmitter molecules, both of which can activate the receptors, an exaggerated response in the receiving cell will occur. However, if the autoreceptors on the sending neuron are also activated, it may reduce its production of the neurotransmitter. This reduction may necessitate that larger amounts of the drug be given in order to maintain the drug's effect. Should the drug then not be given, the amount of neurotransmitter that the sending neuron can release will be lower than normal, the receiving cell will receive insufficient stimulation, and withdrawal symptoms will be experienced.

All the mechanisms resulting in tolerance that I have just described might be termed physiological or **pharmacodynamic** mechanisms because they are due to drug-induced changes in cellular enzymes, membranes, or receptors, which then decrease the ability of the drug to induce its effects. The rate at which tolerance develops is dependent upon drug dosage and the time between doses; the larger the dose and the shorter the time between doses, the more rapidly tolerance would be expected to develop. Furthermore, there is a threshold dose for each drug below which tolerance would not be expected to occur.

Although there is a great deal of research support for many of the pharmacodynamic models of tolerance, there has been increasing recognition that many forms of drug tolerance come about because of learning processes and behavioral adaptations that may occur in the presence of the drug and that are highly task- or situation-specific. Such tolerance is called **context-specific tolerance**. Several mechanisms through which this form of tolerance can develop have been proposed.

Mechanisms of Context-Specific Tolerance

The term **context-specific** or **behavioral tolerance** is applied when an organism is exposed to a drug in one context, displays tolerance to the drug in that context, but then loses the tolerance when it is exposed to the drug in another context. The most common processes involved in this form of tolerance are *habituation, Pavlovian conditioning,* and *instrumental conditioning.*

Habituation is perhaps the most fundamental of these. When an organism is first exposed to a novel stimulus, the stimulus often induces a reaction. A *stimulus* is any event—external or internal—that is capable of activating receptors in one of the senses. A *response* is any measurable reaction in an organism, such as skeletal, smooth, and cardiac muscle contractions; glandular secretions and excretions; neurotransmitter release; EEG pattern changes; or emotional reactions. When the stimulus is presented repeatedly to an organism without variation, there generally is a decrease in the magnitude of the reaction to the stimulus, a phenomenon referred to as habituation. (As noted later in this chapter, habituation is sometimes used in the field of drug abuse as a synonym for psychological dependence, or the process of forming a drug habit, which is very different from the process being described here.)

By definition, psychotropic drugs have both stimulus and response-eliciting properties. When a psychotropic drug is first administered to an organism, it introduces the organism to a new stimulus complex and, much like a novel sound or visual stimulus, it may interrupt or alter ongoing behavior. However, after repeated exposures to the drug-induced stimulus complex with no further consequences, behavior is going to be less and less affected. This is habituation; it is also a form of tolerance (Kesner & Cook, 1983). Evidence that the decreased sensitivity to the drug is due to habituation, and not to pharmacodynamic mechanisms, is provided when the organism is subsequently given the drug in a different environment and the drug again induces a reaction (Baker & Tiffany, 1985).

The preceding discussion does not explain what happens physiologically (psychologists are just now beginning to delineate what the physiological mechanisms are behind habituation in simple organisms like marine mollusks), but this description does place drugs in the same domain as that involving the effect of external stimuli on behavior. The difference is that with drugs internal stimuli are involved.

It has been proposed that Pavlovian conditioning is another process through which behavioral tolerance develops (Stewart & Eikelboom, 1987). Most of you have probably heard or read about how the Russian physiologist Ivan Pavlov conditioned dogs to salivate to tones or lights when these stimuli were paired with food. However, you probably remember little else about this form of conditioning and were not particularly impressed with the process in terms of its potential impact on you and other people around you. However, this process may be a factor in developing tolerance, and it can have a profound impact with respect to the induction of psychological dependence on drugs. In some cases, it can induce conditioned reactions that appear to be similar to the abstinence symptoms associated with physical dependence. Because of its potential role in the areas of tolerance and dependence, this process will be explored in some detail here.

Pavlovian conditioning begins when an organism is exposed to a stimulus that automatically (i.e., innately) elicits one or more reactions in the organism. The stimulus is called an *unconditioned stimulus* (UCS) and the responses it elicits are called *unconditioned responses* (UCRs). Examples of these stimulus-response cause-and-effect relationships, called reflexes, are the withdrawal of your hand (UCR) from a hot stove (UCS), the elicitation of tears (UCR) by onion fumes (UCS), sneezing (UCR) elicited by pepper in the nose (UCS), bronchial constriction (UCR) elicited by pollen (UCS), and increased heart rate, blood pressure, and sweating, and fright (UCRs) elicited by a loud unexpected sound (UCS). Because psychotropic drugs induce a number of automatic reactions, they also constitute unconditional stimuli. Thus we can say that administration of morphine (UCS) elicits, among other reactions, constriction of the pupils, drying up of secretions, constipation, respiratory depression, analgesia, and euphoria, as UCRs. As another example, nicotine (UCS) elicits increased heart rate and blood pressure, and altered cortical arousal (UCRs).

When a stimulus that generally does not produce much of a reaction by itself occurs prior to a UCS so that it reliably signals or predicts the occurrence of the UCS, conditioning may take place. We recognize that conditioning has occurred when the signal stimulus begins to elicit its own responses, which in many (but not all) cases resemble the UCRs elicited by the UCS. Because the new responses' occurrences are conditional upon the stimulus being paired with the UCS, they are termed *conditioned responses* (CR), and the stimulus now eliciting them is termed a *conditioned stimulus* (CS).

In most cases CRs elicited by a CS prepare the organism for dealing with the impending UCS (Holland, 1984; Hollis, 1984; Lennartz & Weinberger, 1992). For example, if food is put in the mouth, it is a UCS for salivation (UCR). Because one sees the food before it enters the mouth, the sight of food is a signal for food entering the mouth. Thus the sight of food becomes a CS that elicits salivation, which serves a function—in this case to enhance the digestion and chewability of the food. However, food (the UCS) may also decrease hunger (a UCR) because it satisfies a bodily need. In contrast the sight of food may actually increase hunger (a CR)—in this case to produce incentive motivation so the person will approach and consume the food. In the same fashion, signals for impending drug actions come to elicit CRs that prepare the body for the impending drug actions. Unfortunately, as we shall see, some of these CRs may, in the long run, actually be maladaptive for the person—for example, creating a conditioned incentive motivational state that leads the person to take the drug more and more frequently and in larger and larger amounts.

It appears that a wide variety of external stimuli (for instance, the smell of a "joint" or the sight of a syringe), as well as internal stimuli (those of an emotional state such as depression, for example), can take on the properties of a CS. The number of pairings of a CS with a UCS that are required for conditioning to take place are dependent on many factors, but to some extent the species' particular characteristics play a role. For example, rats can associate a novel taste with nausea after only one exposure, even if there is a gap of several hours between experiencing the novel taste and receiving the nausea-inducing stimulus. Chickens, on the other hand, do not appear to associate these events, even after many pairings. Birds can associate novel visual stimuli with sickness after only a few pairings, whereas rats do not appear to do so even after many pairings of these events. I mention these esoteric little facts because, in a similar fashion, humans may vary in their tendency to associate certain events with the drug effects they experience. Therefore, they may vary in their tendency to experience conditioned reactions that play a role in their becoming psychologically dependent on the drug.

How can Pavlovian conditioned responses play a role in many types of tolerance phenomena? In most of the studies that have dealt with this question, animals were exposed to a drug like morphine or alcohol (UCS) on several occasions in a specific environmental context (CS) (Hinson & Siegel, 1982). Some of the animals were then given a behavioral test following exposure to the drug in this same (CS) environmental context, while the other animals were given the same drug dose but were tested in a different context (no CS). Usually, the animals tested in the no-CS context exhibited larger drug effects than the animals tested in the CS context. One explanation is that in the CS environment a CR was elicited that was opposite to the drug-induced effects (UCRs); thus it was termed a *compensatory CR*. The net outcome was that the effectiveness of the drug (UCS) appeared to be reduced. However, in the no-CS context, there would be no compensatory CR to counteract the drug-induced UCR. The interesting implication of these studies is that if the organism is exposed to the CS, but without the drug being given, a compensatory CR should occur. Such a reaction would appear withdrawal-like. However, in the few cases where attempts have been made to directly observe compensatory-type CRs under laboratory conditions (that is, when the organism is exposed to the CS without the drug UCS being present), they appear weak and extinguish rapidly, if they occur at all (Tiffany et al., 1983; Sobrero & Bouton, 1989). Because the withdrawal symptoms associated with chronic use of many drugs are often quite severe and persist for several days, it is likely that other mechanisms, which may act synergistically with compensatory CRs, are involved in their production. In any case, compensatory CRs may be a factor in drug tolerance and drug dependence. As will be discussed later on, other types of CRs may also be involved in producing drug dependence.

A third behavioral mechanism through which drug tolerance can develop is *instrumental conditioning* (Ferraro, 1976). Whereas Pavlovian conditioning occurs without the organism necessarily doing anything— that is, the process occurs by the simple pairing of two different types of stimuli—instrumental conditioning begins with responses that are originally emitted without any apparent stimulus needed to produce them. The form and frequency of their subsequent occurrence are then altered depending upon the consequences of those responses. (The term "instrumental" is used to indicate that the behavior is instrumental or necessary for the conditioning process to occur. Common examples of instrumental behaviors are those involved in driving a car, hitting a golf ball, lighting a cigarette, snorting cocaine, and writing a letter.) These consequences are generally referred to as reinforcers and punishers. Stimuli that follow behavior and subsequently increase the probability of occurrence of that behavior in similar settings are termed *reinforcers*. Stimuli that follow behavior and decrease the probability of occurrence of that behavior in similar settings are called *punishers*.

Reinforcers can be either "primary" or "secondary." Primary reinforcers are stimuli that either reduce physiological needs or have inherent hedonic properties (for example, food, sex, and water). Secondary (also called conditioned) reinforcers are stimuli that predict or are associated with the increased probability of obtaining primary reinforcers (for instance, getting money increases one's chances of obtaining food, sex, and water). Drug-taking behavior is instrumental behavior. Drugs may have primary reinforcing value, and the environmental context cues in the presence of which the drugs are taken may become secondary reinforcers. Therefore, it should be obvious that instrumental conditioning plays a role in drug dependence and, as will now be discussed, in the development of tolerance to drugs.

Drugs that affect performance may also affect the organism's ongoing behavior and the contingencies of reinforcement and punishment, thereby bringing instrumental conditioning processes into the picture (Ferraro, 1976). In most cases the introduction of a psychotropic drug will interfere with the ability of the organism to maintain control over its reinforcement and punishment. For example, people who drive a car well without drugs may find themselves, under the influence of a few drinks, crossing median lines, hitting curbs, being honked at, running red lights, or getting into an accident. In other words, the drug is detrimental to the relationship between the behavior of driving and its consequences. However, with more and more exposure to this set of circumstances, these same people may learn how to compensate for these detrimental effects. For example, they may learn to look at the speedometer more frequently, keep a greater distance between themselves and other cars, and make adjustments in simple motor skills.

This learning model for tolerance applies to all drugs that affect behavior, and there are a number of implications for this form of tolerance (Ferraro, 1976). First, in order for it to occur, the organism must perform the task under the influence of the drug; that is, if two identical organisms are given identical doses of the drug on several occasions, only the organism performing a specific task under the influence of the drug will develop tolerance through this process. In this case, if the organism that had been given the drug without exposure to the task were subsequently given the drug, and then it attempted to perform the task, the effects initially induced in the other organism would be evident.

Second, the tolerance developed in this fashion should be task-specific. In other words, learning to compensate for the detrimental effects of alcohol on driving will probably not alter alcohol's detrimental effects on typing, because the two tasks require entirely different psycho-motor skills and involve different consequences. However, should two tasks involve similar components, tolerance developed in one should generalize to the other. For example, the development of compensatory responses allowing one to maintain one's balance on a bicycle when intoxicated with alcohol should transfer when the person attempts to ride a motorcycle under the influence of alcohol.

Third, while drug-induced detriments in performance will result in tolerance, alterations in the organism's behavior that do not hinder its ability to achieve reinforcement (or escape or avoid aversive events) will not show tolerance, because with the latter effects there is nothing for which the organism must learn to compensate. The same principle applies if the drug facilitates performance.

Fourth, the rate of tolerance development should be a function of the difficulty of the task or the availability of compensatory responses. That is, just as in learning how to do any task, the fewer components there are to learn, the faster one learns how to perform the task properly.

Fifth, once compensatory responses are learned under the influence of a drug, they should be available for use over relatively long periods of time without further exposure to the drug or the task. This would be expected simply because learning is generally defined as a relatively permanent change in behavioral potential as a function of practice or experience. What is learned should not dissipate simply through disuse or time, although, of course, forgetting may occur.

Finally, behavioral tolerance established to one drug should transfer to other drug states that produce similar behavioral effects because of either stimulus or response generalization. For example, while alcohol and marijuana may have quite dissimilar pharmacological actions in the CNS, the effects of low doses of alcohol and marijuana may be sufficiently similar that behavioral tolerance developed to one may generalize to the other.

Tolerance due to the development of instrumental compensatory responses that counteract a drug's effects has been demonstrated to occur with a variety of psychotropic drugs, including amphetamine, cocaine, morphine, alcohol, and barbiturates. Interestingly, the compensatory responses need not be overtly behavioral; they can also be cognitive. For example, it has been shown that tolerance to some of alcohol's behaviorally disruptive properties is facilitated even in persons who merely mentally rehearsed performing a task while under the influence of alcohol (Sdao-Jarvie & Vogel-Sprott, 1986).

It should be added that learning has also been suggested to be a process by which increased drug sensitivity with previous exposure can come about (a phenomenon referred to earlier as *reverse tolerance* or sensitization). For example, marijuana has the reputation of not inducing much of an effect the first time a person tries it, but with more exposure to the drug the person begins to experience more of an effect from the same amount. Similar statements have been made by cocaine users. It has been suggested that low doses of these drugs do not induce particularly noticeable effects in the user, but that with continued usage the person learns to recognize the effects that have been labeled by users as pleasurable. It is also possible, through Pavlovian conditioning, that CRs, which are like the UCRs produced by the drug, summate with the drug-induced effects to induce a larger overall subjective effect.

Clearly there are many mechanisms through which drug tolerance occurs. No single mechanism can account for the phenomena associated with tolerance—that is, the fact that some drug effects dissipate with successive drug exposures, while others remain unchanged or increase in magnitude. We have discussed tolerance in two main frameworks: learning models and pharmacodynamic models. Yet, from a reductionistic perspective, both pharmacodynamic and behavioral forms of tolerance may come about because of the same physiological mechanisms. Learning models simply emphasize the stimulus context, the task requirements, and the behavioral effects of drugs as factors in tolerance development. Pharmacodynamic models emphasize the drug concentration and time between drug exposures as the primary factors in tolerance development.

What Is Dependence?

Like tolerance, drug dependence per se may not be detrimental to an individual or society, but once it occurs, it may lead the individual to do things that are behaviorally maladaptive, physiologically hazardous, or socially unacceptable. **Drug dependence** is a general term indicating that a person's drug use has led to the user's experiencing uncontrollable and unpleasant mood states that in turn lead the user to use the drug compulsively despite obvious adverse consequences. This is distinguished from **drug abuse**, which commonly refers simply to a person's use of drugs in doses or ways that result in adverse consequences (Newcomb & Bentler, 1989).

To a certain degree, the consequences of drug dependence are sometimes related to the laws and social norms of one's culture (Brecher, 1972). For example, because of laws limiting heroin's availability, one can argue that the consequences of heroin dependency in the United States are much more severe for the dependent person than they might be without those laws (this topic will be discussed in Chapter 10). The point is, we are all dependent upon numerous substances and activities (food, water, sex, etc.), but we do not normally think of these dependencies as problems unless we are deprived of them.

There are two basic forms of drug dependence: psychological (or psychic) dependence and physical (or physiological) dependence. Neither of these is particularly easy to define, and it is sometimes difficult to distinguish between the two, not only because the symptoms associated with them can be confused, but because the two often occur together. **Psychological dependence** refers to a strong compulsion or desire to experience the effects of a drug because it produces pleasure or reduces psychic discomfort. This type of dependence can be termed **primary psychological dependence** in order to distinguish it from the secondary form to be discussed shortly. Generally it leads to regular or continuous administration of the drug, so that taking the drug becomes habitual. Because of these characteristics, some authors in the area of drug abuse refer to psychological dependence as habituation. However, since this term can be confused with the phenomenon of habituation described earlier in this chapter, I do not view it as an appropriate term.

In a sense, psychological dependence is the counterpart to context-specific tolerance because the affective states underlying it are heavily influenced by the context the person is in and because it is primarily the result of learning and memory processes. Similarly, physiological dependence is the counterpart to pharmacodynamic tolerance because some of the mechanisms behind the latter are the likely causes of the manifestations of physiological dependence.

Psychological dependence comes about because drug-taking behavior is regularly followed by the rewarding effects of a drug. Several lines of evidence suggest that virtually all recreational and abuse-prone drugs derive their rewarding properties by directly or indirectly activating brain reward circuits. The complex reward system in the brain, which includes a variety of hindbrain, midbrain, and forebrain loci, was discovered when studies indicated that animals would engage in various behaviors (e.g., pressing a lever) if these behaviors resulted in the delivery of a mild electrical current to some areas in the brain but not others (Olds & Milner, 1954). Virtually all abuse-prone drugs, including widely disparate pharmacologically acting drugs like morphine, cocaine, alcohol, and marijuana, have been found to enhance brain stimulation reward or lower brain reward thresholds in these circuits. Animals will also work for microinjections of most of these drugs into these reward circuits but not other brain areas. Finally, virtually all abusable drugs enhance basal neuronal firing or basal neurotransmitter release in these reward circuits (Gardner & Lowinson, 1991). However, because this reward system depends on a variety of neurotransmitter systems, primarily dopaminergic and enkephalinergic and secondarily noradrenergic and GABAergic systems (among others), the mechanism(s) through which abusable drugs act may differ greatly. These pharmacodynamic mechanisms will be discussed in subsequent chapters.

How does one go about determining whether a drug has reinforcing properties prior to its compulsive use by humans? A common laboratory technique used to assess the psychological dependence liability of a drug, removed from social, cultural, or expectancy factors, involves determining whether or not nonhumans (for example, monkeys or rats) will self-administer the drug. A small catheter (tube) is permanently implanted in a laboratory animal. The catheter goes directly into the blood going into the heart, and is connected to a pump outside the animal. The animal can activate the pump, and thus self-administer a dose of the drug, by performing some learned behavioral response, like pressing a lever. The dependence liability of the drug is determined by how frequently the animal responds when the drug is injected versus when an inert substance is injected. Animals will readily perform the response in order to administer most drugs that are abused by humans. For example, morphine, heroin, cocaine, and amphetamine, drugs that can induce a strong psychological dependence in humans, are very readily self-administered by rats and monkeys with this procedure, but caffeine, which is not readily abused by humans, is not reliably self-administered by animals (Woods, 1978). This technique is not an infallible approach to determining the potential dependence liability of a drug, because some drugs that may induce psychological dependence in humans are not self-administered by nonhumans—for example, LSD and marijuana compounds.

This technique is also useful in illustrating how habitual drug taking can become. Monkeys allowed to administer morphine in this fashion eventually develop stable patterns of responding so that the amount of morphine administered on a daily basis is fairly constant. In other words, while they can self-administer as much morphine as they wish, they stabilize at an amount considerably below that which they could receive (this phenomenon has been shown not to be due to the animal's becoming so intoxicated that it cannot perform the response). However, if the monkey is administered the amount of morphine that it normally stabilizes on without having to do anything, it will continue to respond and administer even more morphine (Leavitt, 1982).

Physical (or physiological) dependence is said to occur when a state, termed an **abstinence syndrome**, characterized by physical disturbances develops when the administration of a drug is suspended after prolonged use or its actions are terminated by the administration of a specific antagonist. In almost all cases, the effects of withdrawal are the opposite of the direct effects induced by the drug. Thus, for example, withdrawal from barbiturates, which normally exert a calming, sleep-inducing, anticonvulsant action, is characterized by anxiety, inability to sleep, and convulsions (which can be lethal). Withdrawal from opiates, which cause constipation, dry up the nasal passages, induce sleep, reduce sex drive, and reduce pain (among many other effects), is characterized by diarrhea, runny nose, inability to sleep, spontaneous ejaculations (men) or orgasms (women), and hypersensitivity to pain (Jaffe, 1985).

The duration and intensity of an abstinence syndrome are also highly correlated with the duration and intensity of a drug's direct effects (see Figure 6–2). For example, a drug with a short plasma half-life (say, 4 hours) will likely induce a relatively intense but short-lasting behavioral effect. If given infrequently, cessation of its use will not likely result in abstinence symptoms. However, if taken frequently, so that the CNS is continuously exposed to the drug, its withdrawal will likely result in a relatively intense abstinence syndrome that dissipates fairly quickly (that is, over a few days). Conversely, a drug with a long plasma half-life (say, 24 hours) will likely induce relatively weak but long-lasting behavioral effects. If taken frequently enough so that the CNS is continuously exposed to the drug, its withdrawal is likely to result in a relatively weak abstinence syndrome that dissipates slowly (that is, over a few weeks). Also, as one might expect, the more frequently a drug is administered and the greater the dose, the more extensive the abstinence syndrome will be (Jaffe, 1985; Okamoto et al., 1986).

In Figure 6–2, we see that in case A with a short-acting drug administered at spaced intervals, there is likely to be no pharmacodynamic tolerance and no withdrawal. In case B, in which a short-acting drug is administered at a constant dosage and at closely spaced intervals, there is likely to be pharmacodynamic tolerance and a mild, but short-lasting, abstinence syndrome. In case C, in which the short-acting drug is administered at closely spaced intervals and the dose is increased (indicated by X), there is likely to be a relatively more intense and longer-lasting abstinence syndrome than in case B. In case D, with a longer-lasting drug administered at spaced intervals, pharmacodynamic tolerance will not be readily apparent, and the abstinence syndrome (if evident at all) will be mild. In case E, in which the longer-lasting drug is administered at more closely spaced intervals, pharmacodynamic tolerance and the abstinence syndrome will be somewhat more apparent than in case D. Furthermore, while the abstinence syndrome in case E may be less severe than in case C, it is likely to be more protracted.

If a person becomes physically dependent on a drug, a second form of psychological dependence can develop. That is, once physical dependence exists and the person becomes familiar with the symptoms of abstinence, the person may develop a craving for the drug that is based on the person's fear or anxiety of experiencing the abstinence syndrome. Therefore, the person seeks out and administers the drug to alleviate the fear or anxiety. This type of psychological dependence is sometimes referred to

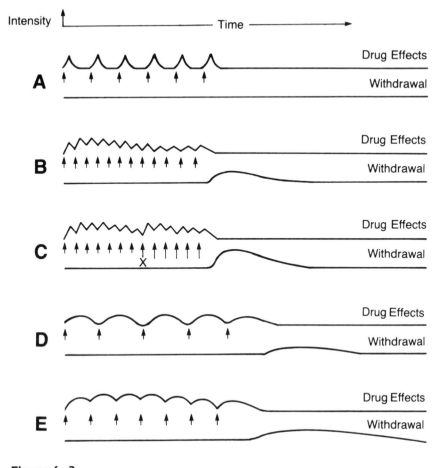

Figure 6–2

Relationships between the intensity of a drug's effects and the intensity of the abstinence syndrome when the drug is no longer administered. The arrows indicate when the drug is administered.

as **secondary psychological dependence**, in order to distinguish it from the primary psychological dependence described earlier, which can occur whether or not the person is physically dependent on the drug.

Although tolerance and physical dependence often accompany each other, they are not necessarily related. At least some degree of drug tolerance inevitably precedes physical dependence, but physical dependence does not always follow when tolerance to a drug develops. In other words, if someone is physically dependent on a drug, that person will have developed tolerance to many of its effects. However, if a person has developed tolerance to a drug's effects, it does not mean that the person is physically dependent on the drug. This is most likely due to the fact there are many mechanisms for inducing tolerance, and only some of them may also result in physical dependence (Wuster et al., 1985).

We might note at this point that before the terms "psychological dependence" and "physical dependence" were in vogue, the term **drug addiction** was used. Over 30 years ago the World Health Organization (WHO) defined drug addiction as a state of periodic or chronic intoxication detrimental to the individual or society, produced by the repeated consumption of a drug. Its characteristics were described as an overpowering desire or need (compulsion) to continue taking the drug, because of either psychological or physical dependence on the effects of the drug, and a tendency to increase the dose or frequency of use (Hoffman, 1983).

Prior to the 20th century, the term "addiction" meant simply a strong inclination toward certain kinds of conduct, with little or no stigma associated with it. Often it referred to a habit—good or bad, but more often good, such as an addiction to reading. However, as the term came to be more and more associated with drugs, the term became stigmatic. Furthermore, it often became synonymous with physiological dependence, in spite of the WHO definition indicating that either psychological dependence or physical dependence (or both) may be involved. For these reasons, many experts today try to avoid using the term addiction with respect to drugs. However, because the term has become so ingrained in our language, it will continue to be used. When, on occasion, it is used in the remainder of this book, it will be used in the sense of the WHO definition. In this context, whenever the term "addict" is used in this text it will refer to someone who has a strong compulsion to use a particular substance.

Some psychotropic drugs have a relatively strong potential for producing both physical and psychological dependence; others appear capable of inducing one without the other; and still others do not appear to induce either to any significant degree. I would hesitate to say that any psychotropic drug is incapable of inducing either or only one kind of dependence; it is just that there is no clear evidence one way or another in some cases. However, the argument has been made that just about any psychotropic drug, if the organism is exposed to it in large enough doses and for a long enough period of time, will provoke abstinence symptoms when the drug is rapidly eliminated from the body (Hollister, 1987).

Classes of drugs for which there is clear evidence of a moderate to strong potential for both physical and psychological dependence would include all drugs with sedative-hypnotic properties. Among them are alcohol, barbiturates, nonbarbiturate sedative-hypnotics, antianxiety drugs (sometimes called "minor tranquilizers"), and the narcotics, such as heroin, morphine, codeine, and methadone. Drugs that have a high potential for inducing psychological dependence, but for which physical dependence is either questionable or relatively mild, would include the psychostimulants, such as cocaine, amphetamines, and related compounds, and psychosis-mimicking drugs, such as LSD, mescaline, psilocybin, and marijuana.

Some drugs have minimal potential for inducing psychological dependence, but if taken for a period of time, will induce physical dependence and provoke withdrawal symptoms if the person ceases taking them. (Nasal spray, although not a psychotropic drug, is capable of having this effect.) Certain narcotics with mixed agonist-antagonist properties are in this category.

Finally, drugs used in the treatment of major mental and emotional disturbances, such as lithium, antidepressants, and antipsychotics, have minimal potential for inducing psychological dependence or signs of abstinence. In fact, many patients would prefer to stop taking these types of drugs because of the unpleasant side effects associated with them.

As stated earlier, even drugs that traditionally have not been recognized as being capable of inducing physical dependence (cocaine, for instance) may, if given in large enough quantities and for a long enough period of time, upon cessation of drug administration induce physiological and psychological disturbances opposite to the drug-induced effects. Perhaps we have not recognized these symptoms as withdrawal because they do not resemble, quantitatively or qualitatively, the symptoms associated with the sedative-hypnotics and the narcotics. This issue will be dealt with more fully when these drugs are discussed in later chapters. (Several years ago, when I pointed out the possibility of physical dependence with all psychotropic drugs, a student suggested that if this were true, giving LSD chronically in large amounts to schizophrenics might result in their becoming rational and nondelusional upon withdrawal. I quickly pointed out that although it was an intriguing hypothesis there are exceptions to every generalization.)

Factors in Dependence

A multitude of sociological, psychological, and genetic factors have been suggested to be involved in the abuse of drugs (see National Institute on Drug Abuse monographs edited by Harris, 1980, 1981, and Thompson & Johanson, 1981, for extensive reviews of this topic). Genetics has been one of the most consistent factors in the etiology (the study of the causes or origins of diseases) of alcoholism. For example, children of alcoholic parents are much more likely to become alcoholics than children of nonalcoholic parents, whether they are raised by their biological parents or adoptive parents (Cloninger, 1987). Although there is no clear evidence for it as yet, genetic differences in endorphin levels or receptors have been suggested to be a factor in the development of narcotic addiction (Khantzian, 1985). In general, only environmental and intrapsychic factors have so far been implicated in drug use and abuse among children and teenagers, although it seems likely that genetic factors may contribute more to drug abuse than to use, which appears to be initiated in social settings (Newcomb & Bentler, 1989).

Sociological factors in drug involvement have been discussed at length by a multitude of authors (Harris, 1980, 1981). With respect to extensive illicit drug use, the strongest and most direct factor is the user's selling of drugs, which in turn is strongly related to factors such as drug availability, significant others' labeling of the person as deviant, peer influence, early childhood deviance, poor school adjustment, and weak family influence (Clayton & Voss, 1981). For example, when one's family influence (defined in terms of family control, closeness of mother, and communication with parents) is weak, there is a higher likelihood during the early teens that the person will (1) exhibit signs of early deviance (i.e., be involved in unconventional or deviant activities); (2) be strongly influenced by peers who are delinquent, steal, engage in gang fights, drink alcohol, smoke marijuana, or use other drugs; and (3) exhibit poor school adjustment (i.e., dislike school and get low grades). Early deviance will also tend to increase the degree of peer influence and decrease the person's school adjustment. These factors then increase the person's likelihood of becoming "labeled" as a troublemaker and increasing the person's drug availability. These then make the person more likely to sell and use illicit drugs.

Generally ignored as a factor in drug abuse, but one of the most consistently replicated correlates of nonabuse, is religion (Gorsuch, 1988). With respect to alcohol use, for example, people in all religious denominations use less alcohol than nonreligious people, with those denominations traditionally opposed to alcohol using it less. Of those who do drink, the religious abuse alcohol less than do the nonreligious.

Although racial factors are often assumed to play a role in drug abuse in the United States, the available evidence indicates that, with the exception of heroin use, alcohol and other drug use is actually lower among African-American adolescents than among whites (Austin, 1990). African-Americans, however, may have greater secondary problems arising out of substance abuse than whites—for example, liver damage, cancer, pulmonary disease, malnutrition, hypertension, and birth defects.

Exposure to licit substances, such as alcohol and tobacco, is also a major factor in abuse of both licit and illicit substances. In fact, numerous studies have demonstrated that there has been a reasonably consistent sequence of stages of drug involvement in North American and similar cultures over the last 30 years or so (Blaze-Temple & Lo, 1992; Fleming et al., 1989; Kandel, 1975). Generally the sequence begins with the use of more socially accepted substances like tobacco and beer, and is followed by an increased likelihood of using "hard" liquor and marijuana; for example, in one recent study less than 2% of middle school students reported trying marijuana without trying cigarettes first (Fleming et al., 1989). This stage then leads to an increased likelihood of using other illicit drugs such as cocaine, heroin, and LSD. (Note the use of the words "increased likelihood of using." These words should not be construed as meaning "a likelihood of using.") In other words, it is very rare in American culture for a person to start using hard liquor or marijuana without first using tobacco or beer, or other illicit drugs without first using marijuana or hard liquor.

The developmental processes of substance use are complex. Some abstainers progress to drug use, others remain abstinent, and still others shift from a pattern of use to nonuse (Coombs et al., 1986). Thus escalation into more extensive patterns of drug use is not inevitable, nor is it always a gradual, progressive occurrence.

A number of hypotheses for predisposing factors in chronic drug use have emphasized personality characteristics, such as sensation- or novelty-seeking traits, extroversion and introversion, antisocial personality characteristics, anxiety, and other social motives. The most consistent finding is that many substance abusers exhibit a history of antisocial behavior (e.g., nonconformity, acting out, and impulsivity) and a high level of depression or low self-esteem (Marlatt et al., 1988). Another consistent observation is that high sensation seekers are much more likely to abuse all types of psychotropic drugs than low sensation seekers (Zuckerman, 1979).

Some authorities have speculated that drug abusers, at least those who tend to select their drugs in a nonrandom manner, are predisposed to addiction because they suffer from painful affective (mood or feeling) states or related psychiatric disorders. In these cases, their drug of choice is presumed to be the result of an interaction between a specific drug's effects and their particular psychological discomfort (Alexander & Hadaway, 1982; Khantzian & Treece, 1985).

Unfortunately, recent empirical studies attempting to verify this hypothesis have either been methodologically flawed or have failed to support them. For example, in chronic drug users who use one drug predominantly, one would expect that those using cocaine would exhibit characteristics similar to those using amphetamine, that sedative-hypnotic users would be similar to opiate users, and that the characteristics of cocaine or amphetamine users would be considerably different from those of sedative-hypnotic or opiate users. However, these predictions have not been supported in methodologically sound research (Spotts & Shontz, 1986). Needless to say, there are a wide variety of potential and probable predisposing factors leading to chronic drug use and dependence.

In addition to preexisting motivational variables associated with drug dependence, once drug taking begins, a number of physiological and conditioning factors enter into the process (Marlatt et al., 1988). If drug taking is shortly followed by the reinforcing effects of the drug, instrumental conditioning is involved and leads to drug seeking and further drug taking. Since drugs serve as unconditioned stimuli, the environmental context in which one takes drugs can come to serve as conditioned stimuli for *conditioned drive states*, that is, drug craving. As discussed earlier in this chapter, conditioned responses that are compensatory to the drug-induced effects (that is, are opposite to the drug effects) may also occur. Thus exposure to these environmental cues will potentially lead to drive states and withdrawal-like effects, which will further increase the desire to engage in drug-taking behavior (Stewart & Eikelboom, 1987). Furthermore, if the drug is capable of inducing pharmacodynamic physical dependence, it can create a physiological drive state most conducive to continuing drug-taking behavior. Once this condition has been created, secondary psychological dependence may be an additional motive for drug taking.

Perhaps a few examples will enhance your appreciation of the potency of these conditioning factors in drug dependence. It has long been recognized that individuals who self-administer drugs are more likely to abuse them than are passive recipients of drugs. For example, doctors who administer narcotics to themselves show a much higher incidence of narcotic abuse than do their patients, to whom narcotics are administered (Leavitt, 1982). Because there are many reasons why this result might occur (for example, doctors have easy access to pharmaceutical-grade narcotics), we cannot say for sure that it is the act of self-administering the drug that is the primary factor in this differential abuse rate.

Studies with rats have shown that they are more likely to exhibit signs of withdrawal following a few days of alcohol exposure if they have previously been administered alcohol chronically and have undergone withdrawal. That is, rats that have not previously experienced withdrawal will not exhibit withdrawal signs following only a few days exposure to alcohol (Leavitt, 1982). In humans undergoing narcotic detoxification, the severity of withdrawal symptoms has often been shown to be more closely related to the patient's anxiety and degree of expected distress than to the amount of narcotic used or the length of narcotic use (Phillips et al., 1986).

A number of studies have shown that an animal's tendency to self-administer narcotics depends upon how similar the environmental cues are to those that were present during the initial stages of addiction (Schuster & Johanson, 1981). Others have shown that rats, if placed in the same environment in which they were previously withdrawn from morphine, will show signs of withdrawal (sudden, brief body twitches), even though they have been drug-free for several months. A similar *conditioned withdrawal* phenomenon has been established in the laboratory with patient volunteers maintained on a methadone regimen by pairing naloxone, a drug (UCS) that induces withdrawal (UCR) in opiate addicts, with a novel stimulus (CS). Upon injecting a placebo instead of naloxone (the injection procedure is the CS), the resulting CRs resembled the withdrawal UCRs. Similar behavioral withdrawal and subjective craving responses (a CR similar to, but not identical to, the withdrawal-type CR) have been shown to occur in abstinent narcotic users watching videotapes of themselves or others administering drugs or seeing other drug-related stimuli. These responses can be virtually eliminated through extinction procedures—that is, continued exposure to the CS alone over a period of a few weeks (Childress et al., 1986a, 1986b).

These are just a few examples indicating the power of conditioning processes, both instrumental and Pavlovian, in the development of drug dependence. Figure 6–3 summarizes the involvement of these processes in drug-taking behavior in terms of the following steps:

1. Predisposing factors motivate the individual to try a drug.
2. With drug availability, drug-taking behavior is initially modeled after drug-taking behavior in parents, peers, etc.
3. The individual experiences primary reinforcing and physiological effects of the drug.
4. Pairing of the environmental context with drug effects constitutes a Pavlovian conditioning trial.
5. Drug-taking behavior is followed by primary (or secondary) reinforcing effects of the drug in the environmental context, which constitutes instrumental conditioning.
6. Postdrug motivational states induced through Pavlovian processes (6a), or because continued exposure to drug effects results in physiological dependence (6b) and fear of undergoing withdrawal (6c), leads to further drug seeking and drug taking.

Note that genetic predispositions may interact or be involved in most, if not all, of the steps.

A number of lessons can be gained from all of this. First of all, there are many predisposing factors leading to initial drug use. Second, once drug taking begins, there are many additional factors that can lead to the maintenance of drug-taking behavior. Third, conditioned withdrawal-type effects can often be confused with pharmacodynamic withdrawal effects. Fourth, although there has long been a concern that physical dependence is a factor in the maintenance of drug-taking behavior, it may be a relatively minor aspect in the maintenance of an addict's habit. Therefore, methods that simply focus on the control of physiological withdrawal are not going to work in the long run (Schuster & Johanson, 1981).

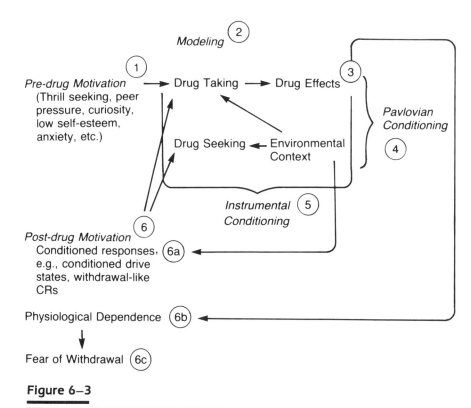

Figure 6–3

Summary of the basic steps and factors involved in the drug dependence process.

General Factors in Treatment for Drug Dependency

The first step in the treatment for drug dependency involves recognizing that a person's drug use is a problem. This recognition is not always easy to make. Once dependence processes begin with drug use, they almost always lead to numerous detrimental consequences for the user, the user's significant others, and, potentially, society in general. (Some specific consequences of drug dependency will be discussed more fully in subsequent chapters.) One would think that these consequences would be recognized by the users, or their friends and family, and would be sufficient reason to get the users to stop or at least seek help. However, two psychological processes generally prevent these things from happening: *denial* and *enabling.*

One of the symptoms of alcoholism and other chemical dependencies is denial, a defense mechanism that prevents users from consciously recognizing that they have a problem. Others may see the problem, but the users cannot. Perhaps at some level the users know their drug use is a problem, but they make excuses, minimize the magnitude of the problem, and blame others for their unpleasant feelings instead of blaming their relationship with mood-altering chemicals.

On the other hand, many of us do well-meaning things for our drug-dependent friends that actually encourage their drug use. Doing such things is called enabling, since it enables drug use to continue. We allow them to keep denying their problem whenever we do anything to help them escape the harmful consequences of their drug use. We do it out of love or concern, but it only makes things worse. We enable when we lie or make excuses for them to friends or employers, lend them money after they have spent their own on drugs, deny that they have a compulsive disorder, drink or take other drugs along with them, stop talking about their drug use because they become angry when we do so, or join them in blaming others for their own bad feelings. In short, any action we take to rescue them from the harmful consequences of their drug use is enabling. It sounds irrational, but when we take away their discomfort, we take away the only thing that might help them see that they are in trouble.

Therefore, the two essential keys to any effective treatment for drug abuse and dependence are these: (1) The person must recognize or be convinced that his or her drug use is a problem; and (2) he or she must have the incentive to change. These statements do not mean that these two conditions must be met before treatment can begin. In most cases, even voluntary patients submit themselves to treatment initially only because of strong social pressure or external coercion; their primary goal is to convince everyone (including themselves) that they do not have a problem (Cummings, 1979).

Any treatment program for addiction will probably have to deal with the predisposing sociological factors that originally led to drug taking. This can be a very difficult task when dealing with a person who has a poor self-image, has labeled himself or herself as a drug user, has a history of deviance, comes from a broken home, or has few education-related skills.

To deal with cue-dependent cravings that may lead to relapse, a treatment program might include permanently removing the addict from drug-associated environmental stimuli. However, because this approach would rarely be feasible for most people, a more practical approach would be to expose the addict to the original drug-taking environment without allowing him or her to experience the rewarding effects of the drug so that the conditioned craving can be extinguished (Childress et al., 1986a). Such a program could involve therapy sessions in which patients listen to audiotapes and watch videos of drug deals, handle drug paraphernalia, and look at or handle anything else that triggers their craving for the drug. It has been suggested that the extinction procedure should resemble actual drug-taking conditions as closely as possible, even to the extent of providing the real possibility of consuming the drug one is dependent on, in order to elicit conditioned reactions that can then be adequately extinguished (Corty et al., 1988). (Unfortunately, Pavlov demonstrated many years ago that even with extensive extinction training the spontaneous recovery of CRs can occur with the simple passage of time).

Another tactic would be to allow addicts to self-administer their drugs but have the effect blocked by a specific antagonist, if there is one. (Specific antagonists are now available for clinical use for narcotics and for experimental use for alcohol and benzodiazepines.) One of the more common treatments for narcotic addiction involves the routine administration of a long-acting narcotic (for example, methadone), which both reduces the psychological craving for narcotics and blocks the effects of all but very large doses of other narcotics. Alternatively, a drug could be given so that when the addict takes the drug of abuse it leads to aversive bodily reactions. For example, disulfiram (Antabuse) has been used in the treatment of alcoholism. If persons who are taking disulfiram consume alcohol, they experience nausea and severe headaches.

Numerous therapeutic interventions have been attempted in order to deal with drug addiction. All of them appear to work some of the time with some individuals. Unfortunately, none of them work for a significant majority of individuals, perhaps because their efficacy is contingent upon the patient's voluntary participation in the treatment. Furthermore, even when treatment appears successful, relapse is common. However, the likelihood of relapse is reduced when the drug user (1) is under compulsory supervision or experiences a consistent aversive reaction related to drinking or other drug use (e.g., use of disulfiram or suffering from a painful ulcer); (2) finds a substitute dependency to compete with drug use (e.g., meditation, compulsive gambling, overeating, running); (3) obtains new social supports (e.g., a grateful employer or new significant other); and (4) becomes a member of an inspirational group (e.g., a religious group, Alcoholics Anonymous, Narcotics Anonymous) (Vaillant, 1988; also see Brownell et al., 1986, for another excellent discussion of the natural history of relapse, its determinants and effects, and methods for prevention).

State-Dependent Learning

The phenomenon to be described in this section is normally discussed in the context of how drugs may influence learning and memory. However, because it can have a profound influence on the maintenance of drug-taking behavior, it seems appropriate to discuss it here in the context of drug dependence. Approximately 20 years ago, some studies were performed in which animals learned tasks under one set of drug conditions and then were tested for their retention of the behavior under another set of drug conditions. The results indicated that the animals did not perform the tasks during the test as well as they would have if the retention test had been conducted under the same drug conditions as those present during the learning phase. This was found to be the case whether a drug was present during the acquisition phase and a nondrug condition was present during the retention phase, or vice versa. In other words, if learning was accomplished under nondrug conditions, retention was best under nondrug conditions; and if learning was accomplished under a drug, retention was best when the drug was present. The phenomenon was noted to occur with a wide variety of drugs and tasks, and it was found to occur in humans (Horton & Mills, 1984). It became known as **state-dependent learning** (also known as **drug-dissociative learning** or **drug-state learning**). In essence, it can be defined as learning under one set of drug (or nondrug) conditions that does not completely transfer to another set of drug conditions.

The usual explanation for the phenomenon is that certain cues—in this case, drug-related cues (perhaps internally produced)—present during the acquisition of information or behaviors become associated with the information or behaviors. Therefore, in order to successfully retrieve that information or perform that behavior during retention, those cues must be present. The more the context cues change between learning and retention, the greater the difficulty in exhibiting the information or behavior.

It should not be difficult now to see how state-dependent learning can become a factor in the continuation of drug-taking behavior. That is, if a person is exposed to a drug on a number of occasions, he (or she) is bound to acquire some new strategies or skills for dealing with the world. If the person then tries to perform those skills at a later time without the drug, he may experience difficulty in doing so and feel that he must be under the influence of the drug in order to perform appropriately. This experience starts a vicious cycle in which the more the person engages in the behavior under the drug's influence, the more likely he will be to feel the need to administer the drug in order to perform the behavior. For example, there are many anecdotal reports of alcoholic writers who have discovered that they are no longer able to write while sober, in spite of the fact that we generally expect people to think and write better without alcohol (particularly large doses). Thus, in order to maintain their success as writers, they continue to expose themselves to a chemical that will eventually lead to a great deal of psychological, neurological, and physiological damage.

State-dependent learning may also play a role in the potential benefits of psychotherapy in a patient who is also taking psychotropic medications. That is, patients may develop new coping strategies during therapy that may be lost or diminished when the patients' drug state changes or they go off their medication. A patient may feel that the therapy was a failure or may become dependent on the medication. Therapists should be aware of this possibility.

Bibliography

Alexander, B. K., & Hadaway, P. F. (1982). Opiate addiction: The case for an adaptive orientation. *Psychological Bulletin, 92,* 367–381.

Austin, G. A. (1990). *Substance abuse among black youth.* Madison: Wisconsin Clearing House.

Baker, T. B., & Tiffany, S. T. (1985). Morphine tolerance as habituation. *Psychological Review, 92,* 78–108.

Blaze-Temple, D., & Lo, S. K. (1992). Stages of drug use: A community survey of Perth teenagers. *British Journal of Addiction, 87,* 215–225.

Brecher, E. M. (Ed.). (1972). *Licit and illicit drugs.* Boston: Little, Brown.

Brownell, K. D., Marlatt, G. A., Lichtenstein, E., & Wilson, G. T. (1986). Understanding and preventing relapse. *American Psychologist, 41,* 765–781.

Childress, A. R., McLellan, T., & O'Brien, C. P. (1986a). Abstinent opiate abusers exhibit conditioned craving, conditioned withdrawal and reductions in both through extinction. *British Journal of Addiction, 81,* 655–660.

Childress, A. R., McLellan, T., & O'Brien, C. P. (1986b). Conditioned responses in a methadone population. *Journal of Substance Abuse Treatment, 3,* 173–179.

Chin, J. H., & Goldstein, D. B. (1977). Drug tolerance in biomembranes: A spin label study of the effects of ethanol. *Science, 196,* 684–685.

Clayton, R. R., & Voss, H. L. (1981). *Young men and drugs in Manhattan: A causal analysis* (NIDA Research Monograph No. 39). Rockville, MD: National Institute on Drug Abuse, Department of Health and Human Services.

Cloninger, C. R. (1987). Neurogenetic adaptive mechanisms in alcoholism. *Science, 236,* 410–416.

Cochin, J. (1970). Possible mechanisms in development of tolerance. *Federation Proceedings, 29,* 19–27.

Coombs, R. H., Fawzy, F. I., & Gerber, B. I. (1986). Patterns of cigarette, alcohol, and other drug use among children and adolescents: A longitudinal study. *International Journal of the Addictions, 21,* 897–913.

Corty, E., O'Brien, C. P., & Mann, S. (1988). Reactivity to alcohol stimuli in alcoholics: Is there a role for temptation? *Drug and Alcohol Dependence, 21,* 29–36.

Cummings, N. (1979). Turning bread into stones. *American Psychologist, 34,* 1119–1129.

Ferraro, D. P. (1976). A behavioral model of marihuana tolerance. In M. C. Braude & S. Szara (Eds.), *The pharmacology of marihuana tolerance* (pp. 475–486). New York: Raven Press.

Fleming, R., Leventhal, H., Glynn, K., & Ershler, J. (1989). The role of cigarettes in the initiation and progression of early substance use. *Addictive Behaviors, 14,* 261–272.

Gardner, E. L., & Lowinson, J. H. (1991). Marijuana's interaction with brain reward systems: Update 1991. *Pharmacology Biochemistry & Behavior, 40,* 571–580.

Gold, M. S., & Dackis, C. A. (1984). New insights and treatments: Opiate withdrawal and cocaine addiction. *Clinical Therapeutics, 7,* 6–21.

Gorsuch, R. L. (1988). Psychology of religion. *Annual Review of Psychology, 39,* 201–221.

Grilly, D. M., & Gowans, G. C. (1986). Acute morphine dependence: Effects observed in shock and light discrimination tasks. *Psychopharmacology, 88,* 500–504.

Harris, L. S. (Ed.). (1980). *Problems of drug dependence, 1980.* Rockville, MD: National Institute on Drug Abuse.

Harris, L. S. (Ed.). (1981). *Problems of drug dependence, 1981.* Rockville, MD: National Institute on Drug Abuse.

Hinson, R. E., & Siegel, S. (1982). Nonpharmacological bases of drug tolerance and dependence. *Journal of Psychosomatic Research, 26,* 495–503.

Hoffman, F. G. (1983). *A handbook on drug and alcohol abuse.* New York: Oxford University Press.

Holland, P. C. (1984). Origins of behavior in Pavlovian conditioning. *The Psychology of Learning and Motivation, 18,* 129–173.

Hollis, K. L. (1984). The biological function of Pavlovian conditioning: The best defense is a good offense. *Journal of Experimental Psychology: Animal Behavior Processes, 10,* 413–425.

Hollister, L. E. (1987). Postmarketing surveillance of psychotherapeutic drugs: Concluding comments. *Psychopharmacology Bulletin, 23,* 405–406.

Horton, D. L., & Mills, C. B. (1984). Human learning and memory. *Annual Review of Psychology, 35,* 361–394.

Jaffe, J. H. (1985). Drug addiction and drug abuse. In A. G. Gilman, L. S. Goodman, T. W. Rall, & F. Murad (Eds.), *The pharmacological basis of therapeutics* (pp. 532–581). New York: Macmillan.

Kandel, D. (1975). Stages in adolescent involvement in drug use. *Science, 190,* 912–914.

Kesner, R. P., & Cook, D. G. (1983). Role of habituation and classical conditioning in the development of morphine tolerance. *Behavioral Neuroscience, 97,* 4–12.

Khantzian, E. J. (1985). The self-medication hypothesis of addictive disorders: Focus on heroin and cocaine dependence. *American Journal of Psychiatry, 142,* 1259–1263.

Khantzian, E. J., & Treece, C. (1985). DSM-III psychiatric diagnosis of narcotic addicts. *Archives of General Psychiatry, 42,* 1067–1071.

Leavitt, F. (1982). *Drugs and behavior.* New York: John Wiley & Sons.

Lefkowitz, R. J., Kobilka, B. K., & Caron, M. G. (1989). The new biology of drug receptors. *Biochemical Pharmacology, 38,* 2941–2951.

Lennartz, R. C., & Weinberger, N. M. (1992). Analysis of response systems in Pavlovian conditioning reveals rapidly versus slowly acquired conditioned responses: Support for two factors, implications for behavior and neurobiology. *Psychobiology, 20,* 93–119.

Mahan, L. C., McKernan, R. M., & Insel, P. A. (1987). Metabolism of alpha- and beta-adrenergic receptors in vitro and in vivo. *Annual Review of Pharmacology and Toxicology, 27,* 215–235.

Marlatt, G. A., Baer, J. S., Donovan, D. M., & Kivlahan, D. R. (1988). Addictive behaviors: Etiology and treatment. *Annual Review of Psychology, 39,* 223–252.

Nathanson, N. M. (1987). Molecular properties of the muscarinic acetylcholine receptor. *Annual Review of Neuroscience, 10,* 195–236.

Newcomb, M. D., & Bentler, P. M. (1989). Substance use and abuse among children and teenagers. *American Psychologist, 44,* 242–248.

Okamoto, M., Rao, S., & Walewske, J. L. (1986). Effect of dosing frequency on the development of physical dependence and tolerance to pentobarbital. *Journal of Pharmacology and Experimental Therapeutics, 238,* 1004–1008.

Olds, J., & Milner, P. (1954). Positive reinforcement produced by electrical stimulation of septal area and other regions of rat brain. *Journal of Comparative and Physiological Psychology, 47,* 419–427.

Pellis, N. R., Kletzly, N. E., Dougherty, P. M., Aronowski, J., & Dafny, N. (1987). Participation of lymphoid cells in the withdrawal syndrome of opiate dependent rats. *Life Sciences, 40,* 1589–1593.

Phillips, G. T., Gossop, M., & Bradley, B. (1986). The influence of psychological factors on the opiate withdrawal syndrome. *British Journal of Psychiatry, 149,* 235–238.

Pohorecky, L. A., Brick, J., & Carpenter, J. A. (1986). Assessment of the development of tolerance to ethanol using multiple measures. *Alcoholism: Clinical and Experimental Research, 10,* 616–622.

Redmond, D. E., & Krystal, J. H. (1984). Multiple mechanisms of withdrawal from opioid drugs. *Annual Review of Neuroscience, 7,* 443–478.

Rosen, O. M. (1987). After insulin binds. *Science, 237,* 1452–1458.

Ross, E. M. (1990). Pharmacodynamics: Mechanisms of drug action and the relationship between drug concentration and effect. In A. G. Gilman, T. W. Rall, A. S. Nies, & P. Taylor (Eds.), *The pharmacological basis of therapeutics* (pp. 33–48). New York: Pergamon Press.

Schuster, C. R., & Johanson, C. E. (1981). An analysis of drug-seeking behavior in animals. *Neuroscience and Biobehavioral Reviews, 5,* 315–324.

Sdao-Jarvie, K., & Vogel-Sprott, M. (1986). Mental rehearsal of a task before or after ethanol: Tolerance facilitating effects. *Drug and Alcohol Dependence, 18,* 23–30.

Seiden, L. S., & Dykstra, L. A. (1977). *Psychopharmacology: A biochemical and behavioral approach.* New York: Van Nostrand Reinhold.

Sobrero, A. P., & Bouton, M. E. (1989). Effects of stimuli present during oral morphine administration on withdrawal and subsequent consumption. *Psychobiology, 17,* 179–190.

Spotts, J. V., & Shontz, F. C. (1986). Drugs and personality: Dependence of findings on method. *American Journal of Drug and Alcohol Abuse, 12,* 355–382.

Stewart, J., & Eikelboom, R. (1987). Conditioned drug effects. In L. L. Iversen, S. D. Iversen, & S. H. Snyder (Eds.), *Handbook of psychopharmacology* (Vol. 19, pp. 1–57). New York: Plenum Press.

Thompson, T., & Johanson, C. E. (Eds.). (1981). *Behavioral pharmacology of human drug dependence.* Rockville, MD: National Institute on Drug Abuse.

Tiffany, S. T., Petrie, E. C., Baker, T. B., & Dahl, J. L. (1983). Conditioned morphine tolerance in the rat: Absence of a compensatory response and cross-tolerance with stress. *Behavioral Neuroscience, 97,* 335–353.

Vaillant, G. E. (1988). What can long-term follow-up teach us about relapse and prevention of relapse in addiction? *British Journal of Addiction, 83,* 1147–1157.

Woods, J. H. (1978). Behavioral pharmacology of drug self-administration. In M. A. Lipton, A. DiMascio, & K. F. Killam (Eds.), *Psychopharmacology* (pp. 595–607). New York: Raven Press.

Wuster, M., Schulz, R., & Herz, A. (1985). Opioid tolerance and dependence: Re-evaluating the unitary hypothesis. *Trends in the Pharmacological Sciences, 6,* 64–67.

Zuckerman, M. (1979). *Sensation seeking: Beyond the optimal level of arousal.* Hillsdale, NJ: Erlbaum.

Chapter Seven

Psychotropic Drug Classification

Classifying drugs is no easy task, since in most cases no sharp distinctions can be made among them. Drugs with almost identical molecular structures may induce entirely different effects, while other drugs whose molecular structures are quite different may induce almost identical effects (Barden & Mason, 1977; Weissman & Milne, 1979). Some drugs may have one effect at one dose and an entirely different effect at another. A drug may have multiple psychological effects in a certain dose range, and depending on the population taking them (or the persons prescribing them), some of these effects may be viewed as desirable in one person and undesirable in another. For example, certain marijuana-like substances may effectively reduce nausea in cancer patients undergoing chemotherapy but may lead to an undesirable clouding of consciousness. In other groups of individuals, these "side effects" are the effects desired. Therefore, it is not surprising that different textbooks may classify drugs in a number of different ways.

Molecular Structure–Activity Relationships

One classification scheme that appears to be intuitively reasonable involves grouping drugs according to their chemical structure (Biel et al., 1978; Petracek, 1978). Although this scheme may often group together drugs that have very similar behavioral effects, in many cases what appear to be relatively minor changes in the molecular structure of a drug can considerably change its basic activity in the body.

Figure 7–1 displays the molecular structures of six different compounds. The first is simply the structure of one of the basic neurotransmitters, dopamine. The second structure is that of amphetamine. As will be described in Chapter 9, the actions of certain doses of amphetamine are very similar to the actions of dopamine. This similarity is not surprising because amphetamine has several biochemical actions that essentially amplify dopamine's actions. One of amphetamine's biochemical actions is to temporarily inhibit the enzyme monoamine oxidase (MAO). The third structure in Figure 7–1 is that of tranylcypromine, a drug with antidepressant properties. While its structure is quite similar to that of amphetamine, it is several thousand times more potent in its ability to inhibit MAO. The fourth structure is that of mescaline. Both mescaline and amphetamine have structural similarities, elevate mood in low doses, and are capable of inducing psychosis-mimicking effects, such as profound distortions in perceptions and in some cases hallucinations. However, the "psychosis" associated with mescaline is readily distinguishable from naturally occurring psychoses, whereas the "psychosis" induced by amphetamine is not. The fifth structure in Figure 7–1 is that of a drug with mescaline-like effects, but it is 10 to 100 times more potent than mescaline. The sixth structure is that of lysergic acid diethylamide (LSD). Although LSD is considerably more potent than mescaline, it is capable of inducing effects that are practically indistinguishable from those of mescaline. To summarize, in the first five relatively similar structures we see actions that in some ways are quite similar and in other ways are quite dissimilar. We also see very similar actions in two drugs with very dissimilar structures.

There are many cases in which molecules that are identical except for their being mirror images of each other often have very different effects on the body. Such molecules are called *optical isomers* (or more technically *enantiomers*), which are commonly differentiated by the prefixes *levo* (or simply *l*, as in *l*-dopa) and *dextro* (or simply *d*, as in *d*-amphetamine) because the two forms in solution rotate plane-polarized light in different directions—to the left with the *levo* isomer and to the right with the *dextro* isomer. When the two isomers display differential receptor-binding properties (for instance, when one isomer binds and the other does not) and therefore induce different effects, they are said to be **stereospecific**.

Parts (a) and (b) of Figure 7–2 show skeleton molecular structures for the levo (active) and dextro (inactive) isomers of morphine. They are mirror images (isomers) of the morphine molecule; one produces analgesia, and the other does not. A slight modification of the active molecule produces the molecular structure shown in part (c), nalorphine, an antagonist of morphine. However, nalorphine still has some weak, narcotic-like effects. It has mixed agonist-antagonist properties. It is thought that when the chain attached to the nitrogen atom is in the "down" position it acts as an antagonist, whereas when it swings around and "up"—indicated by the dashed lines—it acts as an agonist (note the similarity to the active morphine molecule in this position). Another modification of the active molecule produces naloxone, shown in part (d), a narcotic antagonist without any narcotic action at all. It has only antagonist properties. In this

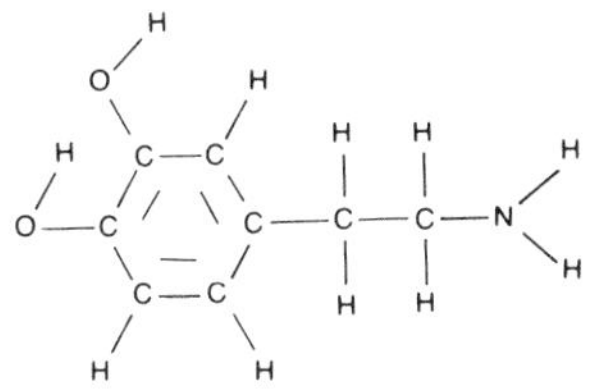

Dopamine

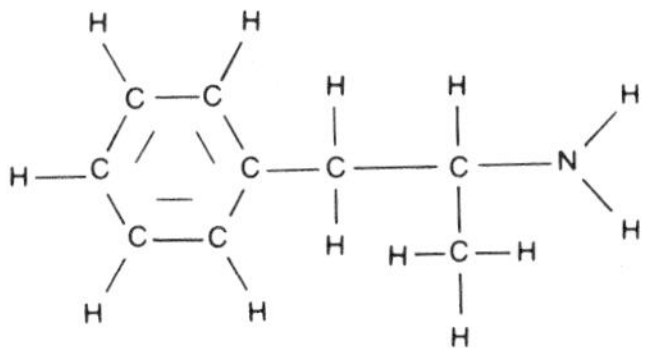

Amphetamine

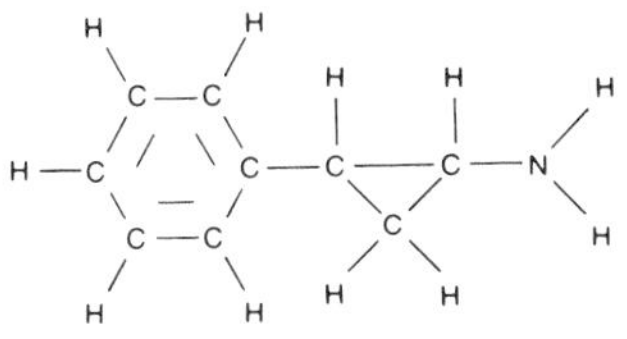

Tranylcypromine

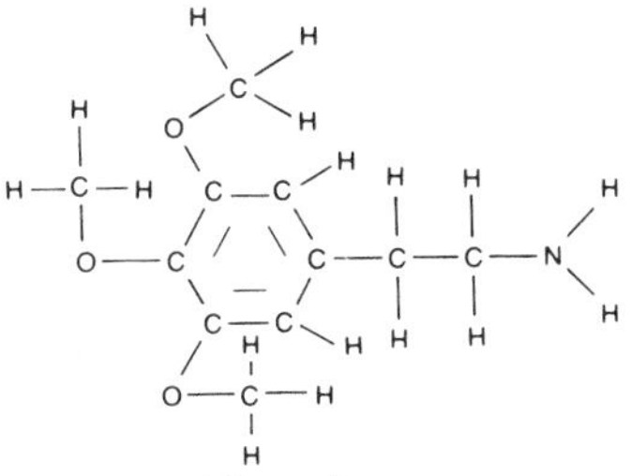

Mescaline

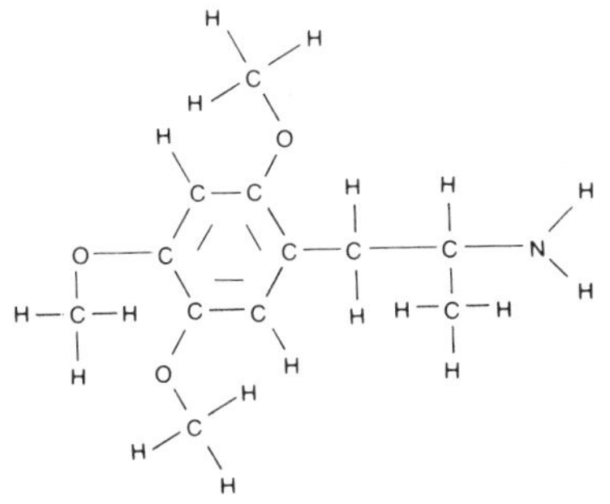

2, 4, 5-trimethoxyamphetamine

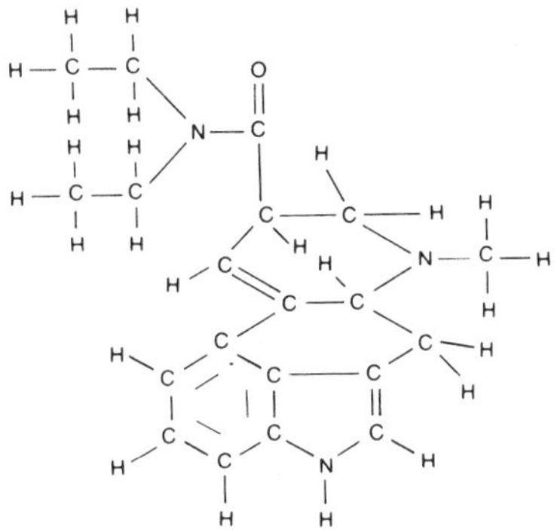

LSD

Figure 7–1

Examples of drugs with similar molecular structures and similar effects; similar structures and qualitatively different effects; and different structures but qualitatively similar effects.

case, the added OH group may prevent the chain attached to the nitrogen atom from swinging into an agonist conformation.

Thus we see that slight modifications in a molecule can change it from an active molecule at its receptor into an inactive molecule, a mixed agonist-antagonist, or a "pure"antagonist. On the other hand, the structure shown in part (f) of the figure—that of the peptide leu-enkephalin—has actions very similar to those of morphine (e). Despite the dissimilarity of their molecular structures, recent studies have indi-

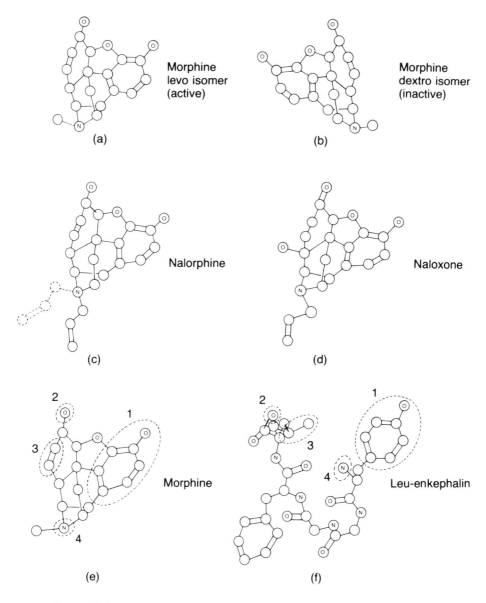

Figure 7–2

Skeleton molecular structures of the isomers of the opiate morphine,
two opiate antagonists (one with opiate properties), and one of the
enkephalins. (O = oxygen, N = nitrogen, unlabeled atoms are carbon, and hydrogen atoms are not shown.)

cated that they do possess analogous regions that probably allow them to both bind to and activate opioid receptors (Barden & Mason, 1977). The peptide can be "twisted" so that critical components of the molecule necessary for receptor occupation correspond to analogous regions on the morphine molecule.

Despite the apparent inconsistencies between drug molecule structures and their activities in the nervous system, recently a great deal of progress has been made toward understanding structure-activity relationships (Pool, 1992). Biologists, using sophisticated molecular computer modeling programs and visualization software, can now easily create proteins on a computer screen and experiment with them— bringing other molecules up close to them and determining which drugs will fit best into their active sites. This capability is particularly valuable for pharmaceutical companies, whose drug designers can test thousands of potential drugs on a computer to find the most promising candidate for producing a specified effect.

Depressant versus Stimulant Classifications

Another way that many authors attempt to classify drugs is according to the activation dimension (Leavitt, 1982; Wallace & Fisher, 1991). In this context, drugs are often described as (CNS) depressants or stimulants. Unfortunately, classifying drugs as stimulants or depressants can often be misleading. One might expect a depressant to decrease mood, motor activity, and the body's metabolic and physiological activities, reduce alertness and induce sleep, decrease brain activity and neurotransmitter turnover, and shift the EEG toward lower frequencies and higher amplitude waves (a physiological correlate of becoming less aroused). One might expect stimulants to do just the reverse. However, it is not that simple. As you will see in the upcoming chapters, drugs rarely do any of these things simultaneously. Thus the terms "depressant" and "stimulant" do not mean much unless one specifies at which biological level the depression or stimulation is occurring, or the dose of the drug.

For example, a drug may stimulate the receptors of a particular set of neurons, but if these receptors allow the influx of negative ions and hyperpolarize the cells, the excitability of the neurons will decrease. Alternatively, the drug may increase the firing rate of one set of neurons or stimulate the release of a particular type of neurotransmitter. However, if the neurotransmitter released happens to be at inhibitory synapses, the drug, in effect, would decrease the excitability of the receiving cells, decrease their firing rate, and decrease the neurotransmitter they release. Conversely, a drug may depress a particular set of neurons in terms of their excitability and their rate of firing. However, if these neurons play an inhibitory role with respect to other neurons, the latter neurons' excitability may increase.

One may talk about a drug's depressant or stimulant role with respect to behavior or emotion, but, again, if one does not specify a particular set of behaviors or emotions and the dose of the drug, the terms "depressant" and "stimulant" impart little information. Although a drug may decrease the relative frequency of one set of behaviors, it may increase the relative frequency of other sets of behaviors. A drug at one dose may elevate mood, but at another dose it may depress mood. For example, alcohol and barbiturates (drugs commonly referred to as depressants) act as depressants biochemically, in that they decrease neurotransmitter turnover rate, and neuropharmacologically, in that they decrease the excitability of individual neurons. However, in low doses, these drugs increase the general activity and mood of many individuals. In high doses, a general suppression of activity and mood will probably occur. Amphetamine (a drug commonly referred to as a stimulant) increases the rate of firing of some neurons while simultaneously decreasing the rate of firing of others. It increases the production of some behaviors and reduces the frequency of others. Furthermore, behaviors that are increased at low doses of amphetamine may be depressed with much higher doses (see, for example, Figure 2–1).

Drug Use Classification

For these reasons, most authors (including this one) in this field prefer to classify drugs according to what they are predominantly used for (Leavitt, 1982; Usdin, 1978; Wallace & Fisher, 1991). Unfortunately, though, this system is far from perfect, because drugs may be used for different purposes in different doses and in different individuals. Nevertheless, in this textbook, drugs will be classified in this context. Before we begin, note that a single drug has many names: chemical, generic, and brand. Furthermore, if it is used recreationally, the drug may have several "street" names as well. The **chemical** name gives a complete description of a particular molecule according to specific rules of organic chemistry. The **generic** name of the compound indicates its legal, official, or nonproprietary name. Once it has been approved for marketing, the drug will have a **brand** name, given to it by its manufacturer. After 17 years, when the patent on a compound runs out, anybody can market it, so it may then have several other brand names. Finally, if the drug is marketed illicitly or used recreationally, it may have a variety of "street" names. So, for example, the chemical name 1-(1-phenylcyclohexyl) piperidine may be referred to by its generic name, phencyclidine, or its brand name, Sernylyn, or its street names—for example, PCP, angel dust, dust, hog, peace pill, and THC, (among many others).

Since most students reading this text are more likely to recognize various drugs by their brand names, along with their generic names, they will be referred to by their most common or initially used brand names the first time they are mentioned. Use of "street" names for drugs has generally been avoided because there are so many—as soon as one becomes popular, another is generated to take its place.

Sedative-hypnotics (sometimes referred to as depressants) sedate, calm, or relax most individuals at low doses and, at somewhat higher doses, induce sleep in most individuals. It should be pointed out that the hypnotic effect of these drugs—sleep—is very different from the phenomena associated with hypnosis. The confusion comes about because it was once believed that hypnosis induced a sleeplike trance. However, we now know that hypnotized people are very much awake. Drugs included in the sedative-hypnotic category are ethyl alcohol (ethanol); barbiturates, such as secobarbital, phenobarbital, and pentobarbital; chloral hydrate; and numerous drugs with barbiturate-like effects, such as glutethimide (Doriden) and methaqualone (Quaalude). Many drugs in this class (for example, phenobarbital) are effective in reducing seizure activity and may be termed **anticonvulsants**. They may also be used as muscle relaxants, although muscle relaxation is secondary to their effects on the CNS.

Anxiolytics, or **antianxiety drugs**, are used in treating disorders where the prevailing symptom is anxiety—for instance, neuroses. The term "minor tranquilizers" is sometimes used to describe the drugs in this category. However, because these drugs are sometimes confused with the major tranquilizers (see the subsequent discussion of antipsychotics), and the word "minor" is often misinterpreted as meaning mild (it actually refers to the fact that these drugs are used to reduce less severe symptoms of psychological dysfunction), it is deemed an inappropriate term by many authors. Prior to the 1900s, several sedative-hypnotics were used to calm anxious and disturbed patients (for example, bromide, chloral hydrate, paraldehyde, urethan, and sulfonal). For the most part, these were replaced by the barbiturates in the early 1900s. Fewer than a dozen other sedatives were successfully marketed before 1960. The nonbarbiturate meprobamate (Miltown) was introduced as an antianxiety agent with great fanfare in 1955. However, over the past 25 years a class of drugs referred to as **benzodiazepines** has pretty much replaced all of these. Common examples of this class of drug would be chlordiazepoxide (Librium) and diazepam (Valium). Many of the drugs in this class may also be effective anticonvulsants. The properties of these drugs are quite similar to those of the sedative-hypnotics, except that with many of the benzodiazepines the sedative and hypnotic doses are supposedly quite different.

The newest member of the anxiolytic category is buspirone (BuSpar). Its molecular structure is uniquely different from the rest of the anxiolytics. It also lacks their hypnotic, anticonvulsant, and muscle-relaxant properties. It does not appear to act synergistically with alcohol, and it is likely to possess a much lower potential for abuse and dependence than the sedative-hypnotics and other anxiolytics. However, such judgments have often been wrong in the past, and further clinical trials will be required in order to substantiate these findings.

Psychostimulants (sometimes referred to as stimulants), in low to moderate doses, increase alertness, reduce fatigue, and elevate mood in most individuals. Drugs in this category include the amphetamines, cocaine, caffeine, and phenylpropanolamine (a common ingredient in over-the-counter appetite suppressors). Note that for drugs in this category, the use context is a recreational one, because these drugs are not presently medically prescribed for these uses. In a medical context, some of these drugs may be used as appetite suppressants (**anoretics** or **anorectics**); others may be used in the treatment of *narcolepsy* (a disorder in which the person has sudden, uncontrollable tendencies to sleep at irregular intervals, such as during the day) or the *attention deficit* (hyperactivity) disorder. In some very special cases, psychostimulants may be prescribed for mild depression.

Antipsychotics are drugs used in the treatment of major mental and emotional disturbances (psychoses). Other authors often refer to these as major tranquilizers, because these drugs calm highly excited schizophrenics and manics. However, the term may be inappropriate in certain cases; for instance, they may also enhance the social interactions and increase the activity of catatonic patients. The term may also lead to their being confused with the so-called minor tranquilizers, a class of drugs which differ greatly from antipsychotics. Therefore, most practitioners prefer not to refer to these drugs as major tranquilizers. Another term often used for these drugs is **neuroleptic**. However, since this term technically means a drug capable of inducing severe neurological symptoms ("lepsis" is Greek for seizure), it is obviously inappropriate in the present classification context. Commonly used antipsycotics include chlorpromazine (Thorazine), thioridazine (Mellaril), and haloperidol (Haldol). Reserpine (Serpasil), a drug that will be mentioned in several contexts in this text, was one of the first of this category of drugs to be introduced, but it is no longer used in the treatment of psychotic disorders.

Humans normally exhibit wide variations in mood states, or affective states, as they are technically called. In some individuals, however, these are so chronic or become so extreme that the individuals become dysfunctional, and in some cases suicidal. In most of these individuals, their exaggerated mood is predominantly one of depression, and such individuals are diagnosed as having a *unipolar disorder*. Others may exhibit depressed episodes at times; at other times, they may exhibit episodes of mania, characterized by frenzied psychomotor activity, excitement, a rapid passing or flight of ideas, exaltation, exaggerated confidence, and unstable attention. Such individuals are commonly diagnosed as having *manic-depression* or a *bipolar disorder*. Drugs used to treat these affective disorders are commonly referred to as **antidepressants** and **antimanics**.

Antidepressants are used in severe, unremitting cases of depression, generally for those depressions for which there appear to be no outstanding causal events. Classic examples of these drugs are imipramine (Tofranil), amitriptyline (Elavil), tranylcypromine (Parnate), and phenelzine (Nardil). Although, as mentioned, the psychostimulants generally raise mood in normal individuals, psychostimulants have not proven to be useful in the treatment of depression (except for some very unusual cases), for several reasons to be discussed later.

Antimanics are most useful in the treatment of manic symptoms, but they may also be useful in the treatment of other symptoms that appear to be only tangentially related to mood. The drug of choice is generally a lithium salt, such as lithium carbonate. An alternative to lithium is carbamazepine (Tegretol). Since these drugs are generally successful in decreasing rapid mood swings—from mania to depression—they are also sometimes referred to as mood stabilizers. Although the antipsychotics are quite effective in reducing manic symptoms and are often used for the initial treatment of mania, they are generally not used for chronic treatment in affective disorders because of their potentially severe side effects.

Drugs taken specifically to severely distort one's perception of reality, disturb cognitive processes, or induce hallucinations are referred to by many names. They are most commonly called **hallucinogens** (for hallucination-generating), **psychotomimetics** (for psychosis-mimicking), or **psychedelics** (for mind-manifesting). However, as discussed in Chapter 11, none of these terms is entirely appropriate in that most substances in this category do not produce the types of psychoses naturally found in humans, nor do they always produce true hallucinations. The third term has even less functional meaning than the other two; nobody really understands what the mind is, or what is meant by the term "manifested" when applied to the mind.

Although these types of drugs are presently used predominantly in a recreational context, some of them, such as LSD, have been used in medical contexts or are presently being used experimentally in medical contexts (for example, compounds related to those found in marijuana). Examples of these types of drugs are LSD, mescaline, psilocybin, phencyclidine (PCP), and cannabinoids (those compounds found in *Cannabis sativa*, more popularly known as marijuana). Anticholinergic compounds, including scopolamine and atropine, may also be included in this category, although several unpleasant characteristics of these latter drugs probably account for their infrequent recreational use.

A wide variety of psychotropic compounds used in the treatment of pain are called either **anesthetics** (without feeling) or **analgesics** (without pain). These include the narcotics (morphine, heroin, codeine, meperidine [Demerol], and methadone [Dolophine]); inhalants like ether and nitrous oxide; many of the sedative-hypnotics (generally given in large doses); cocaine (as a local anesthetic); and ketamine (Ketalar), a phencyclidine-like drug. Many of these drugs are also used recreationally, usually for purposes quite unrelated to medical treatment.

The fact that a drug may have many uses is of particular concern to those in the area of drug therapeutics. When a drug has been shown to be reasonably safe and effective for some specific symptoms, it is approved for medical use by the Food and Drug Administration (FDA) and officially labeled. This labeling includes the information that appears both on the container the drug comes in and on the package insert. The FDA is legally responsible for ensuring that all statements made by the drug manufacturer in labeling the drug are backed by substantial evidence. The FDA has final approval over what the manufacturer may recommend the drug for and what it may say in its advertisements and marketing publications.

However, the FDA does not have any authority over the practice of medicine. There is no federal law prohibiting physicians from prescribing an approved drug for anything they choose, although some states place restrictions on what certain drugs can be prescribed for. As a result, many drugs that have been approved for specific symptoms or disorders are commonly prescribed for entirely different purposes (or unlabeled uses) than those stated by the manufacturer (Pugh & Pugh, 1987). For example, drugs approved for use in the treatment of cardiovascular disease (propranolol), high blood pressure (clonidine), nausea associated with cancer chemotherapy (metaclopramide), and depression and bed-wetting (imipramine) can also be found being prescribed for stage fright, morphine withdrawal, tardive dyskinesia (see Chapter 12), and chronic pain, respectively.

The primary problems with the use classification scheme are readily apparent. First, a drug may be used for several widely disparate symptoms (Zung, 1987). For example, phenobarbital may be used as an anticonvulsant, a sedative, or a hypnotic, and some antidepressants are increasingly being used in the treatment of pain, eating disorders, and phobias. Some anxiolytics appear equally effective in the treatment of certain types of depression. Cannabis may be used recreationally to alter "consciousness," or medically to reduce nausea in cancer patients undergoing chemotherapy (in which case the altered consciousness may be deemed an undesirable side effect). Second, some drugs that would seem to have the ideal properties for alleviating certain symptoms do not work in the long run. For example, amphetamine, which enhances mood in normal individuals, does not usually do so in depressed individuals. Even if it did, it would likely worsen their depression shortly after the person stopped taking it, and it should not be used to treat depression. Third, in many cases, the qualitative effects of a drug are dependent upon dosage or on how long the drug has been taken. For these reasons, even authors who categorize drugs using the same basic rationale as that used in this text tend to have somewhat different classification schemes.

Schedule-Controlled Drugs

One final classification system is provided by the United States government. Ever since the Harrison Narcotic Act of 1914, the federal government has classified psychoactive drugs for legal purposes. The most recent of such drug classification schemes came out of the Controlled Substances Act of 1970, which was designed by the government to improve the administration and regulation of manufacturing, distributing, and dispensing of potentially dangerous drugs. The present branch of the government responsible for this task is the Drug Enforcement Administration (DEA).

The drugs that come under the jurisdiction of the Controlled Substances Act are divided into five schedules and are referred to as **controlled substances**. Schedule I drugs are those that have no currently accepted medical use in treatment in the United States and are presumed to have a high potential for abuse. Schedule II drugs are those that have some currently accepted medical uses in the United States but have a high abuse potential. Schedule III, IV, and V drugs are those with current medical uses and successively lower abuse potentials than those of Schedules I and II. As one might expect, the penalties for nonprescription possession or sale of schedule-controlled drugs increase dramatically as one goes from Schedule V to Schedule I.

Table 7–1 provides some examples of different controlled substances according to schedule. Note that in several cases drugs are placed under different schedules, not so much because of differences in their mechanisms of action, but because of differences in pharmacokinetics. For example, the narcotic drugs heroin and morphine have the same action in the brain; they differ only in terms of their ability to penetrate the blood-brain barrier. The barbiturates secobarbital and phenobarbital both exert basically the same action in the brain, but again differ in how rapidly they penetrate the blood-brain barrier. Placement in these schedules may also be dependent on what a drug is combined with (e.g., codeine with aspirin as opposed to codeine with Actifed) or the concentration of the drug (mg/ml); for example, opium-containing compounds can be placed in Schedules II–V depending on the concentration of opium in them.

The fact that small alterations in a drug molecule can produce minimal changes in its effects has led to considerable problems for the DEA, which is responsible for controlling illegal drugs. By slightly altering the structure of an already illegal drug, "underground chemists" attempted to produce new compounds—often referred to as **designer drugs**—with

Table 7–1

Examples of Controlled Substances According to Schedule

Schedule I
Bufotenine
Dimethyltryptamine
Heroin
Lysergic acid diethylamide—LSD
Marijuana
Mescaline
Psilocybin

Schedule II
Cocaine
Dextroamphetamine (Dexedrine)
Meperidine (Demerol)
Methadone (Dolophine)
Morphine
Secobarbital (Seconal)

Schedule III
Glutethimide
Nalorphine
Phendimetrazine (Adipost)
Some codeine-containing compounds

Schedule IV
Alprazolam (Xanax)
Chloral hydrate
Chlordiazepoxide (Librium)
Diazepam (Valium)
Fenfluramine (Pondimin)
Phenobarbital
Propoxyphene (Darvon)

Schedule V
Buprenorphine (Buprenex)
Some codeine-containing compounds
Some opium-containing compounds

Note. Common brand name is in parentheses.

the same properties as the illegal drug. Until the new chemical structure was specifically designated by the DEA as illegal, its manufacture, sale, and use were legal. Most designer drugs have been analogues (that is, drugs with similar structures) of amphetamine, fentanyl (a very potent synthetic narcotic), meperidine (a synthetic narcotic), or phencyclidine. Although these designer drugs gained the attention of the mass media, it appears that their production and use has declined significantly over the past several years. This decline has been attributed to reports of lethal and toxic reactions to some of these compounds (see the discussion of MPTP in Chapter 10), prosecution of the few individuals with the biochemical expertise and equipment necessary to develop them, and the passing of the Controlled Substance Analogues Enforcement Act in 1986, which essentially treats any controlled substance analogue intended for human consumption as a Schedule I controlled substance (Frank Sapienza, DEA agent, 1988, personal communication).

Laypersons and the mass media often refer to drugs as "hard" or "soft," although it is never clear what characteristics of drugs are being referred to when these terms are used. One might expect that the hard-drug category would correspond to Schedule I and II drugs, and soft drugs would correspond to legal drugs or Schedule IV and V drugs. However, if hard drugs are those with high abuse potential, or those that are relatively toxic to the body, or those that are likely to produce notable behavioral or emotional disturbances, as discussed in later chapters, alcohol and nicotine certainly fit this description. On the other hand, marijuana, a Schedule I drug, is often viewed as one of the soft drugs. Thus describing drugs as hard or soft really does not provide one with any useful information about them. It should be made clear that all psychotropic drugs can be safe or harmful depending on the circumstances in which they are used, how frequently they are used, or how much is used.

Bibliography

Barden, J. A., & Mason, P. (1977). Conformation of (leu^5)enkephalin from x-ray diffraction: Features important for recognition at opiate receptor. *Science, 199,* 1214–1215.

Biel, J. H., Bopp, B., & Mitchell, B. D. (1978). Chemistry and structure-activity relationships of psychotropic drugs: Part 2. In W. G. Clark & J. del Guidice (Eds.), *Principles of psychopharmacology* (pp. 140–168). New York: Academic Press.

Leavitt, F. (1982). *Drugs and behavior* (2nd ed.). New York: John Wiley & Sons.

Petracek, F. J. (1978). Chemistry and structure-activity relationships of psychotropic drugs: Part 1. In W. G. Clark & J. del Guidice (Eds.), *Principles of psychopharmacology* (pp. 134–139). New York: Academic Press.

Pool, R. (1992). The third branch of science debuts. *Science, 256,* 44–47.

Pugh, M. C., & Pugh, C. B. (1987). Unlabeled uses for approved drugs. *American Druggist, 195,* 127–138.

Usdin, E. (1978). Classification of psychotropic drugs. In W. G. Clark & J. del Guidice (Eds.), *Principles of psychopharmacology* (pp. 193–246). New York: Academic Press.

Wallace, B., & Fisher, L. E. (1991). *Consciousness & behavior* (3rd ed.). Boston: Allyn & Bacon.

Weissman, A., & Milne, G. (1979). Cannabinoids: Definitional ambiguities and a proposal. *Neuroscience and Biobehavioral Reviews, 3,* 171–174.

Zung, W. W. K. (1987). Effect of clorazepate on depressed mood in anxious patients. *Journal of Clinical Psychiatry, 48,* 13–14.

Chapter Eight

Sedative-Hypnotics and Anxiolytics

The sedative-hypnotic drugs are perhaps the most commonly used and abused drugs in American society, with alcohol topping the list (Barnes, 1988). Despite the fact that they possess all the qualities that society deems unacceptable with respect to drugs (namely, toxicity, lethality, social disruptiveness, and psychological and physical dependence), and despite the fact that they are more destructive to individuals and society than all other drugs combined, they are readily accepted in both recreational and medicinal contexts. It has been estimated that alcoholics alone represent approximately 20% of the patients seen in psychiatric facilities (Guze, Cloninger, Martin, & Clayton, 1986). Therefore, it is imperative that everyone in American society be fully aware of what these substances can do to cognitive functioning, behavior, and the body.

The term "sedative-hypnotic" is used because, in most individuals, the lower doses of these drugs have a psychological calming effect and somewhat higher doses have a hypnotic, or sleep-inducing, effect. As mentioned in Chapter 7, the term "hypnotic" in this context should not be confused with the state induced by hypnosis, which is a state in which the individual is actually very much awake. These drugs are also commonly called **CNS depressants**, because their predominant tendency is to inhibit the excitability of neurons. However, as indicated on several earlier occasions, the term "CNS depression" may not be appropriate when one is describing the net effect of a drug on all the neurons of the CNS, since not all neurons decrease their rate of firing, particularly at the lower doses. In fact, while many neurons decrease their rate of firing with these drugs, others may increase their rate of firing because of the removal of the inhibitory influence of other neurons—an inhibition of inhibition.

Alcohol (technically ethanol) is the most used and abused recreational sedative-hypnotic drug in American society, and barbiturates and benzodiazepines are among the most frequently abused prescription sedative-hypnotics. In addition, there are many drugs with very similar properties, including chloral hydrate, ethchlorvynol (Placidyl), glutethimide (Doriden), and methaqualone (Quaalude). For the most part, all of these drugs differ primarily in their quantitative aspects—that is, the latency of onset, the intensity of effect, and the duration of action—without having any distinct qualitative differences. Their qualitative effects are directly dose related. Lower doses induce sedation; moderate doses induce sleep somewhat similar to natural sleep, in which the person is still responsive to pain; high doses induce sleep to the point of anesthesia; and successively higher doses can cause coma, respiratory arrest, and death. In the lower dose range, excitement, increased activity, gregariousness, and aggression may occur in some individuals. This phenomenon has commonly been attributed to the disruption of neural pathways of higher cortical origin that play an inhibitory function on subcortical centers of the brain (a phenomenon commonly referred to as **disinhibition**).

To some extent the anxiolytics (minor tranquilizers or antianxiety drugs) share a similar spectrum of effects, although their effects tend to be somewhat more selective in their ability to reduce anxiety without significantly altering other cognitive or perceptual processes or bodily activities like respiration. For example, whereas Seconal (a barbiturate) significantly depresses respiration at hypnotic doses and can induce anesthesia with 10 times the hypnotic dose, the benzodiazepines have minimal effects on respiration in hypnotic doses, and true anesthesia, sufficient to allow surgery, is very difficult to achieve with them. Furthermore, benzodiazepine anxiolytics have considerably higher therapeutic indices than other compounds with sedative-hypnotic qualities.

Alcohol (Ethanol)

Pick 20 American adults at random and the odds are that 15 of them drink moderately or occasionally, two drink to the point at which their drinking may be considered by others to be a problem, and one drinks excessively and chronically to the point where we can consider him or her an **alcoholic** (a compulsive alcohol user). Because of alcohol's prevalent use and potential abuse in American society, I will discuss the properties and characteristics of this drug at some length.

Alcohol has a number of characteristics that make it somewhat unique in comparison to most other drugs (Ritchie, 1985). First, it is a rather bulky drug, requiring several grams to exert noticeable effects, rather than the milligram amounts needed with other drugs. It takes somewhere between 25 and 50 mg of ethanol per 100 milliliters of blood (a blood alcohol content or BAC of 0.025 to 0.05%) to exert measurable effects in most individuals. A BAC of 0.1% is considered legal intoxication in terms of driving in most states. A person can achieve this level by consuming one drink (0.6 ounce ethanol) for every 40 pounds of body weight in one hour. (In this context a drink equals 1.5 ounces of 80 proof liquor, 5 ounces of wine, or 12 ounces of beer).

Alcohol also has somewhat different pharmacokinetic properties than most other drugs. Unlike many drug molecules, the ethanol molecule is a relatively small, neutrally charged particle. These characteristics make it readily absorbed from all compartments of the G.I. tract. In contrast to many psychoactive drugs, it is highly water-soluble. Its oil/water partition coefficient is just high enough for it to readily pass the blood-brain barrier, but low enough so that it is not fat-soluble. Therefore, its onset of action is rather quick and its duration of action rather short. Its low fat solubility also generally results in females achieving somewhat higher plasma concentrations than males, even when the same amount of alcohol is ingested and they weigh the same, because females have more body fat proportionally than males. Unlike most other drugs, whose rate of metabolism is proportional to their concentration, alcohol is metabolized at a fairly constant rate (i.e., it exhibits zero-order kinetics). Furthermore, with most drugs where there is considerable first-pass metabolism, the liver is responsible. With alcohol, it occurs mostly at an upper G.I. tract site (DiPadova, Worner, Julkunen, & Lieber, 1987).

Finally, alcohol is a high-calorie liquid that is almost always ingested orally as a beverage. Thus it provides the body with a ready source of calories. The alcohol in wine is derived through the interaction of yeast and sugar (fermentation) in fruits, whereas beer and distilled spirits are derived through the interaction of yeast and sugar in grains (after the starch in the grain is converted enzymatically to sugar). The alcohol content of these beverages is generally specified in terms of **proof**, which is exactly double the actual percentage of ethyl alcohol (ethanol) they contain. For example, 90 proof whiskey is 45% ethanol.

To some extent, these characteristics contribute to some of the unique problems associated with alcohol. For example, chronic users of alcohol often suffer from liver damage, partially because the liver spends a lot of time and energy trying to metabolize alcohol, and brain damage, partially because the individuals are consuming a large portion of their calories in alcohol and neglecting to eat proper amounts of other foods containing proteins, vitamins, and minerals essential for neuron maintenance (Rao, Larkin, & Derr, 1986; Ritchie, 1985).

Ethanol Pharmacokinetics

It takes approximately one hour for 90% of the alcohol in a drink to get into the bloodstream. However, because alcohol is rapidly and readily absorbed from the stomach, its accumulation in the brain is rapid enough to exert noticeable effects within minutes. Carbonated alcoholic beverages tend to enhance the absorption of alcohol because the carbonation forces the alcohol into the small intestine, where there is greater surface area for the absorption to take place and, thus, more rapid accumulation of alcohol in the brain.

Alcohol is metabolized at a rate of approximately 12 to 18 ml/hour, or 1.0 to 1.5 ounces of 80 proof vodka per hour (Ritchie, 1985). The liver accounts for approximately 90% of the alcohol metabolized. The first metabolite is acetaldehyde, a highly toxic substance capable of inducing nausea, headache, and high blood pressure. Acetaldehyde is then rapidly metabolized into acetic acid, which is further metabolized into carbon dioxide and water, which are then excreted. Approximately 5% of alcohol is excreted by way of the lungs, and a minimal amount of alcohol is directly eliminated in the urine.

Alcohol also interferes with the normal metabolic activities of the liver because of its own metabolism. Alcohol reduces the rate at which the liver forms glucose, oxidizes fats, and releases complex fats. As a result, when there is extensive exposure to alcohol, the liver accumulates fat, and blood sugar levels are depressed. Free fatty acids are not broken down and are deposited in the liver cells themselves. Eventually, the cells may rupture or become isolated and die. Cell death is followed by the formation of fibrous connective tissue (fibrosis), which is nonfunctional, at least with respect to what the liver is supposed to do.

Thus early stages of chronic alcohol consumption are characterized by fatty livers; some individuals eventually develop *cirrhosis* (severe hardening and contraction of the liver). Until recently, it was believed that the poor dietary practices of alcoholics were responsible for cirrhosis, and bad diet may indeed contribute to the problem. However, studies with baboons and other animals exposed to alcohol levels equivalent to those of human alcoholics but having a nutritionally adequate diet have indicated that good dietary practices do not prevent this damage. Whether the diets in these animal studies were in fact nutritionally adequate with respect to carbohydrate ingestion has recently been questioned (Rao et al., 1986).

Although there is some relationship between plasma level of alcohol and its behavioral effects, there is also a considerable lack of correspondence between the peak plasma levels of alcohol in the blood and the peak behavioral and subjective effects induced (see Figure 8–1). That is, it has long been recognized that the behavioral effects of alcohol are far greater when plasma levels are on the rise than when they are falling (Ritchie,

1985). At one time, it was believed that this effect was due to the fact that it takes considerably longer for alcohol levels in the forearm veins (where blood for alcohol analysis was drawn) to equal concentrations in intracranial arteries. However, recent studies assessing the time course for actual brain levels of alcohol found this belief to be unfounded. The fact that the same brain concentrations of ethanol during the rising and falling portions of the time-concentration function (a matter of an hour or two) induce substantially different effects suggests the development of rapid tolerance (tachyphylaxis). This is probably due to some homeostatic adjustments in the neuronal membranes in the presence of alcohol.

Considering its widespread use, one would hope that the relative margin of safety of alcohol would be high. Unfortunately, it is not. The BAC of persons who have died from acute alcohol exposure is typically around 0.5% (a level achieved in a 165-pound male drinking 23 drinks in four hours). Since responsible social drinking generally results in BACs of around 0.05% (achieved in the same man drinking four drinks in four hours), the therapeutic index of alcohol is around 6—not very high. Fortunately, there are two built-in mechanisms that generally prevent lethal levels from being reached. If one approaches a BAC of around 0.12% rapidly enough, vomiting may occur, because of local irritation of the G.I. tract, disturbances in vestibular functioning, or the accumulation of acetaldehyde in the brain. If one gets past this point, most persons become stuporous or pass out when a BAC of around 0.35% is reached. Therefore, the lethal limit would only be achieved in those who consume alcohol rapidly enough to achieve higher concentrations before they pass out.

Ethanol Pharmacodynamics

Whereas most psychoactive drugs directly alter functions at the synapse, alcohol alters practically every aspect of conduction and synaptic neurotransmission. At the neuropharmacological level, alcohol is believed to act directly on neuronal membranes by altering their basic semisolid structure and making them more "fluid" (Chin & Goldstein, 1977). At high doses this fluidizing action may inhibit the movements of the Na^+ and K^+ ions across the membranes and interfere with the ability of the neuron to generate and conduct action potentials. At lower doses that lead to intoxication, alcohol has been shown to enhance the activity of GABA at its receptors, which, in turn, hyperpolarizes neurons by allowing more Cl^- to enter (Zorumski & Isenberg, 1991). This action, which may be related to the just-mentioned fluidizing action on the membrane, can be completely blocked by a benzodiazepine derivative (Ro15–4513), which may be acting as an inverse agonist (Britton, Ehlers, & Koob, 1988). Although Ro15–4513 blocks alcohol's intoxicating properties, it does not reduce the lethal effects of high doses of alcohol. Therefore, the drug is unlikely to come into clinical use because if people drink to get drunk and they take the

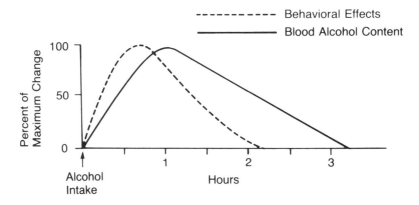

Figure 8–1

Percentage change in BAC levels and behavioral variables as a function of time since alcohol is administered. Note that the peak behavioral effects of alcohol occur prior to attaining peak BAC levels and that the behavioral effects dissipate considerably before all the alcohol has left the body.

drug beforehand, they could end up drinking so much alcohol in order to override the drug's effect that they could die (Kolata, 1986). Furthermore, there is evidence that Ro15–4513 by itself may induce seizure activity in primates (Miczek & Weerts, 1987).

Another action of alcohol, which also occurs with intoxicating doses, is to inhibit the excitatory effects of glutamate and aspartate at the NMDA receptor-ion complex. This action results in less Ca^{++} and Na^+ ion flow into neurons and a decreased ability for the cell to depolarize (Lovinger, White, d&e Weight, 1989). The net result of all these actions is that individual neurons become less excitable and exhibit reduced spontaneous electrical activity, and they repolarize more slowly after firing. In turn, the release of neurotransmitters and the subsequent activation of their receptors decrease.

The effect of ethanol is not always that of depressing neuronal functions (Pohorecky, 1977). Although alcohol has the ability to disrupt all neuronal membranes, some neurons may be more sensitive to its effects than others, so lower doses of alcohol may decrease the excitability of some neurons while leaving others unaffected except at higher concentrations. Thus, if the neurons whose excitability is decreased normally play an inhibitory role in the activity of those neurons that are not affected by low doses of alcohol, the latter's rate of firing may increase due to the loss of inhibitory control. However, once concentrations of alcohol reach higher levels, these neurons may also become less excitable, and their rate of firing will decrease.

Psychological Effects of Ethanol

Alcohol has been used for centuries, and by many cultures, for a variety of effects. Some of these effects are due to pharmacology, but a great many of the "effects" of alcohol are due to set and expectancy (Critchlow, 1986; Cutter et al., 1986; Hull & Bond, 1986). The most notable and global expectancy about alcohol is that it serves as a positive transforming agent that enhances social and physical pleasure; enhances sexual performance and responsiveness; increases power, social assertiveness, and aggression; and reduces tension (Marlatt et al., 1988). Individuals may acquire these beliefs even before beginning to drink, and they appear to be powerful predictors of both adolescent drinking status and adult alcoholism. Heavy drinkers generally expect more positive and fewer negative consequences than do light drinkers.

Because some individuals become more active, excited, and aggressive under low to moderate doses of alcohol (Pihl & Zacchia, 1986), the common view among laypersons is that alcohol is a stimulant. However, as mentioned earlier, the apparent stimulation is due to the loss of inhibitory control by those parts of the brain (such as the reticular activating system and the cortex) involved in the most highly integrated mental functions, which are dependent on social conditioning and experience, and which generally lead to sobriety and self-control (Ritchie, 1985).

These effects, in turn, are reflected in more of the undesirable consequences of alcohol, such as engaging in criminal activity (for example, homicide, robbery, rape, and arson) and family violence (like spouse beating and child abuse) and getting involved in traffic accidents. Statistically, alcohol consumption is the single most common denominator to all of these activities; in approximately half of all these examples, either the perpetrators or the victims were determined to be under the influence of alcohol (Guze et al., 1986; Peele, 1984; Quayle, 1983). (It should be noted that numerous surveys indicate that undesirable effects of alcohol are believed to be much more likely to occur in others—that is, people are much less likely to report that they occur in themselves.)

Alcohol tends to disrupt ongoing psychological processes in a dose-dependent manner. In general the types of faculties affected by increasingly larger doses of alcohol are depressed in the reverse order in which they were originally developed: first, complex cognitive skills (e.g., planning and problem solving); then fine learned motor skills (golfing); then gross learned motor skills (walking); and finally, visual accommodation and unconditioned reflexes (hand jerk upon touching a hot surface, breathing).

Various processes involved with learning and memory are also disrupted by alcohol (Mello, 1978; Nelson et al., 1986) (see Figure 9–2 for a summary of the various stages involved in learning and memory). Attention to relevant stimuli, ability to encode new information, and short-term memory (ability to maintain new information in storage for several seconds) all decrease. In the most extreme case, these processes may be so affected that the person may experience *blackouts*—that is, complete amnesia regarding events that took place over much of the period of intoxication. More often, long-term memory is affected, primarily with respect to our ability to retrieve information from storage, possibly because of state-dependency. Although there is some evidence that alcohol given immediately after learning new information may actually facilitate its retrieval at a later time (Hashtroudi et al., 1981), this finding has not been verified and should not be personally acted upon. Although alcohol induces sleep, it is not exactly a natural sleep, since REM (the sleep stage in which rapid eye movements and vivid dreams are most pronounced) is considerably reduced (Ritchie, 1985).

Alcohol has numerous effects on tissues other than the brain. It increases blood circulation to the skin, causing a warm, flushing sensation. However, this change increases the rate of loss of body heat when exposed to the cold. The galvanic skin response or GSR (actually a measure of sweat gland activity) is suppressed, and heart rate decreases, although in some individuals the initial effect of alcohol is to increase blood pressure, heart rate, and blood sugar level. These increases are probably related to an elevation in catecholamine blood levels stemming from a decrease in their clearance from the blood, possibly due to alcohol's disruption of norepinephrine neuronal reuptake (Ritchie, 1985). After an hour or so, these activities often decline below normal. Alcohol stimulates production of acid and pepsin in the stomach (potentially leading to ulcers), and this effect could explain why some people's appetites are enhanced by alcohol. Alcohol inhibits the release of antidiuretic hormone from the hypothalamus, causing water to be eliminated at a high rate. Thus drinking alcoholic beverages to relieve thirst is counterproductive.

Chronic Effects of Alcohol Use

It should be apparent from the preceding discussion that the liver is one of the organs most likely to be affected by chronic alcohol consumption. Alcohol-induced liver disease is primarily restricted to the fatty liver and is a benign and asymptotic condition. However, after years of alcohol abuse, a minority of alcoholics (heavy alcohol users) suddenly develop the potentially lethal condition called *alcoholic hepatitis*, characterized by cellular death and organ inflammation (Schanne et al., 1981). Although it is not clear what mediates the transformation of fatty liver into cirrhosis, there is evidence that some general physical effects of alcohol on cellular membranes render cells susceptible to otherwise nonlethal injuries. In other words, normally random exposure of the liver to membrane-active toxins (such as viruses and products of intestinal bacteria), which are normally well tolerated, overwhelm the homeostatic mechanisms of the cells in the presence of chronic alcohol exposure. This mechanism may also account for alcohol-induced disease in other organs, including the heart, the pancreas, and the nervous system (Laposata & Lange, 1986). Another likely mechanism for cellular damage involves the reduced ability of liver mitochondria to metabolize acetaldehyde, which in turn may promote the perpetuation of liver damage (Hasumura et al., 1975). Whatever the mechanism, once the liver cells lose their ability to metabolize alcohol, the individual's reaction to alcohol and other drugs actively metabolized by the liver is considerably exaggerated with respect to both duration and accumulation (Mazoit, Sandouk, Zetlaoui, & Scherrmann, 1987).

A wide variety of studies have indicated that, as a group, chronic alcoholics develop a relatively enduring pattern of cognitive and motor deficits (McEntee & Mair, 1978; Oscar-Berman, 1980; Svanum & Schladenhauffen, 1986). These deficits are generally not large, nor are they consistent across studies. Some of the lack of consistency is likely due to differences in how alcoholism is defined (to be discussed shortly), the ages of the subjects, the number of years of drinking, and how soon the tests were administered after abstinence. In general, global I.Q. scores of alcoholics are in the normal range. Although most studies have indicated that nonverbal I.Q. is somewhat lower than verbal I.Q. among alcoholics, other studies have not found such differences. Impairments are often displayed in abstract reasoning ability, new learning, problem solving, and perceptual motor functions. Inability to shift cognitive and attentional sets may also occur (for example, a person who has developed one strategy for a task or who attends to one type of stimulus may continue using that strategy when it is no longer appropriate or may not perceive a new type of stimulus if one is suddenly presented).

Unfortunately, all of the studies attempting to assess physiological or neurological dysfunction in alcoholics are retrospective; that is, they are done only after the diagnosis of alcoholism. Thus it is not clear to what extent the deficits noted may have existed prior to the alcoholism phase and may, in fact, have contributed to the person's becoming alcoholic in the first place. As yet, research has not demonstrated a clear and consistent relationship between levels of alcohol consumption and neuropsychological deficits.

A considerable body of evidence suggests that right-hemisphere functions (e.g., visual-spatial skills and visual-perceptual analysis) are more impaired in alcoholics than left-hemisphere functions (e.g., verbal-linguistic abilities). Because this pattern of cognitive decline in chronic heavy drinkers is similar to that observed in aged individuals, some have suggested that alcoholism is associated with "premature aging" of cognitive capabilities (Ryan, 1982). However, a recent review of empirical research findings on cerebral asymmetries in alcoholics indicates that, although general information-processing mechanisms may decline in alcoholics, particularly for tasks that stress the person's acquired skills and abilities, there is probably no change in the balance of hemispheric specialization that accounts for the cognitive deficits observed (Ellis & Oscar-Berman, 1989).

It has generally been assumed that the disturbance to cognitive functions in alcoholics is the result of what alcohol does to the brain. However, a recent study of alcoholics who received liver transplants has challenged this assumption (Arria et al., 1991). A year after receiving new livers, all but two of the 13 alcoholics assessed returned to basically normal functioning in tests assessing psychomotor, visual, and perceptual abilities. The main exception, a lack of improvement in memory capacity, could be related to the results of other studies suggesting that chronic alcohol intake irreversibly damages the hippocampus—a brain structure heavily involved in memory formation (Wilson et al., 1987).

Chronic alcohol consumption has also been associated with cerebral atrophy and a number of functional deficits in cerebral and cerebellar function (Carlen et al., 1978; Golden et al., 1981). People suffering from these conditions can show some recovery when abstinence is maintained over periods of weeks to many months (Carlen et al., 1978). Rapid recovery may be attributed to the resolution of the alcohol withdrawal syndrome—a biochemical process—whereas gradual functional improvement may have a structural basis—a reversible atrophy indicative of the plasticity in the CNS.

The mechanisms for cellular death with respect to the CNS are also not well understood, although there is clear evidence that a great deal of damage is indirectly due to alcohol consumption. Much of the alcohol-associated brain damage (*Wernicke's disease*) and the resulting impairment in learning and memory (*Korsakoff's syndrome*) have traditionally been attributed to malnutrition, especially thiamine deficiency, rather than to the direct neurotoxic effect of ethanol (Rao et al., 1986; Ritchie, 1985). These problems come about because a large portion of the alcoholic's diet is derived from alcohol, which happens to be very high in calories but contains no other essential nutrients, and the consumption of proper amounts of proteins, vitamins, and essential nutrients is low. Poor diet associated with chronic alcohol intake can also depress appetite and prevent proper absorption of nutrients from the G.I. tract (Pezzarossa et al., 1986). Therefore, treatment of these neurological disorders with thiamine and glucose is generally helpful, although it will not reverse symptoms that are the result of neuronal losses, because neurons in the brain do not regenerate.

Although the relationship between diet and neuropathy is clear, it is nevertheless the case that both neuropathological and neuropsychological deficits have been observed in some alcoholic patients who have no history of malnutrition. In some cases, these deficits can be traced to head injuries stemming from falls, fights, or car accidents (Svanum &

Schladenhauffen, 1986). A genetic predisposition may be involved in other cases. Finally, studies with animals maintained on nutritional diets and given large quantities of alcohol chronically have reported significant loss of specific CNS neurons, such as those in the hippocampus (Riley & Walker, 1978; Walker et al., 1980). The functional significance of these findings for human alcoholics is not clear, because the concentrations of alcohol used in these studies is much higher than those sustained in humans.

Chronic alcohol consumption can also severely affect numerous sexual functions. Male alcoholics, with or without overt liver disease, exhibit certain underactive gonadal functions, including testicular atrophy, impaired sperm production, impotence, and decreased libido, as well as abnormalities in the metabolism of sex hormones. Much of the evidence suggests that these deficits are due to increased activities of the drug-metabolizing enzymes in the liver resulting from chronic alcohol exposure, which, in turn, severely reduces testosterone levels (Van Thiel et al., 1974).

Beneficial Effects of Alcohol

As discussed earlier, alcohol (or expectations about it) induces a variety of effects that users find pleasurable or beneficial to them. Furthermore, despite all that I have said about alcohol up to this point, there is no evidence that chronic exposure to less than 2 ounces of ethanol per day (approximately four drinks) is associated with any untoward health consequences for the user. (As discussed a little later on, this statement probably does not apply to a developing fetus.) In fact, many studies have indicated that drinking of these amounts—often described as moderate drinking—may have some health benefits (Turner et al., 1981). For instance, longevity and other signs of physical health tend to be greatest in moderate drinkers, although no causal link between moderate drinking and these variables has been established. Statistically, longevity is somewhat shorter in abstainers and is shortest in heavy drinkers. The beneficial effects of moderate alcohol use have been attributed to lowered risk of cardiovascular disease (Rimm et al., 1991). Enhanced quality of life and decreased arousal from stress may also be a factor in this phenomenon.

Tolerance, Dependence, and Alcoholism

As is the case with most drugs, tolerance to ethanol develops at different rates, depending on the measures one employs to evaluate it, and there is no uniform underlying mechanism responsible (Cicero, 1978; Pohorecky et al., 1986). In addition to the tachyphylaxis phenomenon described earlier, a low to moderate degree of tolerance develops to most of the behavioral and mood-altering effects of alcohol, such that the chronic user must take larger and larger amounts in order to obtain the desired effects. Minimal tolerance develops to the lethal effects of alcohol, so that, in effect, the therapeutic index for the drug gets smaller and smaller. There is cross-tolerance among alcohol and all the sedative-hypnotic drugs.

Just about all of the mechanisms described in Chapter 6 for the development of tolerance seem to operate with alcohol. There is some metabolic tolerance in that the drug-metabolizing enzymes of the liver may be increased by approximately 15–30% with chronic use (Ritchie, 1985). Because less neurotransmitter is being released, because of the effect of alcohol on conduction, there is the possibility that numerous neurotransmitter postsynaptic receptors become more sensitive with prolonged exposure to alcohol. Thus higher concentrations of alcohol are needed to continue to depress the activation of these receptors.

Most of the tolerance to alcohol is believed to be due to behavioral compensation; that is, the individual learns to compensate for the detrimental effects of the drug on behavior (Wenger et al., 1981). Finally, some recent studies indicate that some tolerance is due to the development of Pavlovian conditioned compensatory responses, which may counter the direct actions of alcohol (Crowell et al., 1981). Both of these mechanisms imply that the degree of intoxication with alcohol is very situationally dependent; that is, the effects of alcohol are most pronounced in novel situations or tasks.

Alcohol, like other sedative-hypnotics, has a strong potential for inducing both psychological and physiological dependence. When either or both of these occur with alcohol, the term **alcoholism** is used, and the individual is referred to as an **alcoholic**. It is not clear exactly what is so positively reinforcing about alcohol. Its taste is obnoxious to practically everybody at first, and nonhumans are somewhat equivocal in their tendency to self-administer it. Most strains of rats and monkeys avoid drinking alcohol unless they are positively reinforced for doing so, or unless the catheter infusion method is used (Woods, 1978).

There is a great deal of variability in humans' reactions to alcohol and in their tendency to develop alcoholism (Reed & Hanna, 1986). Some get physically ill after drinking and will not continue to drink. Others apparently experience neither pleasurable nor unpleasant reactions. These individuals may drink socially but will not become alcoholic. Another group of individuals experience pleasurable reactions to alcohol but rarely become alcoholic. The final group of people derive an unusually pleasurable reaction from alcohol, can drink a lot, and are highly likely to become alcoholic.

Although physical dependence on alcohol generally requires several months or years of exposure to alcohol to develop, many experts believe that a single day's exposure to a large quantity of alcohol can induce physical dependence, which is commonly experienced as a **hangover** (Cicero, 1978). The fact that reexposure to alcohol can "cure" a hangover ("the hair of the dog that bit you") supports this belief. Some of the symptoms of a hangover may be related to a buildup of acetaldehyde in the brain, depletion of norepinephrine, lack of sleep, dehydration, and low blood sugar. In addition, alcohols other than ethanol (referred to as congeners) may enhance a hangover, which is probably why some alcoholic beverages induce greater hangovers than others.

Withdrawal from chronic use of greater than moderate doses of alcohol (say, a pint of whiskey per day for several weeks) may be limited to prolonged disturbances in the EEG during sleep. The abstinence syndrome after cessation of larger doses may be evidenced as a high degree of arousal associated with weakness, tremor, anxiety, and elevated blood pressure, pulse rate, and respiratory rate. In severe reactions, 12 to 48 hours after the person stops drinking, convulsions may occur, and a toxic psychosis may appear with symptoms such as irritability, headaches, fever, nausea, agitation, confusion, and visual hallucinations. This latter syndrome is referred to as **delirium tremens** or the D.T.s, which typically appear 2 to 4 days after drinking stops (Romach & Sellers, 1991). Because of the convulsions and the associated respiratory arrest, withdrawal from alcohol and other short-duration sedative-hypnotics can be lethal. Therefore, medical treatment is strongly advised.

What Is Alcoholism?

There has been a considerable amount of discussion as to exactly what constitutes alcohol dependence, or alcoholism, and definitions of this disorder vary (Barnes, 1988). The idea that alcoholism is a disease dominates American treatment programs, with advocates of such a model hypothesizing an underlying process based on physical dependency, genetic disposition, and the assumption that it is progressive (Marlatt et al., 1988). Other experts are critical of such a view because it depends on how one defines a disease. This model also fails to account for commonalities among addictions that do not involve substance use (e.g., compulsive gambling), and it does not explain how and why many people appear to overcome their addictions without any treatment or why they seem to benefit from a variety of treatment approaches (Marlatt et al., 1988).

Some authorities prefer to view alcoholism as a compulsive drug-use disorder, arguing that until the chronic exposure to alcohol induces physiological damage there is nothing distinctive about alcoholics except for their inability to regulate their use of alcohol in spite of experiencing adverse consequences. In 1988 the U.S. Supreme Court ruled that the government may continue viewing alcoholism as "willful misconduct" rather than an uncontrollable disease when awarding veterans' education benefits. However, the disease designation—adopted by the American Medical Association in 1957—is commonly accepted, if only to counteract the disorder's social stigma and to establish that it is treatable and arrestable (Guze et al., 1986). Some experts describe alcoholism in terms of the amount of alcohol consumed, whereas others feel the consequences of alcohol and the attendant behaviors associated with it, whatever the amount ingested, should be emphasized. With so many different criteria, determining the incidence of alcoholism is difficult, but a ballpark figure for the number of alcoholics in the United States would be around 10 million, or 1 out of 12 drinkers (Barnes, 1988).

Alcoholism is characterized by continuous or periodic: impaired control over drinking, preoccupation with alcohol, use of alcohol despite numerous adverse consequences, and distortions in thinking, most notably denial. For example, there may be one or more unsuccessful efforts to cut down on or control alcohol use, or the person may continue to use alcohol despite knowledge of having persistent or recurrent social, psychological, or physical problems that are caused by their alcohol use. The person may have numerous driving accidents under the influence of alcohol, physically abuse the spouse or children, spend a great deal of money on alcohol, miss work because of drinking alcohol or recovering from its effects, or experience ulcers or high blood pressure. Alcoholics may also display a marked tolerance to alcohol and a characteristic withdrawal syndrome when alcohol use ceases. It should be emphasized that physical dependence is not a necessity in order for a person to be deemed an alcoholic; many individuals who are not physically dependent on alcohol are still considered alcoholic if the other characteristics are evidenced. However, if one is physically dependent on alcohol, then the person is definitely an alcoholic. The prevailing view is that even after such persons stop drinking for some length of time, they are still considered to be alcoholic because, should they return to drinking alcohol, the likelihood of the noted characteristics being evidenced is quite high.

Loss of control over one's consumption of alcohol is one factor that is highly debated (Fingarette, 1988). Some experts in the area of alcoholism view alcoholics as being qualitatively different from nonalcoholics in this dimension, as if alcohol acts like an "on-off" switch for them. Others view loss of control along a continuum of degrees of control. This is not a subtle distinction, as it has important bearing on the type of treatment prescribed for alcoholism. For those who believe that alcohol acts like an "on" switch, the primary treatment goal is complete abstinence from alcohol (Mello, 1978). For those who believe that there is a continuum of control, drinking in moderation is not only feasible but is perhaps a more appropriate goal in many individuals with an alcohol problem (Robertson et al., 1986). The reasoning here is that some individuals will avoid all treatment modalities, such as Alcoholics Anonymous, that emphasize complete abstinence, because they cannot see themselves going through life without ever taking another drink. Presently, there is much greater acceptance of the controlled drinking treatment goal in Britain than in the United States, where there is considerable resistance to this idea.

Etiology of Alcoholism

Alcoholism is found in all classes of society and in all walks of life. The ratio of male to female alcoholics is approximately 6:1 (Guze et al., 1986). There is no consistent evidence to indicate that a particular personality type develops the disorder; however, individuals high in antisocial characteristics, as measured by a variety of personality tests, have been consistently shown to be prone to alcoholism (Cadoret et al., 1987; Cloninger, 1987). Such individuals are generally males whose pattern of drinking is fairly continuous. They often engage in thrill-seeking behavior, fights, and criminal activities, rarely binge drink, display little guilt or anxiety over their drinking, and are low in the need for social rewards. Conversely, female alcoholics are much more likely to abstain from drinking for periods of time and then binge once they start drinking. They tend not to engage in thrill-seeking and antisocial activities, they have high social reward dependence, and they often feel guilty or fearful about their alcohol dependence. Many male alcoholics also share these characteristics (Cloninger, 1987).

Many studies have indicated that genetics is probably involved in this disorder (Cadoret et al., 1987; Cloninger, 1987; Vaillant & Milofsky, 1982). First of all, numerous studies assessing the acute responses of normal humans to alcohol have shown some degree of genetic control in a wide variety of responses (Reed & Hanna, 1986). Differences between races (Orientals and Caucasians) have been shown to occur with respect to facial flushing and dysphoria (a state of feeling unwell or unhappy), rate of metabolism, levels of alcohol-metabolizing enzymes, and heart and blood pressure responses. Within-race genetically controlled differences have been shown to occur with respect to rates of absorption, metabolism, EEG alterations, heart rate, and blood pressure.

Second, with respect to alcoholism per se, several studies have noted that the *concordance rate** for alcoholism in identical twins is double that obtained in fraternal twins (approximately 55% versus 28%) (Kendler et al., 1992). People whose biological parents (one or both) display alcoholism and who were adopted as children by nonalcoholic parents have a

*Concordance rate refers to the percentage of pairs of individuals who share some trait or characteristic. If the concordance rate for alcoholism was 1% in pairs of genetically unrelated people raised apart, and was 100% in pairs of identical twins raised apart (that is, in every case either both members of a pair were alcoholic or neither member was alcoholic), then there would be overwhelming evidence that genetics was the sole determinant of alcoholism. Conversely, if the concordance rates were 1% in both unrelated and genetically identical sets, the evidence would be overwhelmingly in favor of environmental factors.

significantly higher incidence of alcoholism than adoptees whose biological parents were not alcoholics (Cloninger, 1987; Vaillant & Milofsky, 1982). This finding appears to be particularly true for the pattern of alcoholism discussed earlier involving antisocial characteristics (von Knorring et al., 1987). In general, most of the recent evidence suggests that genetic factors account for about half of the variance in liability to alcoholism and that they are of similar etiologic importance for alcoholism in women and men (Kendler et al., 1992; Pickens et al., 1991).

For the past two decades, researchers have been trying to identify biological characteristics or even actual genes that are associated with a predisposition to alcoholism—so far without much success. Although there is general agreement that many genes are involved in the disorder and that they are different for different groups of individuals, many scientists suspect that there are no specific genes for alcoholism per se (Holden, 1991). More likely there are a variety of genes that lead to a susceptibility to a number of compulsive behaviors—for example, alcohol or other drug addictions, gambling, or eating disorders—in which the type of disorder is shaped by environmental and temperamental factors. This suggestion is supported by the fact that there is a tremendous variability among alcoholics. Though close to a third of alcoholics also exhibit symptoms of other mental disorders—such as anxiety, depression, manic-depression, childhood conduct disorder, and antisocial personality—most alcoholics do not. Also, alcoholism can set in early and fast or gradually develop over decades; some are binge drinkers while others are chronic maintenance drinkers. Thus it is likely to be some time before we can fit all the disparate pieces of the puzzle together so that the predisposing factors behind this disorder are established with some certainty.

Over the years several studies have suggested that there are a number of biological and behavioral characteristics or markers of alcoholics. For example, studies have suggested that alcoholics metabolize alcohol into acetaldehyde at a faster rate and convert acetaldehyde into acetic acid at a slower rate than nonalcoholics do. A genetic basis for these metabolic differences was indicated by studies showing that similar differences occur between relatives of alcoholics (relatives who drank little or no alcohol) and relatives of nonalcoholics (Schuckit & Rayses, 1979; Watterlond, 1983).

Most studies looking for biological differences between alcoholics and nonalcoholics have been retrospective; that is, these characteristics were noted after alcoholism was evidenced. Thus it is not clear whether these characteristics preceded heavy alcohol use or were caused by it. To circumvent the problem, researchers have attempted to determine whether non-alcohol-abusing young adults with a family history of alcoholism differ, in terms of their reactions to alcohol, from those without a family history of alcoholism (Schuckit & Gold, 1988). There is general agreement in these studies that, when given alcohol, young adults with a family history of alcoholism exhibit (1) lower scores on many subjective scale items (e.g., dizziness, floating feelings, and level of perceived drug effects); (2) less decrement in motor performance (e.g., body sway); and (3) less change in prolactin and cortisol (hormones that have been noted to change after drinking alcohol). Other studies have noted that brain wave deficits that are often seen in alcoholics also appear in the sons of alcoholics before the boys have ever used alcohol (Begleiter et al., 1984). These results, in addition to supporting the view that some of the variation in the propensity for alcoholism is biologically based, suggest that it may be possible to determine which individuals are prone to alcoholism prior to their becoming heavy users of alcohol and to warn such individuals about their predisposition to developing the disorder.

Environmental factors also are implicated in the vulnerability to alcoholism (Zucker & Gomberg, 1986). As noted above, even in identical twins the concordance rates are nowhere close to 100%. Furthermore, one-third of alcoholics have no family history of alcoholism, and only 30–40% of sons of alcoholics become alcoholics (Kolata, 1988). For years environmental factors have been assumed to explain the findings of studies showing that different cultures have different alcoholism rates that are not easily tied in with per capita consumption of alcohol. For example, in France, where per capita consumption of alcohol is high, there is a high rate of alcoholism. However, in Italy and Greece, where per capita alcohol consumption is high, the rate of alcoholism is low. In the United States and Sweden, which have relatively low per capita consumption of alcohol, alcoholism is relatively high. In viewing the drinking habits and attitudes of these cultures, it appears that the lowest incidence of alcoholism occurs when (1) the children are exposed to alcohol early in life in a family or religious setting, with parents presenting an example of moderate drinking; (2) alcohol is served in small or diluted quantities, usually with meals; (3) abstinence is socially acceptable and excessive drinking is not; (4) drinking is not viewed as proof of adulthood or virility; and (5) there are well-established ground rules for drinking behavior (Aronow, 1980).

Despite the apparent cultural differences in alcoholism rates, no specific environmental factors have been shown to correlate with alcoholism. Some studies have shown that adoptees of adoptive parents who display alcohol-related problems are no more likely to become alcoholics than the general population. Others have shown that alcohol-related problems in the adoptive family do predict increased adoptee alcohol abuse. Still others have shown that alcohol-related problems in the adoptive family only predict adoptee alcohol abuse if there was a concomitant genetic disposition—that is, the adoptee had a biological parent who was alcoholic (Cadoret et al., 1987; Cloninger, 1987). Although considerably speculative, there is some evidence that environments that contribute to alcoholic vulnerability (1) do not promote impulse control; (2) view drunkenness as acceptable behavior; (3) reduce a person's cognitive ability to appraise information that might limit alcohol consumption; or (4) do not provide nondrug alternative sources of gratification (Heilbrun, et al., 1986; Mello, 1978).

Obviously, there are numerous factors, many of which have probably not even been considered, that contribute to the induction of alcoholism. Perhaps the only thing that is certain is that impurities in alcoholic beverages, vitamin deficiencies, and hormonal changes are not factors (when hormonal changes occur, they are probably an effect of the disorder rather than a cause) (Ritchie, 1985).

Treatment of Alcoholism

Along with a multitude of potential interacting causes of alcoholism, there are a multitude of ways of treating the problem, none of which has had universal success with all individuals. One thing is clear: for any of them to work, the alcoholic must not be physically dependent, because the motivational forces for continuing to drink are just too great in the physically dependent alcoholic. Since withdrawal from alcohol can be lethal, medical intervention is advisable. This generally entails substituting a long-acting anxiolytic—for example, diazepam (Valium)—and then gradually reducing the dose over several days. However, anxiolytics that remain in the body for a shorter period of time, such as oxazepam (Serax), may be preferable because they allow physicians to more easily adjust dosages as needed. Carbamazepine (Tegretol), a medication commonly prescribed to control epileptic seizures, is currently being tested for treatment of alcohol withdrawal (Romach & Sellers, 1991).

Once the physical dependence phase is over with, other interventions can be applied (chemical, psychological, or both). Chemical treatments for maintaining abstinence have ranged from drugs that induce nausea when accompanied by alcohol to drugs that attempt to promote insight into the causes of one's drinking. One of the most common chemical interventions involving disulfiram (Antabuse) has been used for over 20 years (Fuller et al., 1986). This drug competes for the same enzyme that normally metabolizes the alcohol metabolite acetaldehyde into acetic acid. Thus, with the intake of alcohol, there is a buildup of acetaldehyde in the body, and a toxic reaction occurs, consisting of nausea and a headache. The patient is either told of these unpleasant reactions or is given small test amounts of alcohol to precipitate the reaction, so that he or she will know what to expect.

Theoretically, this approach should keep the alcoholic abstinent. Unfortunately, however, most well-controlled studies on the efficacy of disulfiram treatment have indicated that the drug is no more effective than a placebo (Fuller et al., 1986). One of the basic problems with disulfiram is that its effectiveness as a drinking deterrent depends entirely on the person's willingness to comply with the treatment regimen or even accept it in the first place—both of which are rare (Brubaker et al., 1987). Furthermore, since the craving for alcohol is still present, the person needs only to stop taking the disulfiram for a few days in order to start drinking again. There are other problems associated with disulfiram treatment. One is that the person must be very careful to avoid all substances that might contain alcohol, such as cough medicine. Another is that several side effects—for example, psychotic-like reactions—can occur with chronic disulfiram exposure.

Anthropological reports have suggested that American Indians belonging to the Native American Church, which uses the mescaline-containing peyote plant in their religious ceremonies, have a lower incidence of alcohol problems than other Indian groups. In the early 1960s, a few pilot studies with LSD were conducted with alcoholics to see if the supposedly insight-promoting properties of this drug would be useful in reducing their alcohol problem (Brecher, 1972). These generally involved one or two exposures to LSD under medical supervision. Although there was some indication of an initial reduction in alcohol consumption, six-month follow-ups showed no greater improvement with LSD than with a placebo. However, before more extensive research could be conducted with LSD, governmental restrictions became so difficult for researchers that no further studies were attempted.

More recently, efforts to identify drugs that may reduce the desire to drink alcohol have led to the discovery that serotonin-enhancing agents appear to diminish ethanol preference and consumption (Tollefson, 1989). Serotonin precursors (e.g., tryptophan), reuptake inhibitors (e.g., fluoxetine, zimelidine, fluvoxamine), and postsynaptic agonists have all been reported to reduce ethanol intake in humans and nonhumans. Although several of these treatments may also be effective in the treatment of depression, their effect on alcohol intake appears to be unrelated to their ability to reduce depression symptoms, since they work in non-depressed alcoholics and their effect on alcohol intake occurs more rapidly than their antidepressant effects. Naltrexone (Trexan), an opiate antagonist currently used to treat heroin addiction, and buspirone (BuSpar), a drug used to treat anxiety disorders, are also being explored as possible treatments for curbing alcohol craving. Further clinical work on the long-term consequences and efficacy of these treatments is needed before they can be considered to be useful in the treatment of alcoholism. Lithium, commonly used in the treatment of manic-depression, has been periodically touted as an effective treatment for alcoholism since the 1970s, but a recent exhaustive study of this treatment failed to support its efficacy in this regard (Dorus et al., 1989).

Among the psychologically based treatments, a number of traditional psychodynamic approaches, behavior modification techniques, and group therapies have been applied in the treatment of alcoholism. Psychodynamic therapy does not seem to work, and support for the efficacy of behaviorally based therapies has been equivocal (Jaffe, 1990).

Perhaps one of the most controversial of these studies was conducted with 20 alcoholics who had been physically dependent on alcohol (Holden, 1980). Through behavior modification techniques, they were taught to drink alcohol moderately. Follow-ups conducted one or two years later seemed to indicate that the vast majority of these individuals were still drinking moderately and functioning within normal levels. However, a follow-up 10 years later, conducted by another group of researchers, indicated that only one of the 20 was drinking moderately (Pendery et al., 1982). Some of the subjects in the study had died of alcohol-related problems, because they had continued to drink heavily, while others were either drinking excessively or were forced to abstain completely in order to be functional. Although the original investigators were severely criticized for their methodological techniques, and for promoting a way of dealing with alcoholism that was antithetical to traditional beliefs about alcoholism, they subsequently responded by pointing out that despite the admittedly dismal outcome of their interventions with the experimental subjects, the individuals were still better off than the subjects who served as untreated controls.

Controlled-drinking training may still be a viable alternative for problem drinkers who have not developed a heavy physical dependence on alcohol (although I'm sure many experts will cringe at such a suggestion) (Elal-Lawrence et al., 1987; Robertson et al., 1986). The fact is, many individuals who receive extensive treatment for their alcoholism return to what can be considered controlled drinking (defined as less than 64 and 48 grams of ethanol per day for men and women, respectively) following the period of abstinence required while they are in treatment. Those who do are more likely to have received some type of training in controlled drinking, such as setting frequency-quantity targets, learning about the antecedents of drinking, keeping diaries, learning how to refuse drinks, changing from high- to low-alcohol beverages, changing drinking environments and companions, and learning alternatives to drinking (Alden, 1988). How many of these individuals return to their former destructive patterns of drinking is still unknown, because few researchers have the time or money to follow their subjects for more than a year or two.

Perhaps one of the most accepted approaches to dealing with alcoholism is the one taken by Alcoholics Anonymous (AA). This organization, founded by a group of alcoholics, believes that alcoholism is a disease, that abstinence is required to deal with the disease, and that faith in a higher spiritual being is important in the recovery process. From a psychological perspective, this group provides peer education about alcoholism and its consequences for the individual, and provides support through the testimonials of many individuals who share the problems of alcoholism (Jaffe, 1990). These individuals also serve the vital function of being able to respond to the denials and rationalizations that inevitably occur in the alcoholic and that prevent the person from accepting the fact that he or she has a problem. Unfortunately, there is considerable difficulty in determining the actual effectiveness of AA, since the group is reluctant to give researchers access to their records or members. Furthermore, participation in AA is almost always voluntary, raising questions of how self-selection might be a factor in the efficacy of AA. In one study, less than half of those treated for alcoholism in formal settings (discussed next) chose to attend AA meetings (Elal-Lawrence et al., 1987). In another study, it was found that those who chose to participate in AA were less pathological in their personality profile than those who did not voluntarily participate (Thurstin et al., 1986).

Over the past 20 years, a number of treatment centers for chemical dependency have sprung up around the United States. These generally involve several days of assessment and several weeks of inpatient and outpatient treatment. The environment is highly structured, activities are regimented, and there is a heavy emphasis on peer-group therapy. It is probably still too early to determine the overall impact of these treatment centers in dealing with the age-old problem of alcoholism, particularly because these centers are selective in terms of the clients they accept and the treatment is expensive.

The ability to select one's clients greatly influences the outcome of any treatment, because there is strong evidence that there are a number of characteristics of alcoholics that predict successful treatment (Holden, 1987). Alcoholics who respond well, regardless of treatment, are those with jobs, stable family relationships, minimal psychopathology, no history of past treatment failures, and minimal involvement with other drugs. Unfortunately, however, most alcoholics do not fall into this favored category. Furthermore, alcohol abusers whose history suggests a primary diagnosis of depression have been found to respond to treatment better than substance abusers with a diagnosis of antisocial personality.

In short, it is important to take with a grain of salt any claim of effective alcoholism treatment unless the characteristics of the clients are indicated. The fact is, on the basis of recent reviews of controlled comparisons among treatment settings (where different types of patients have been clumped together), there is little evidence that there is an overall advantage for residential over nonresidential settings, for longer over shorter inpatient programs, for more cost-intensive over less cost-intensive programs, or for inpatient over outpatient programs (Holden, 1987; Miller & Hester, 1986).

However, a recent study comparing minimal versus intensive controlled-drinking treatment interventions for low to moderate dependence problem drinkers indicated that the intensive group reduced consumption and increased abstinent days significantly more than the minimal group (Robertson et al., 1986). Similar benefits were noted in a more recent study of employed problem drinkers randomly assigned to one of three rehabilitation regimens: compulsory inpatient treatment, compulsory attendance at AA meetings, or a choice of options. Though the estimated costs for the hospital group were about 10% higher than for the other two groups, the other two groups required more subsequent treatment (inpatient) and evidenced lower rates of abstinence and continuous sobriety two years after initial treatment (Walsh et al., 1991).

Only about 15% of alcoholics ever receive formal treatment; many end up in jail, die from traffic or other accidents, or die from medical complications of their alcoholism. Depending on the criteria used for assessing treatment outcomes, somewhere between one-third and two-thirds of the alcoholics who are treated can be viewed as successes; that is, the person becomes abstinent or engages in nonproblem drinking (Marlatt et al., 1988). Interestingly, numerous studies have indicated that many alcohol abusers are able to positively change their use patterns without the assistance of formal treatment. Factors associated with successful self-change include a high level of motivation and commitment to change, public announcements, social support, alterations in one's social and leisure-time activities, general life-style changes that decrease exposure to conditioned craving cues, development of stress-coping strategies, and the generation of negative expectations over continued use and positive expectations concerning continued abstinence (Marlatt et al., 1988).

Fetal Alcohol Syndrome

Pregnant women who consume alcohol should be aware of the potentially serious consequences of their drinking on their offspring—one of the most severe consequences being the **fetal alcohol syndrome** (FAS). First described in 1968, FAS is commonly characterized by mild to moderate mental retardation, small head circumference, absence of the groove between the nose and upper lip, inordinate profusion of hair on the face at birth, folds on eyelids, underdeveloped jaw area, cleft palate, joint anomalies, and cardiac irregularities. Behavioral characteristics, reported in more than 50% of the cases, include irritability in infancy and hyperactivity in childhood (Clarren & Smith, 1978).

It is generally accepted that the adverse effects of prenatal alcohol exposure exist along a continuum, with complete FAS at one end of the spectrum and incomplete features of FAS, including more subtle cognitive-behavioral deficits, at the other. Thus infants with suboptimal neurobehavioral responses may exhibit later deficits in such aspects of daily life as judgment, problem solving, and memory (Streissguth et al., 1989). Many of the symptoms of FAS decline as the children get older, but in most cases, these children remain at a considerable disadvantage in comparison to normal children (Steinhausen & Spohr, 1986). For example, a recent study of I.Q. in FAS patients indicated that I.Q. remained stable from a mean age of 8 years, 4 months (mean I.Q. of 66) to a mean age of 16 years, 7 months (mean I.Q. of 67) (Streissguth et al., 1991).

The incidence of FAS and the severity of the symptoms are directly related to the amount of alcohol consumed by the mother during the first trimester. Numerous mechanisms have been proposed for the production of FAS (Keir, 1991). The most recent studies have pointed to ethanol's ability to disrupt the synthesis of retinoic acid, a metabolite of vitamin A, as a mechanism for inducing FAS, since an optimal level of retinoic acid is needed for normal development of the limbs and CNS. As yet, there is no clear association between the incidence and severity of FAS and other factors that may be confounded with extensive maternal alcohol use in humans, such as maternal malnutrition, other drug use, intellectual functioning, and socioeconomic level (Steinhausen & Spohr, 1986). The risk of FAS has been reported to be sevenfold higher in blacks than in whites, even after adjustment for the frequency of maternal alcohol intake, occurrence of chronic alcohol problems, and number of children borne (Sokol et al., 1986), raising the question of some kind of genetic susceptibility to FAS.

The minimal amount of alcohol necessary for inducing FAS has not been determined, but most of the evidence suggests that it can occur when more than one ounce of ethanol is consumed per day. One cannot assume, however, that smaller amounts do not have any adverse effect on fetal brain growth and differentiation. Nor can one assume that such effects will not occur during the last trimester of pregnancy, when the fetus is generally considered to be least susceptible to environmental influence. In fact, one study indicated that pregnant women who drank heavily during the first two trimesters but were able to abstain or significantly reduce their alcohol consumption prior to the third trimester, produced offspring with no significant growth retardation (Rosett & Weiner, 1985). In contrast, more than a third of the neonates of mothers who drank heavily throughout pregnancy exhibited growth retardation. These findings suggest not only that damage can occur in the last trimester, but also that much of the damage that may occur during the first two trimesters may be reduced if drinking stops prior to the third trimester. Very little research has been done on pregnant women to determine the effects of binge drinking on fetuses. However, drinking seven drinks once a week is more likely to induce fetal abnormalities than having one or two drinks on a daily basis.

Barbiturates and Other Sedative-Hypnotics

Barbiturates are rapidly becoming the dinosaurs of drugs; they enjoyed a long period of use as sedative and hypnotic agents, but aside from a few specialized uses today, they have been displaced by the benzodiazepines. Furthermore, these and other drugs in the sedative-hypnotic class have effects so similar to alcohol's effects (Harvey, 1985) that little further discussion of them is needed, except to note that long-term alcohol exposure probably has more toxic physiological consequences (see earlier discussion on alcohol's unique characteristics and chronic effects of alcoholism). Since the mid-1800s, when the first barbiturate was derived (it is believed that the name came about either because the urine of a girl named Barbara was used to derive the compound or because the compound was synthesized on Saint Barbara's Day), more than 2,000 compounds with the same basic structure have been developed. Sedative-hypnotic compounds without the barbiturate structure, such as methaqualone and glutethimide, have been synthesized, but their actions are essentially indistinguishable from those of the barbiturates (Harvey, 1985).

In 1903, Barbitone became the first of these compounds to be used clinically. Since that time, these substances have been used as general anesthetics for surgery, as treatments for anxiety-related symptoms, as sleep aids, and as anticonvulsants. Barbiturates differ from each other primarily in terms of pharmacokinetics, which determines how quickly the drugs act, their intensity of action, and their duration of action. All three of these properties are tied together. The differences in these properties are a major factor in determining what these drugs are used for. Representative barbiturates are thiopental, a fast-acting, ultrashort-duration (approximately 15 minutes) drug used primarily as an anesthetic; secobarbital, a short-duration (approximately 1½ hours) drug used as a sleep inducer; pentobarbital and amobarbital, short- to intermediate-duration (approximately 4 hours) drugs used either for their sedative or sleep-inducing qualities; and phenobarbital, a relatively long-acting (approximately 6 hours) drug used as a sedative or an anticonvulsant.

The medical uses for these drugs have declined considerably over the past 20 years, primarily because of the development of newer compounds with less toxicity or dependence liability (such as the benzodiazepines, which will be discussed shortly) (Harvey, 1985). The primary advantage of the barbiturates at present is their cost. They are no longer under patent, and thus they are very inexpensive.

Despite lacking the barbiturate molecular structure, the substitute sedative-hypnotics mentioned earlier in this chapter have no properties, desirable or undesirable, that distinguish them from the barbiturates. In fact, at least one of these compounds—Quaalude (methaqualone)—was eventually withdrawn from the market because of its almost purely recreational use and abuse potential.

Barbiturates (and the nonbarbiturate alternatives) tend to decrease the excitability of neurons throughout the nervous system (Harvey, 1985). Although barbiturates depolarize some neurons, their predominant action throughout the nervous system is to hyperpolarize neurons. The inhibitory influence of barbiturates has been postulated to be due to their ability to enhance GABA's activity at the $GABA_A$-type receptor, which results in the opening of Cl⁻ channels, allowing Cl⁻ to flow into neurons and hyperpolarizing them. The primary action of barbiturates appears to be one of prolonging the duration that these channels remain open (Cooper et al., 1991). The inhibitory effects of barbiturates may also be due to increases in potassium (K^+) conductance (that is, the flow of K^+ inside neurons to the outside) (O'Beirne et al., 1986). Accompanying these activities is an increase in the levels of most neurotransmitters, in all likelihood because of their decreased utilization. The rate of oxygen consumption and cerebral glucose metabolism in all areas of the brain is reduced with these drugs (Hibbard et al., 1987).

A wide variety of behaviors, perceptual processes, and mental activities are affected by even the low doses of these drugs that are used for their calming and sedating effects. As mentioned previously, these actions are almost indistinguishable from those of alcohol. Although they are all used for enhancing or inducing sleep, the pattern of sleep induced is not really what one would consider normal. In general, during an eight-hour night of sleep, we go through several stages of sleep. These stages differ with respect to how easy it is to wake the person, how physiologically aroused the body is, the mental content, the types of brain waves (EEG) produced, and the person's eye movements. All stages have been presumed to have some functional significance, but there is no consensus as to what specific functions they have. Most nonbenzodiazepine sedative-hypnotics tend to prolong the deeper stages of sleep and reduce the stage known as REM (rapid eye movement) (Harvey, 1985). REM is the stage in which vivid dreams are most common. However, the ability to suppress REM sleep is not restricted to the sedative-hypnotics. This characteristic has been noted to occur with many other types of drugs as well, including psychostimulants and marijuana.

The mechanisms for inducing tolerance to alcohol apply to the barbiturates, although the latter appear to have a greater effect than alcohol on the drug-metabolizing enzymes of the liver (increasing their levels up to five times their normal level) (Harvey, 1985). As indicated earlier, cross-tolerance occurs with all of these substances, and the psychological and physical dependence associated with them is quite similar. The faster-acting compounds, which also have more intense effects and shorter durations, are more likely to be abused, and the abstinence syndrome associated with them is likely to be more intense, but less protracted, than that associated with the longer-acting compounds.

Anxiolytics

Anxiolytics, often referred to as antianxiety drugs or minor tranquilizers (so-called because of their use in minor cases of pathology), have properties very similar to those just described for the sedative-hypnotics. For example, they are effective anticonvulsants and muscle relaxants, they reduce a variety of aggressive tendencies, and they decrease anxiety. However, the actions of these drugs were hypothesized to be more specific than barbiturates and similar compounds in affecting the limbic system (which modulates emotionality, fear, aggression, sexuality, motivation, and pleasure) at doses that do not affect the reticular activating system (involved in maintaining a high level of consciousness and awareness) or the cerebral cortex (involved in higher mental processes like thinking and problem solving).

The first of these compounds that was purported to have these properties was meprobamate (Miltown). However, it did not quite live up to its reputation in subsequent clinical tests and was not found to be significantly different from earlier sedative-hypnotic compounds. A few years later, the first benzodiazepine, chlordiazepoxide (Librium), was developed, and it is this class of drugs that has essentially taken over as the prototypic anxiolytic. Other benzodiazepines that are most commonly prescribed for the treatment of anxiety are diazepam (Valium), oxazepam (Serax), clorazepate (Tranxene), lorazepam (Ativan), prazepam (Centrax), alprazolam (Xanax), and halazepam (Paxipam). For many years the Valium brand of diazepam was the most popular drug of this group, but Xanax has replaced it as the most commonly prescribed anxiolytic, probably because of growing fears of addiction with Valium, competition from generic forms of diazepam, and limited evidence that Xanax may possess somewhat better antidepressant, antipanic, and antiphobic effects (DeVane et al., 1991).

There are a number of differences between the benzodiazepine anxiolytics and earlier compounds (including meprobamate) used in the treatment of anxiety-related disorders. The most striking difference is their high therapeutic index (Harvey, 1985). Very few deaths are attributable to overdoses of these drugs by themselves, although they have been involved in a number of deaths when combined with other sedative-like drugs, because of their additive effects. Their high therapeutic index is probably due to their specific ability to enhance the activity of a normally endogenous inhibitory neurotransmitter (GABA), as opposed to the more generalized neuronal suppressive effects of other sedative-hypnotic drugs. This may also account for why benzodiazepines have minimal general anesthetic effects except at very high doses. Another advantage is that they have minimal effects on the drug-metabolizing enzymes of the liver, and therefore do not enhance the hepatic metabolism of themselves or other drugs.

Part of the more selective action of the benzodiazepines may be due to the fact that there are specific receptors for them, located in the neuronal cell membranes, which mediate their action in the CNS. These benzodiazepine receptors seem to be highly specific for benzodiazepine agonists and antagonists (the latter appear to induce the symptoms of anxiety) and some nonbenzodiazepine compounds with similar psychoactive properties. The highest concentrations of these receptors are found in the cerebral cortex, limbic structures, and the cerebellum. Although the function of these receptors is unclear, the action of benzodiazepines at these receptors has been suggested to be one of facilitating the activity of GABA, which is predominately one of enhancing the flow of Cl^- ions into neurons and hyperpolarizing them (Cooper et al., 1991).

Benzodiazepines are indirect GABA agonists, as they do not bind directly to GABA receptors, but appear to occupy receptors that enhance the activity of GABA at $GABA_A$ receptors (Zorumski & Isenberg, 1991). As a result, the degree of effect of benzodiazepines depends on the concentration of GABA; that is, they produce marked effects at low GABA concentrations and minimal effects when high GABA concentrations are present. The lack of effect on maximal GABA responses may, in part, account for the lower toxicity of benzodiazepines compared with barbiturates in cases of overdose. Some of the endogenous ligands for these "benzodiazepine" receptors, termed DBIs for diazepam-binding inhibitors, have recently been identified (Barbaccia et al., 1988). Some of these may function to exert a natural anxiolytic action, whereas others have been shown to induce anxiety reactions (which presumably may have been adaptive in certain situations at some point in evolution).

The action and thus the effects of benzodiazepines can be blocked completely with flumazenil (Mazicon, a drug currently being tested for clinical use in the United States). Flumazenil acts by competitively displacing benzodiazepines from their specific binding sites. In addition to its valuable use in locating and identifying specific benzodiazepine receptor sites, flumazenil has been used to rapidly reverse the effects of benzodiazepines used in surgical procedures, as an antidote in cases of benzodiazepine poisoning, and to reverse benzodiazepine comas (Ghoneim et al., 1989).

Benzodiazepine Efficacy

The benzodiazepines are effective in reducing anxiety-related symptoms in approximately 70–80% of the persons with these symptoms. Their clinical efficacy must be evaluated against the fact that these symptoms vary considerably across time, and remission of symptoms with a placebo occurs in approximately 25–30% of patients. Perhaps for this reason, physicians who believe in the efficacy of these drugs seem to have greater success with their patients than physicians who do not believe in their efficacy (Leavitt, 1982). The drug's effectiveness may also depend upon its effects on the patients' other defenses for combatting anxiety or behaviors they typically find useful to them. For instance, a professional golfer who takes a benzodiazepine to deal with tournament anxiety may actually play worse, and subsequently feel worse, because the drug disrupts motor abilities. Persons who are least likely to benefit from anxiolytic therapy are those with chronic dissatisfaction or insecurity, and those with character disorders, such as an antisocial personality. Such individuals are more likely to escalate their dosage, engage in impulsive overdosing, and succumb to physical dependence.

Many of the benzodiazepines are good anxiolytics because they are absorbed relatively slowly when given orally, with peak plasma levels occurring after several hours. This allows them to be taken only once or twice a day and induces a smooth, long-lasting effect. Diazepam is rapidly absorbed and reaches peak plasma levels in about an hour, which may account for its popularity both in clinical practice and on the streets. Most of the benzodiazepines are converted into active metabolites, which may partially account for the long duration of their action (Harvey, 1985). Their duration of action may be up to three or four times longer in premature neonates and the elderly than in young adults and children (Kerns, 1986).

Benzodiazepines that are highly lipid-soluble and do not form active metabolites may be useful in treating sleep disorders, because they have a fast onset of action but do not interfere with the next day's activities. However, aside from pharmacokinetic differences, in general there is no evidence that one benzodiazepine is more effective than another or that benzodiazepines labeled as hypnotics are more effective for sleep or less effective for daytime anxiety (Dubovsky, 1990).

As is the case with other drugs with sedative-hypnotic properties, tolerance develops to some of the pharmacological actions of benzodiazepines (File, 1985), and cross-tolerance may occur. However, the rate of tolerance may be slow (for example, to the anxiolytic effects), fast (for example, to sedative and anticonvulsant actions), or nonexistent (as in stimulant-type actions). The tolerance to benzodiazepines does not appear to be critically dependent upon altered metabolism, or Pavlovian or instrumental conditioning processes (Griffiths & Goudie, 1987). As discussed shortly, alterations in the GABA receptor complex may be responsible for some degree of tolerance.

Benzodiazepines have moderate psychological dependence liability. For instance, monkeys may self-administer them but not to the degree to which they self-administer cocaine (Johanson, 1987). Physical dependence may also occur when doses considerably above therapeutic levels are administered. The severity of withdrawal is inversely related to the plasma half-life of the benzodiazepine (DeVane et al., 1991). However, since many benzodiazepines, and their active metabolites, accumulate and persist in the body for several days, withdrawal symptoms after chronic use may not appear for a week or so after abrupt discontinuation of these drugs, and the withdrawal symptoms are generally less intense than those occurring with other sedative-hypnotics. Furthermore, high doses must be given for a considerable length of time before marked withdrawal symptoms (qualitatively similar to those occurring with other sedative-hypnotic agents) develop.

As might be expected, chronic exposure to benzodiazepines is associated with progressive development of GABA receptor down-regulation and desensitization, which is concomitant with the development of tolerance as well as withdrawal symptoms upon discontinuation of these drugs (Zorumski & Isenberg, 1991). Withdrawal following chronic benzodiazepine exposure can also be triggered by the administration of flumazenil (Lukas & Griffiths, 1982). However, both tolerance and dependence can be prevented if flumazenil is given periodically along with the benzodiazepine (Gallager et al., 1986).

The toxic reactions and side effects of benzodiazepines are similar to those of the sedative-hypnotics. In some cases, a paradoxical increase in hostility and irritability, and even anxiety, as well as vivid or disturbing dreams, may accompany benzodiazepine use (Baldessarini, 1985). Confusional states in the elderly are commonly induced with these and other sedative compounds, and these states may be incorrectly attributed to senility. Other potential side effects of these drugs include skin rashes, nausea, headaches, vertigo, light-headedness, sexual impotence, lowered white cell counts, and menstrual irregularities.

Few reasonable clinicians would take the position that anxiety-related symptoms should be treated solely with drugs or solely with psychotherapy. It is difficult to compare efficacy rates between pharmacotherapy and psychotherapy, since there are so many factors determining the efficacy of drugs by themselves and so many different types of psychotherapy. Both seem to be in the same efficacy range in comparison to a placebo; that is, the average treated person is better off than 75% of placebo-treated patients (Smith & Glass, 1977). There is no consensus about combining anxiolytics with psychotherapy. Many clinicians feel that it is impossible to do successful psychotherapy (that is, behavioral, cognitive, or interpersonal therapy) in the presence of drug therapy. They believe the presence of discomfort is a motivating force for psychotherapy and that if the drug lessens the discomfort, patients will avoid dealing with the forces that are making them uncomfortable in the first place. Other clinicians feel that anxiolytics may be useful adjuncts to psychotherapy—if for no other reason than that if one treatment does not work the other might.

Sedative-Hypnotics and Insomnia

In doses somewhat higher than those needed to sedate, the sedative-hypnotics induce sleep. Until recently, barbiturates were the most common treatment for insomnia. (This sleep disorder involves [1] the real or perceived inability to get to sleep or to stay asleep at night, resulting in subjective feelings of fatigue, [2] the chronic inability to maintain the amount and quality of sleep necessary for efficient daytime functioning, and [3] complaints of poor sleep, unrefreshing sleep, and sleep punctuated by abnormal restlessness.) However, the use of barbiturates for this purpose has declined primarily because they are being supplanted by somewhat safer drugs in the benzodiazepine class. It has long been recognized that the barbiturate sedative-hypnotics have numerous liabilities. Among these are their relatively low therapeutic index, their strong tendency to suppress REM sleep, their high psychological dependence potential, and their potentially lethal withdrawal effects when physical dependence develops. Furthermore, there is a relatively fast tolerance development to their sleep-inducing effects. While the functions of REM sleep and the consequences of suppressing it are still being debated, it is clear that, once the suppressing factors have been removed, REM activity increases dramatically for a few days and the dream content tends to be very bizarre and emotionally upsetting (Wallace & Fisher, 1991).

Because of these properties, more and more cases of insomnia are being treated with drugs in the benzodiazepine class, such as flurazepam (Dalmane), which have considerably higher therapeutic indexes, have minimal effects on REM sleep, have less psychological dependence potential, and are less likely to induce severe physical dependence and withdrawal effects. However, benzodiazepines do have characteristics that make them less than ideal treatments for insomnia. They can raise the arousal threshold to such an extent that outside noises that should awaken the person, such as a smoke alarm, do not do so (Johnson, Spinweber, Webb, & Muzet, 1987). Also, there is evidence that benzodiazepines disrupt the deeper stages of sleep (stages 3 and 4) (Harvey, 1985), an effect which may prove to be just as significant as REM inhibition. On the other hand, this may be a factor in the efficacy of benzodiazepines in the treatment of sleepwalking and night terrors (the latter involving a sudden and intense arousal from slow-wave, deep sleep, accompanied by sharp body movements, a rise in heart rate and respiration, mental confusion, and extreme fright), which are most commonly observed to occur during the deeper stages of sleep (Rall, 1990).

Flurazepam and its several active metabolites tend to accumulate in the body over several days of use. This accumulation can produce daytime aftereffects such as lethargy and decreased coordination (also possible with the sedative-hypnotics). A more recently developed drug in this class, temazepam (Restoril), does not appear to have detrimental effects on next-day performance in psychomotor activities. This advantage is primarily due to its having no active metabolites. On the other hand, shorter-acting drugs, like temazepam and triazolam (Halcion), are more likely to induce early-morning insomnia (an increase in wakefulness during the final hours of drug nights), similar to rebound insomnia that occurs after withdrawal from the drug (Kales, Soldatos, Bixler, & Kales, 1983). In fact, recent reports on Halcion's side effects—rebound insomnia, daytime nervousness, panic attacks, and amnesia—have led some experts to suggest that it be removed from the market. Although it is still available for clinical use, prescriptions for it declined considerably from 1988 to 1990.

All of the drugs used in the treatment of insomnia have a number of problems in common. They are all synergistic with alcohol and other CNS depressants; their combination with alcohol or other CNS depressants is one of the major causes of "overdose" deaths. In the elderly, who traditionally complain and suffer from insomnia, the diminished alertness that can come about with the use of these drugs can be confused with senility or dementia. The fact that these drugs do effectively induce sleep may prevent a patient from dealing with the problems causing insomnia. Finally, one must question the use of a potentially hazardous drug for the treatment of a disorder that is not particularly disruptive or hazardous to one's health. The fact is, in many cases, complaints of insomnia are exaggerated, and without knowing the purpose of sleep, it is difficult to determine how much sleep one should get and what represents normality or insomnia.

Buspirone

After 20 years and umpteen different variations on the basic benzodiazepine molecule (resulting in numerous patented drugs with the same properties), pharmacologists have finally synthesized a novel anxiolytic agent unrelated to the benzodiazepines and other sedative-hypnotics in structure and pharmacological profile. The drug is buspirone (BuSpar). As is typical in this field, the drug was originally developed for something other than what it may actually be most useful for. Initially, it looked like it might have antipsychotic properties. However, extensive clinical studies have shown buspirone to be comparable to the benzodiazepines diazepam and clorazepate in the treatment of anxiety (Eison & Temple, 1986; Goa & Ward, 1986). It is also effective in patients with mixed anxiety and depression. Unlike the benzodiazepines, buspirone (1) lacks hypnotic, anticonvulsant, and muscle-relaxant properties; (2) takes one or two weeks of daily treatment before the onset of its anxiolytic effects is noted; (3) is much less likely to induce drowsiness and fatigue; (4) does not impair psychomotor or cognitive function; (5) has minimal potential for abuse and dependence (in fact, it may have dysphoric properties in moderate doses); (6) has no synergistic effect with alcohol; (7) lacks affinity for the benzodiazepine receptor and does not appear to act via GABA mechanisms; and (8) is not cross-tolerant with benzodiazepines and does not help reduce benzodiazepine withdrawal (Lader & Olajide, 1987).

Although its biochemical and electrophysiological properties have not been sufficiently delineated, buspirone appears to affect monoaminergic activity differently than the benzodiazepines do. It suppresses serotonergic activity, primarily because it is a partial agonist at somatodendritic serotonin autoreceptors (termed $5HT_{1A}$ receptors) (Frazer et al., 1990), while enhancing dopaminergic and noradrenergic cell firing. Benzodiazepines tend to suppress all three type of cells (Davis & Gelder, 1991). However, buspirone's proposed mechanism of action regarding its anxiolytic properties is one of down-regulating $5HT_{1A}$ and $5HT_2$ receptors, which may explain why chronic exposure is needed before its benefits are evidenced (Charney et al., 1990).

Buspirone's unique properties have led to its being labeled as "anxioselective." It appears that it will be most useful in anxious patients for whom daytime alertness is particularly important. However, for patients who would benefit from a fast onset of action, or sedative and muscle-relaxant effects, the benzodiazepines would be preferred. Also, because there is no cross-tolerance with benzodiazepines, patients who are switched immediately from a benzodiazepine to buspirone may perceive the drug as ineffective. In fact, in patients who have been on a benzodiazepine for a long time and are then switched to buspirone, withdrawal symptoms may occur. These may be misinterpreted by the patients as an indication of the drug's ineffectiveness, or as side effects.

Overall, buspirone appears to be a fascinating new drug with promising potential. More recent studies with buspirone and other structurally similar $5HT_{1A}$ partial agonists (e.g., gepirone and ipsapirone) have indicated that this class of drug may also be useful in the treatment of clinical depression (Rickels et al., 1990; Heller et al., 1990). Because gepirone and ipsapirone, unlike buspirone, have low affinity for DA receptors, the $5HT_{1A}$ agonist properties of these drugs appear to mediate their antidepressant effects.

Other Novel Antianxiety Drugs

A number of anxiolytics are under study that appear to possess more specific therapeutic actions and fewer side effects than the drugs discussed in the preceding sections. Adinazolam is a type of benzodiazepine that appears to have anxiolytic, antidepressant, and antipanic properties. Nonbenzodiazepines—alpidem and zolpidem (termed imidazopyridines)—have been developed that have selective affinity for limbic but not cortical or spinal benzodiazepine receptors (Dubovsky, 1990). As a result, sedation, muscle relaxation, cognitive or psychomotor impairment, tolerance, and physical dependence are not likely to occur.

Alpidem is as potent an anxiolytic as the benzodiazepines, but improvement may continue for a longer period of time. Zolpidem has sleep-inducing properties but does not appear to disturb sleep stages or produce daytime effects.

Inhalants: Anesthetic Gases and Solvents

Inhalants consist of a wide variety of gases (ether, halothane, nitrous oxide, chloroform) and industrial solvents (e.g., toluene, a component of some glues) that have sedative-hypnotic properties. Some of these are used as general anesthetics to put patients to sleep before surgery. Others are used for their intoxicating and euphoric properties. Although these substances comprise a rather heterogeneous group of drugs, most of them are believed to work indiscriminatively by dissolving in neuronal membranes to somehow modify neuronal ion channel activity, because their potency is highly correlated with their lipid-solubility. However, some anesthetic gases, such as isoflurane, appear to act by binding directly to specific proteins in the CNS, because different isomers exert stereospecific effects on neuronal ion channels (Franks & Lieb, 1991). Whatever the mechanism of action, high doses of most of these substances decrease neuronal activities; at low doses they may increase some types of neuronal activity, most likely as a result of disinhibition (Jaffe, 1990).

Because of the heterogeneity of actions and because few of the many compounds of this nature have been systematically studied, little is known about their intoxicating properties. Some of them have been shown to have addictive qualities; for example, animals will self-administer nitrous oxide, chloroform, and toluene (Jaffe, 1990). Tolerance occurs with those substances that have been tested, but cross-tolerance may occur between some of these but not others. Fatalities have been noted to occur with their use, most commonly resulting from cardiac arrythmias or insufficient oxygen to the brain. CNS atrophy and renal damage have been associated with chronic use of many of these substances—for example, hexane and toluene (Jaffe, 1990).

Bibliography

Alden, L. E. (1988). Behavioral self-management controlled-drinking strategies in a context of secondary prevention. *Journal of Consulting and Clinical Psychology, 56*, 280–286.

Aronow, L. (1980). *Alcoholism, alcohol abuse, and related problems: Opportunities for research.* Washington, DC: National Academy Press.

Arria, A. M., Tarter, R. E., Starzl, T. F., & Van Thiel, D. H. (1991). Improvement in cognitive functioning of alcoholics following orthotopic liver transplantation. *Alcoholism: Clinical and Experimental Research, 15,* 956–962.

Baldessarini, R. J. (1985). *Chemotherapy and psychiatry.* Cambridge, MA: Harvard University Press.

Barbaccia, M. L., Costa, E., & Guidotti, A. (1988). Endogenous ligands for high-affinity recognition sites of psychotropic drugs. *Annual Review of Pharmacology and Toxicology, 28,* 451–476.

Barnes, D. M. (1988). Drugs: Running the numbers. *Science, 240,* 1729–1731.

Begleiter, H., Porjesz, B., Bihari, B., & Kissin, B. (1984). Event-related brain potentials in boys at risk for alcoholism. *Science, 225,* 1493–1495.

Brecher, E. M. (Ed.). (1972). *Licit and illicit drugs.* Boston: Little, Brown.

Britton, K. T., Ehlers, C. L., & Koob, G. F. (1988). Is ethanol antagonist Ro15–4513 selective for ethanol? *Science, 239,* 648–649.

Brubaker, R. G., Prue, D. M., & Rychtarik, R. G. (1987). Determinants of disulfiram acceptance among alcohol patients: A test of the theory of reasoned action. *Addictive Behaviors, 12,* 43–51.

Cadoret, R. J., Troughton, E., & O'Gorman, T. W. (1987). Genetic and environmental factors in alcohol abuse and antisocial personality. *Journal of Studies on Alcohol, 48,* 1–8.

Carlen, P. L., Holgate, R. C., Wortzman, G., & Wilkinson, D. A. (1978). Reversible cerebral atrophy in recently abstinent chronic alcoholics measured by computed tomography scans. *Science, 200,* 1076–1078.

Charney, D. S., Krystal, J. H., Delgado, P. L., & Heninger, G. R. (1990). Serotonin-specific drugs for anxiety and depressive disorders. *Annual Review of Medicine, 41,* 437–446.

Chin, J. H., & Goldstein, D. B. (1977). Drug tolerance in biomembranes: A spin label study of the effects of ethanol. *Science, 196,* 684-685.

Cicero, T. J. (1978). Tolerance to and physical dependence on alcohol: Behavioral and neurobiological mechanisms. In M. A. Lipton, A. DiMascio, & K. F. Killman (Eds.), *Psychopharmacology* (pp. 1603–1618). New York: Raven Press.

Clarren, S. K., & Smith, D. W. (1978). The fetal alcohol syndrome. *New England Journal of Medicine, 298,* 1063–1067.

Cloninger, C. R. (1987). Neurogenetic adaptive mechanisms in alcoholism. *Science, 236,* 410–416.

Cooper, J. R., Bloom, F. E., & Roth, R. H. (1991). *The biochemical basis of neuropharmacology,* 6th ed. New York: Oxford University Press.

Critchlow, B. (1986). The powers of John Barleycorn: Beliefs about the effects of alcohol on social behavior. *American Psychologist, 41,* 751–763.

Crowell, C. R., Hinson, R. E., & Siegel, S. (1981). The role of conditional drug responses in tolerance to hypothermic effects of ethanol. *Psychopharmacology, 73,* 51–54.

Cutter, H. S. G., O'Farrell, T. J., Whitehouse, J., & Dentch, G. M. (1986). Pain changes among men from before to after drinking: Effects of expectancy set and dose manipulations with alcohol and tonic as mediated by prior experience with alcohol. *International Journal of the Addictions, 21,* 937–945.

Davis, J. D., & Gelder, M. (1991). Long-term management of anxiety states. *International Review of Psychiatry, 3,* 5–17.

DeVane, L., Ware, M. R., & Lydiard, R. B., (1991). Pharmacokinetics, pharmacodynamics, and treatment issues of benzodiazepines: Alprazolam, adinazolam, and clonazepam. *Psychopharmacology Bulletin, 27,* 463–473.

DiPadova, C., Worner, T. M., Julkunen, R.J.K., & Lieber, C. S. (1987). Effects of fasting and chronic alcohol consumption on the first-pass metabolism of ethanol. *Gastroenterology, 92,* 1169–1173.

Dorus, W., Ostrow, D. G., Anton, R., et al. (1989). Lithium treatment of depressed and nondepressed alcoholics. *Journal of the American Medical Association, 262,* 1646–1652.

Dubovsky, S. L. (1990). Generalized anxiety disorder: New concepts and psychopharmacologic therapies. *Journal of Clinical Psychiatry, 51* (suppl.), 3–10.

Eison, A. S., & Temple, D. L. (1986). Buspirone: Review of its pharmacology and current perspectives on its mechanism of action. *American Journal of Medicine, 80,* 1–9.

Elal-Lawrence, G., Slade, P. D., & Dewey, M. E. (1987). Treatment and follow-up variables discriminating abstainers, controlled drinkers and relapsers. *Journal of Studies on Alcohol, 48,* 39–46.

Ellis, R. J., & Oscar-Berman, M. (1989). Alcoholism, aging, and functional cerebral asymmetries. *Psychological Bulletin, 106,* 128–147.

File, S. E. (1985). Tolerance to the behavioural actions of benzodiazepines. *Neuroscience and Biobehavioral Reviews, 9,* 113–121.

Fingarette, H. (1988). *Heavy drinking: The myth of alcoholism as a disease.* Berkeley: University of California Press.

Franks, N. P., & Lieb, W. R. (1991). Stereospecific effects of inhalational general anesthetic optical isomers on nerve ion channels. *Science, 254,* 427–430.

Frazer, A., Maayani, S., & Wolfe, B. B. (1990). Subtypes of receptors for serotonin. *Annual Review of Pharmacology and Toxicology, 30,* 307–348.

Fuller, R. K., Branchey, L., Brightwell, D. R., et al. (1986). Disulfiram treatment of alcoholism: A Veterans Administration cooperative study. *Journal of the American Medical Association, 256,* 1449–1455.

Gallager, D. W., Heninger, K., & Heninger, G. (1986). Periodic benzodiazepine antagonist administration prevents benzodiazepine withdrawal symptoms in primates. *European Journal of Pharmacology, 132,* 31–38.

Ghoneim, M., Dembo, J., & Block, R. (1989). Time course of antagonism of sedative and amnesic effects of diazepam by flumazenil. *Anesthesiology, 70,* 899–904.

Goa, K. L., & Ward, A. (1986). Buspirone: A preliminary review of its pharmacological properties and therapeutic efficacy as an anxiolytic. *Drugs, 32,* 114–129.

Golden, C. J., Graber, B., Blose, I., Berg, R., Coffman, J., & Bloch, S. (1981). Difference in brain densities between chronic alcoholic and normal control patients. *Science, 211,* 508–510.

Griffiths, J. W., & Goudie, A. J. (1987). Analysis of the role of behavioural factors in the development of tolerance to the benzodiazepine midazolam. *Neuropharmacology, 26,* 201–209.

Guze, S. B., Cloninger, C. R., Martin, R., & Clayton, P. J. (1986). Alcoholism as a medical disorder. *Comprehensive Psychiatry, 27,* 501–510.

Harvey, S. C. (1985). Hypnotics and sedatives. In A. G. Gilman, L. S. Goodman, T. W. Rall, & F. Murad (Eds.). *The pharmacological basis of therapeutics* (pp. 339–371). New York: Macmillan.

Hashtroudi, S., Parker, E. S., Yablick, L., DeLisi, L. E., & Wyatt, R. J. (1981, November). *Generation is a better "antidote" for alcohol amnesia than semantic elaboration.* Paper presented at the meeting of the Psychonomic Society, Philadelphia.

Hasumura, Y., Tesckle, R., & Lieber, S. S. (1975). Acetaldehyde oxidation by hepatic mitochondria: Decrease after chronic ethanol consumption. *Science, 189,* 727–728.

Heilbrun, A. B., Cassidy, J. C., Diehl, M., Haas, M., & Heilbrun, M. R. (1986). Psychological vulnerability to alcoholism: Studies in internal scanning deficit. *British Journal of Medical Psychology, 59,* 237–244.

Heller, A. H., Beneke, M., Kuemmel, B., Spencer, D., & Kurtz, N. M. (1990). Ipsapirone: Evidence for efficacy in depression. *Psychopharmacology Bulletin, 26,* 219–222.

Hibbard, L. S., McGlone, J. S., Davis, D. W., & Hawkins, R. A. (1987). Three-dimensional representation and analysis of brain energy metabolism. *Science, 236,* 1641–1646.

Holden, C. (1980). Rand issues final alcoholism report. *Science, 207,* 855–856.

Holden, C. (1987). Is alcoholism treatment effective? *Science, 236,* 20–22.

Holden, C. (1991). Probing the complex genetics of alcoholism. *Science, 251,* 163–164.

Hull, J. G., & Bond, C. F. (1986). Social and behavioral consequences of alcohol consumption and expectancy: A meta-analysis. *Psychological Bulletin, 99,* 347–359.

Jaffe, J. (1990). Drug addiction and drug abuse. In A. G. Gilman, T. W. Rall, A. S. Nies, & P. Taylor (Eds.), *The pharmacological basis of therapeutics* (pp. 522–573). New York: Pergamon Press.

Johanson, C. E. (1987). Benzodiazepine self-administration in rhesus monkeys: Estazolam, flurazepam and lorazepam. *Pharmacology, Biochemistry, and Behavior, 26,* 521–526.

Johnson, L. C., Spinweber, C. L., Webb, S. C., & Muzet, A. G. (1987). Dose level effects of triazolam on sleep and response to a smoke detector alarm. *Psychopharmacology, 91,* 397–402.

Kales, A., Soldatos, C. R., Bixler, E. O., & Kales, J. D. (1983). Early morning insomnia with rapidly eliminated benzodiazepines. *Science, 220,* 95–97.

Keir, W. J. (1991). Inhibition of retinoic acid synthesis and its implications in fetal alcohol syndrome. *Alcoholism Clinical and Experimental Research, 15,* 560–564.

Kendler, K. S., Heath, A. C., Neale, M. C., Kessler, R. C., & Eaves, L. J. (1992). A population-based twin study of alcoholism in women. *Journal of the American Medical Association, 268,* 1877–1882.

Kerns, L. L. (1986). Treatment of mental disorders in pregnancy. *The Journal of Nervous and Mental Disease, 174,* 652–659.

Kolata, G. (1986). New drug counters alcohol intoxication. *Science, 234,* 1198–1200.

Kolata, G. (1988, May). Alcoholic genes or misbehavior? *Psychology Today, 22,* 34–37.

Lader, M., & Olajide, D. (1987). A comparison of buspirone and placebo in relieving benzodiazepine withdrawal symptoms. *Journal of Clinical Psychopharmacology, 7,* 11–15.

Laposata, E. E., & Lange, L. G. (1986). Presence of nonoxidative ethanol metabolism in human organs commonly damaged by ethanol abuse. *Science, 231,* 497–499.

Leavitt, F. (1982). *Drugs and behavior.* New York: John Wiley & Sons.

Lovinger, D. M., White, G., & Weight, F. F. (1989). Ethanol inhibits NMDA-activated ion current in hippocampal neurons. *Science, 243,* 1721–1724.

Lukas, S. E., & Griffiths, R. R. (1982). Precipitated withdrawal by a benzodiazepine receptor antagonist (Ro15–1788) after 7 days of diazepam. *Science, 217,* 1161–1163.

Marlatt, G. A., Baer, J. S., Donovan, D. M., & Kivlahan, D. R. (1988). Addictive behaviors: Etiology and treatment. *Annual Review of Psychology, 39,* 223–252.

Mazoit, J.-X., Sandouk, P., Zetlaoui, P., & Scherrmann, J.-M. (1987). Pharmacokinetics of unchanged morphine in normal and cirrhotic subjects. *Anesthetic Analgesics, 66,* 293–298.

McEntee, W. M., & Mair, R. G. (1978). Memory impairment in Korsakoff's psychosis: A correlation with brain noradrenergic activity. *Science, 202,* 905–907.

Mello, R. E. (1978). Alcoholism and the behavioral pharmacology of alcohol, 1967–1977. In M. A. Lipton, A. DiMascio, & K. F. Killman (Eds.), *Psychopharmacology* (pp. 1619–1638). New York: Raven Press.

Miczek, K. A., & Weerts, E. M. (1987). Seizures in drug-tested animals. *Science, 235,* 1127.

Miller, W. R., & Hester, R. K. (1986). Inpatient alcoholism treatment. *American Psychologist, 41,* 794–805.

Nelson, T. O., McSpadden, M., Fromme, K., & Marlatt, G. A. (1986). Effects of alcohol intoxication on metamemory and on retrieval from long-term memory. *Journal of Experimental Psychology: General, 115,* 247–254.

O'Beirne, M., Gurevich, N., & Carlen, P. L. (1986). Pentobarbital inhibits hippocampal neurons by increasing potassium conductance. *Canadian Journal of Physiological Pharmacology, 65,* 36–41.

Oscar-Berman, M. (1980). Neuropsychological consequences of long-term chronic alcoholism. *American Scientist, 68,* 410–419.

Peele, S. (1984). The cultural context of psychological approaches to alcoholism. Can we control the effects of alcohol? *American Psychologist, 39,* 1337–1351.

Pendery, M. L., Maltzman, I. M., & West, L. J. (1982). Controlled drinking by alcoholics? New findings and a reevaluation of a major affirmative study. *Science, 217,* 169–175.

Pezzarossa, A., Cervigni, C., Ghinelli, F., Molina, E., Gnudi, A. (1986). Glucose tolerance in chronic alcoholics after alcohol withdrawal: Effect of accompanying diet. *Metabolism, 35,* 984–988.

Pickens, R. W., Svikis, D. S., McGue, M., Lykken, D. T., Heston, L. L., & Clayton, P. J. (1991). Heterogeneity in the inheritance of alcoholism. *Archives of General Psychiatry, 48,* 19–28.

Pihl, R. O., & Zacchia, C. (1986). Alcohol and aggression: A test of the affect-arousal hypothesis. *Aggressive Behavior, 12,* 367–375.

Pohorecky, L. K. (1977). Biphasic action of ethanol. *Neuroscience and Biobehavioral Reviews, 1,* 231–240.

Pohorecky, L. K., Brick, J., & Carpenter, J. A. (1986). Assessment of the development of tolerance to ethanol using multiple measures. *Alcoholism: Clinical and Experimental Research, 10,* 616–622.

Quayle, D. (1983). American productivity: The devastating effect of alcoholism and drug abuse. *American Psychologist, 38,* 454–467.

Rall, T. W. (1990). Hypnotics and sedatives: Ethanol. In A. G. Gilman, T. W. Rall, A. S. Nies, & P. Taylor (Eds.), *The pharmacological basis of therapeutics* (pp. 345–382). New York: Pergamon Press.

Rao, G. A., Larkin, E. C., & Derr, R. F. (1986). Biologic effects of chronic ethanol consumption related to a deficient intake of carbohydrates. *Alcohol and Alcoholism, 21,* 369–373.

Reed, T. E., & Hanna, J. M. (1986). Between- and within-race variation in acute cardiovascular responses to alcohol: Evidence for genetic determination in normal males in three races. *Behavior Genetics, 16,* 585–598.

Rickels, K., Amsterdam, J., Clary, C., et al. (1990). Buspirone in depressed outpatients: A controlled study. *Psychopharmacology Bulletin, 26,* 163–168.

Riley, J. N., & Walker, D. W. (1978). Morphological alterations in hippocampus after long-term alcohol consumption in mice. *Science, 201,* 646–648.

Rimm, E. B., Giovannucci, E. L., Willett, W. C., et al. (1991). Prospective study of alcohol consumption and risk of coronary disease in men. *Lancet, 338,* 464–468.

Ritchie, J. M. (1985). The aliphatic alcohols. In A. G. Gilman, L. S. Goodman, T. W. Rall, & F. Murad (Eds.), *The pharmacological basis of therapeutics* (pp. 372–386). New York: Macmillan.

Robertson, I., Heather, N., Dzialdowski, A., Crawford, J., & Winton, M. (1986). A comparison of minimal versus intensive controlled drinking treatment interventions for problem drinkers. *British Journal of Clinical Psychology, 25,* 185–194.

Romach, M. K., & Sellers, E. M. (1991). Management of the alcohol withdrawal syndrome. *Annual Review of Medicine, 42,* 323–340.

Rosett, H. L., & Weiner, L. (1985). Alcohol and pregnancy: A clinical perspective. *Annual Review of Medicine, 36,* 73–80.

Ryan, C. (1982). Alcoholism and premature aging: A neuropsychological perspective. *Alcoholism: Clinical and Experimental Research, 6,* 79–96.

Schanne, F.A.X., Zucker, A. H., & Farber, J. L. (1981). Alcohol-dependent liver cell necrosis in vitro: A new model. *Science, 212,* 338–340.

Schuckit, M. A., & Gold, E. O. (1988). A simultaneous evaluation of multiple markers of ethanol/placebo challenges in sons of alcoholics and controls. *Archives of General Psychiatry, 45,* 211–216.

Schuckit, M. A., & Rayses, V. (1979). Ethanol ingestion: Differences in blood acetaldehyde concentrations in relatives of alcoholics and controls. *Science, 202,* 54–56.

Smith, M. L., & Glass, G. V. (1977). Meta-analysis of psychotherapy outcome studies. *American Psychologist, 32,* 752–760.

Sokol, R. J., Ager, J., Martier, S., et al. (1986). Significant determinants of susceptibility to alcohol terotogenicity. *Annals of the New York Academy of Sciences, 477,* 87–102.

Steinhausen, H. C., & Spohr, H.-L. (1986). Fetal alcohol syndrome. In B. B. Lahey, & A. E. Kazdin (Eds.), *Advances in clinical child psychology,* (Vol. 9, pp. 217–243). New York: Plenum Press.

Streissguth, A. P., Randels, S. P., & Smith, D. F. (1991). A test-retest study of intelligence in patients with fetal alcohol syndrome: Implications for care. *Journal of the American Academy of Child and Adolescent Psychiatry, 30,* 584–587.

Streissguth, A. P., Sampson, P. D., & Barr, H. M. (1989). Neurobehavioral dose-response effects of prenatal alcohol exposure in humans from infancy to adulthood. *Annals of the New York Academy of Sciences, 562*, 145–158.

Svanum, S., & Schladenhauffen, J. (1986). Lifetime and recent alcohol consumption among male alcoholics. *The Journal of Nervous and Mental Disease, 174*, 214–220.

Thurstin, A. H., Alfano, A. M., & Sherer, M. (1986). Pretreatment MMPI profiles of A.A. members and nonmembers. *Journal of Studies on Alcohol, 47*, 468–471.

Tollefson, G. D. (1989). Serotonin and alcohol: Interrelationships. *Psychopathology, 22* (suppl.), 37–48.

Turner, T. B., Bennett, V. L., & Hernandez, H. (1981). The beneficial side of moderate alcohol use. *Johns Hopkins Medical Journal, 148*, 53–63.

Vaillant, G. E., & Milofsky, E. S. (1982). The etiology of alcoholism. *American Psychologist, 37*, 494–503.

Van Thiel, D. H., Gavaler, J., & Lester, R. (1974). Ethanol inhibition of vitamin A metabolism in the testes: Possible mechanism for sterility in alcoholics. *Science, 186*, 941–942.

von Knorring, L., Oreland, L., & von Knorring, A.-L. (1987). Personality traits and platelet MAO activity in alcohol and drug abusing teenage boys. *Acta Psychiatrica Scandanavica, 75*, 307–314.

Walker, D. W., Barnes, D. E., Zornetzer, S. F., Hunter, B. E., & Kubanis, P. (1980). Neuronal loss in hippocampus induced by prolonged ethanol consumption in rats. *Science, 209*, 711–713.

Wallace, B., & Fisher, L. E. (1991). *Consciousness and behavior* (3rd ed.). Boston: Allyn & Bacon.

Walsh, D. D., Hingson, R. W., Merrigan, D. M., et al. (1991). A randomized trial of treatment options for alcohol-abusing workers. *New England Journal of Medicine, 325*, 775–782.

Watterlond, M. (1983, June). The telltale metabolism of alcoholics: A new interpretation of standard blood tests may lead to early diagnosis. *Science83*, 72–76.

Wenger, J. R., Tiffany, M., Bombardier, C., Nicholls, K., & Woods, S. C. (1981). Ethanol tolerance in the rat is learned. *Science, 213*, 575–576.

Wilson, B., Kolb, B., Odland, L., & Wishaw, I. Q. (1987). Alcohol, sex, age, and the hippocampus. *Psychobiology, 15*, 300–307.

Woods, J. H. (1978). Behavioral pharmacology of drug administration. In M. A. Lipton, A. DiMascio, & K. F. Killman (Eds.), *Psychopharmacology* (pp. 595–607). New York: Raven Press.

Zorumski, C. F., & Isenberg, K. E. (1991). Insights into the structure and function of GABA-benzodiazepine receptors: Ion channels and psychiatry. *American Journal of Psychiatry, 148*, 162–173.

Zucker, R. A., & Gomberg, E.S.L. (1986). Etiology of alcoholism reconsidered: The case for a biopsychosocial process. *American Psychologist, 41*, 783–792.

Chapter Nine

Psychostimulants

Another category of drugs that, for the most part, were originally derived for their clinical use but are now being used more extensively for recreational purposes, consists of the **psychostimulants**. This term is used because, in low to moderate doses, these drugs produce heightened mood (at its extreme it is described as euphoria), increase vigilance and alertness, and reduce fatigue and the tendency to sleep. Generally, signs of increased sympathetic nervous system activity, such as increased heart rate and blood pressure, are evidenced. As one might expect with such actions, the EEG frequency shifts to higher frequencies.

Other frequently used terms for these drugs are "behavioral stimulants" and "CNS stimulants"; however, these terms do not do justice to the actual common properties of these drugs. Although some behaviors may increase in some individuals with these drugs, others may dramatically decrease, depending on the dose, the frequency of the behavior typically observed without the drug, and the individual (Grilly, 1977; Tecce & Cole, 1974; Wender et al., 1981). Likewise, while some neurons become more excitable and increase their rate of firing, others dramatically reduce their rate of firing. Actually, none of the terms mentioned adequately describes the effects of these drugs if the drugs are used in large amounts acutely or moderate amounts chronically. Some of these effects will be dealt with shortly.

Within this category are several structurally different types of drugs (see Figure 9–1 for their basic molecular structures). By far, the most commonly used psychostimulant is caffeine, which belongs to the xanthine family. Nicotine is another popular drug with psychostimulant properties. The amphetamines, together with other structurally related drugs, comprise another popular class. In a class by itself (no pun intended) is the increasingly popular cocaine. Other classes of drugs that might fit in this category are the antidepressants, some

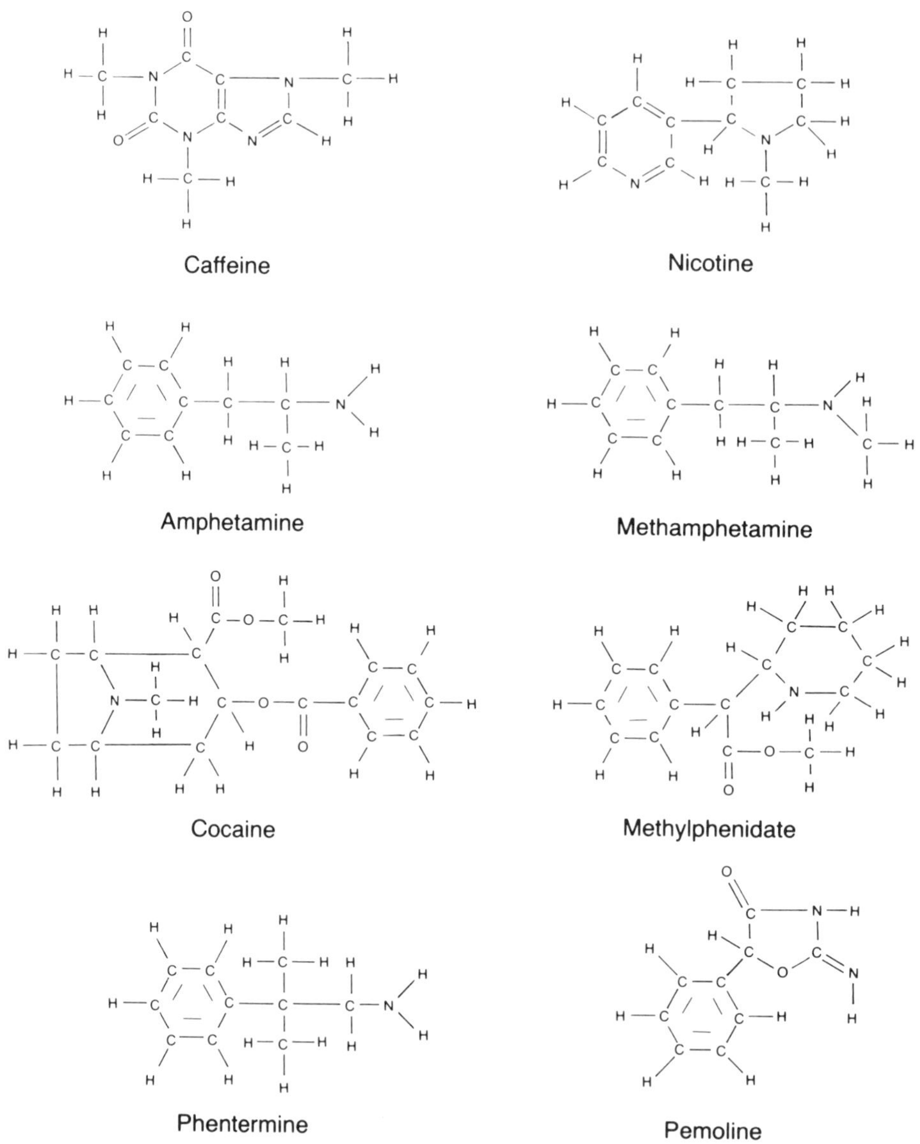

Caffeine

Nicotine

Amphetamine

Methamphetamine

Cocaine

Methylphenidate

Phentermine

Pemoline

Figure 9–1

Molecular structures of some representative psychostimulant drugs.

convulsants, and magnesium pemoline. However, the antidepressants enhance mood only in severely depressed individuals, not in normal individuals. The doses of the convulsants with psychostimulant properties are so close to being toxic that they are unlikely to be used in this capacity. Magnesium pemoline, which has been around for some 20 years, has not established its niche in either clinical or recreational spheres.

Caffeine

Caffeine is the most widely used behaviorally active drug in the world (Griffiths et al., 1986). Your morning cup of coffee, your soda pop at lunch, your afternoon cup of tea, and your chocolate sundae all contain this relatively mild psychostimulant (see Table 9–1). It is one of several substances referred to as methylxanthines. The typical adult in the United States consumes about 400 mg of caffeine a day, with coffee and tea consumption accounting for almost 90% of total caffeine intake (Weidner & Istvan, 1985). Based on typical patterns of use throughout the day and a plasma half-life of approximately 5 hours, peak caffeine plasma levels typically occur in the early evening (Benowitz, 1990). However, owing to variability in absorption, metabolization, and excretion, as well as the fact that numerous metabolites of caffeine are formed that are also psychoactive (e.g., theophylline, theobromine, and paraxanthine), it is difficult to determine the overall time course and impact of caffeine on an individual. It is important to note that cigarette smokers, who generally consume more coffee than nonsmokers, metabolize caffeine at an accelerated rate. Upon smoking cessation, caffeine plasma levels increase on average more than 200%, which could increase the person's "jitteriness" and be a contributing factor in tobacco withdrawal symptoms (Benowitz, 1990).

What makes caffeine or coffee so popular is still unclear. In intravenous drug self-administration experiments with animals, caffeine has been shown to have reinforcing effects in some cases but not in others. Likewise, with humans, the reinforcing effects of caffeine have been variable, and in some individuals caffeine has been found to induce dysphoric effects. The most recent evidence suggests that caffeine is rated as having the most desirable and pleasant reactions in heavy coffee drinkers, particularly after they have not had any coffee for several hours. Coffee abstainers are more likely to report unpleasant and undesirable reactions to caffeine. This finding suggests that many of the reinforcing effects of caffeine stem from its ability to terminate caffeine withdrawal (Griffiths et al., 1986).

The pharmacodynamics of caffeine are complex. The most important

Table 9–1

Caffeine in Beverages and Foods

	Caffeine (milligrams)
Coffee (5-ounce cup)	
Brewed, drip method	60–180
Brewed, percolator	40–170
Instant	30–120
Decaffeinated	2–5
Tea (5-ounce cup)	
Brewed	20–110
Instant	25–50
Cocoa (5-ounce cup)	2–20
Chocolate milk (8 ounces)	2–7
Chocolate (one ounce)	1–35
Soft drinks (12 ounces) (in which caffeine is listed as ingredient)	30–60

Note. From "The Latest Caffeine Scorecard" by C. Lecos, 1984, *Consumer's Research, 67,* 35–36.

mechanism of caffeine's stimulant effects is antagonism of central adenosine receptors (Benowitz, 1990). Since adenosine is a potent inhibitor of synaptic transmission of central and peripheral synapses, its antagonism by caffeine results in an increase in the firing of cortical neurons and the locus coeruleus (a major regulator of arousal and vigilance), and an increase in behavioral activity; at high doses it elicits convulsions (Benowitz, 1990). Some of caffeine's actions also seem to be mediated by the catecholamine norepinephrine, since caffeine has discriminable properties in common with more potent psychostimulants, particularly cocaine and methylphenidate (Holtzman, 1986, 1987). Also, caffeine-induced stimulation of locomotor activity in animals can be prevented with alpha-adrenergic-blocking drugs, or when catecholamine synthesis is inhibited prior to caffeine treatment.

The effects of caffeine vary considerably among individuals in terms of wakefulness, psychomotor coordination, mood alterations, and autonomic nervous system response (Lombardo, 1986). Two cups of coffee, which contains approximately 150 mg of caffeine (unless it is decaffeinated), has the mood-elevating and fatigue-relieving properties of threshold doses of amphetamine (approximately 2 to 5 mg). However, larger doses generally do not have more of a mood-elevating effect, although 7 to 10 cups of coffee may cause insomnia, restlessness, mild sensory disturbances, or muscle tenseness (collectively called caffeinism), or may precipitate anxiety or panic attacks in susceptible individuals (Charney, et al., 1985). Caffeine can raise blood pressure slightly, or it may have no effect. Similarly, heart rate changes are variable and, with some caffeine doses, may actually decrease. Increases in galvanic skin conductance level and reactivity are generally noted (Davidson & Smith, 1991). Thus the evidence suggests that caffeine may not increase all indexes of arousal nor change them in the same way in all persons (Zahn & Rapoport, 1987).

Persons ingesting caffeine or beverages containing caffeine usually experience less drowsiness and fatigue, and more rapid and clearer flow of thought (Zwyghuizen-Doorenbos et al., 1990). As little as 32 mg of caffeine has been shown to significantly improve auditory vigilance and visual reaction time (Leiberman et al., 1987). Caffeine can produce an increased capacity for both muscular work and sustained intellectual effort (Sawyer et al., 1982), but it can also disrupt arithmetic skills and task performance when delicate muscular coordination and accurate timing are required (Rall, 1985). Several studies on efficiency of information processing in humans have shown that the effects of caffeine are dependent upon dose, task demands, the subject's sex, and the subject's typical level of arousal (Anderson & Revelle, 1983; Erikson et al., 1985). Some studies have concluded that extroverts (or high impulsives) tend to show dose-dependent improvements in performance, whereas introverts (or low impulsives) show improvements with lower doses and decrements with higher doses (Eysenck, 1967; Gupta & Gupta, 1990). Others have shown either no change or decrements in information processing, depending on the sex of the subject and the task demands (Erikson et al., 1985). (The dose ranges of caffeine used in these studies were equivalent to zero to four cups of regular coffee.) Thus, other than the conclusion that the behavioral effects of caffeine are quite subtle, there does not appear to be a consensus as to whether or not caffeine improves information processing efficiency in general (Battig, 1991). It may all depend upon whether one is a heavy consumer of coffee in the first place.

It a common belief that caffeine can counteract the effects of sedative-hypnotic type drugs, but the empirical evidence for this belief is equivocal. The equivalent of 2–3 cups of coffee (250 mg caffeine) has been shown to significantly reduce next day benzodiazepine-induced drowsiness (Johnson, et al., 1990). Caffeine has also been shown to reduce the effects of alcohol on various types of complex reaction time. However, for most tasks—such as manual dexterity, balance, numerical reasoning, and verbal fluency—the deleterious effects of alcohol intoxication are not reduced by caffeine (Fudin & Nicastro, 1988). Thus an intoxicated driver after consuming a few cups of coffee might feel more alert—and perhaps notice an apparent reduction in drunkenness. But he or she will still be impaired in terms of the motor coordination and decision-making required for properly driving a motor vehicle.

Tolerance develops to many of the effects of caffeine, most likely due to up-regulation of adenosine receptors in the brain (Benowitz, 1990). Withdrawal symptoms are uncommon, except following heavy use (around 500 mg per day) (Sawyer et al., 1982). Headaches are the most common symptom. They may be due to a rebound effect from caffeine's normal vasoconstrictive properties. (Perhaps this effect explains why so many over-the-counter analgesic preparations combine caffeine with aspirin.) Caffeine withdrawal symptoms may also include increased fatigue, sleepiness, and laziness, and decreased vigor and alertness. A neonatal withdrawal syndrome, consisting of irritability, jitteriness, and vomiting, has been reported in infants born to mothers who consumed large amounts of caffeine during pregnancy (Benowitz, 1990).

Amphetamines and Related Drugs

In contrast to caffeine, amphetamines and structurally related drugs exert more potent and distinct emotional and cognitive effects, which may account for their popular recreational use and abuse potential. From the 1940s through the 1970s, these drugs were a major drug of abuse. Their use has declined somewhat since the 1970s because of governmental changes in their classification (at present they are Schedule II drugs), pressures on manufacturers to reduce the quantities produced, and pressures on physicians to reduce the types of clinical uses for them.

Amphetamine was initially synthesized in the late 1800s, but medical uses for it were not developed until the late 1920s. Although it is quite effective when administered orally, it was initially marketed in the form of inhalers for use in asthma treatment. It quickly gained popularity because of its potent CNS effects (Brecher, 1972). Shortly thereafter, amphetamine (marketed as Benzedrine in the United States) was discovered to be made up of two isomers, l- and d-amphetamine. The latter was found to be considerably more potent and was marketed as Dexedrine. A minor modification in the amphetamine molecule yielded the slightly more potent methamphetamine (Desoxyn, Methedrine). With the recognition of the potential psychopathological toxicity and dependence associated with the amphetamines, other compounds with very similar molecular structures were synthesized, including methylphenidate (Ritalin), pipradol (Meratran), phenmetrazine (Preludin), and phentermine (Ionamin). These amphetamine-related substances exert basically the same qualitative effects as the amphetamines do. (Some of these drugs are no longer on the market or the brand names they are marketed under have changed.)

Minor changes in the chemical structure of the basic amphetamine molecule can significantly alter the particular spectrum of its pharmacological and biochemical activities (Biel, 1970). Some changes may abolish both psychostimulant and appetite suppressant (anorexic) effects. Others may decrease only the anorexic effects, and others may decrease only the psychostimulant effects. Other changes profoundly enhance the MAO-inhibiting properties of the compound; for example, tranylcypromine (Parnate) is some 5,000 times more potent than amphetamine in terms of MAO inhibition. Other modifications result in some psychotomimetic compounds, such as DOM (dimethoxymethylamphetamine), that produce effects similar to those of mescaline, but possess considerably higher potency. Many of these compounds will be dealt with in later chapters.

Pharmacokinetics and Pharmacodynamics of Amphetamines

Amphetamines are relatively high in lipid-solubility and are very well absorbed when taken orally or inhaled as a vapor. Intravenous administration results in brain penetration within seconds. Although most amphetamines are not sufficiently volatile to vaporize when smoked, a new form of methamphetamine hydrochloride (called "ice" because of its transparent, sheetlike crystals) has been developed so that it can be inhaled through smoking. Inhalation allows it to produce a rapid onset of effect, similar to smoking cocaine, but as with other amphetamines its effects last much longer—on the order of several hours (Cho, 1990).

Although the amphetamines and related compounds bear a strong molecular resemblance to the catecholamines (norepinephrine and dopamine), little of their activity appears to be due to a direct agonist action at catecholamine receptors. Instead, they have neuropharmacological properties that enhance the level of catecholamines in the synaptic cleft, which then increases catecholamine receptor activation. Many of the acute effects of amphetamine can be reversed with antidopaminergic drugs, such as the antipsychotics chlorpromazine and haloperidol.

Amphetamine increases both the spontaneous leakage and the stimulated (action potential) release of catecholamines from axon terminals, inhibits their reuptake back into the terminals, and has a mild, temporary, inhibitory action on the enzyme MAO (which, you may recall, normally metabolizes the monoamines intraneuronally into inactive molecules) (Cole, 1978). Most of the catecholamines released appear to be from newly synthesized stores in the axon terminal—that is, outside the vesicles. Presumably, the other amphetamine-like substances have similar biochemical actions, although there appear to be minor differences in degree and type of action. Methylphenidate, for example, has much the same activity as amphetamine except that it seems to release primarily catecholamines that are stored in vesicles (Moore et al., 1977).

Although amphetamine and related psychostimulants (and cocaine) enhance catecholamine activity throughout the nervous system, which then results in a variety of effects on mood and behavior, most studies have indicated that the primary reward properties of these drugs are due to their ability to enhance dopaminergic activity in a part of the limbic system called the nucleus accumbens (Chu & Kelley, 1992).

The actions just described occur with acute drug exposure. However, with chronic drug exposure, some of these actions eventually result in the depletion of the catecholamines (Cole, 1978). This is presumably due to the enhanced rate of extraneuronal metabolization through COMT as well as reduced synthesis, which would be expected because of increased activity of the catecholamines at auto receptors. This process would account for the tolerance developed to amphetamine's behavioral and subjective effects (Rees et al., 1987). Because of the enhanced activity at postsynaptic receptors, there may also be a reduction in the sensitivity of these receptors. Neither of these actions can account for the curious phenomenon whereby chronic exposure to amphetamine can actually sensitize the organism to the psychosis-inducing properties of the drug, a phenomenon to be discussed more extensively later on. With sufficiently high doses of amphetamine, serotonin depletion may also occur and may be a factor in the development of amphetamine-induced psychosis (Segal, 1977).

Psychological Effects of Amphetamines

The specific behavioral effects of amphetamine and related compounds depend to a great extent on the task requirements, the normal frequency of the behavior, the dose, and individual characteristics. Although psychostimulants are commonly believed to have effects in hyperactive children that are different from those observed in normal children or adults, empirical evidence indicates that, other than the magnitude of observed effects, amphetamines produce qualitatively similar effects in all three groups (Rapoport et al., 1980). (For further discussion of this issue see Chapter 14.)

In terms of quality of performance on various tasks, the most striking beneficial effects are noted when the person is fatigued (Lombardo, 1986). Low to moderate doses tend to facilitate performance of tasks dependent on sustained attention (for instance, detecting infrequently occurring objects on radar screens) or those requiring quickness and strength (such as blocking and tackling in football, swimming, and track events) (Jaffe, 1990). High doses generally interfere with performance of these types of tasks. In tasks requiring smooth, accurate motions, low doses induce variable effects in individuals, in some cases enhancing, but in most cases interfering with, performance. In moderate to high doses, performance is hindered. Perhaps these task-drug interactions are the reason football players (at least linemen and linebackers) may be more prone to use these substances, whereas golfers and tennis players invariably avoid them.

Although amphetamine-related drugs often increase many kinds of activity, some kinds of behaviors, particularly those that occur frequently to begin with, are actually reduced by these drugs. Part of the reason for these differential effects is that not all behaviors can be increased simultaneously because one type of activity may compete with another (Grilly, 1977). Thus, for example, undifferentiated motor activity (hyperactivity) observed in many children with attention deficit disorder may be reduced with psychostimulants because on-task activity is enhanced.

In humans, mood and alertness tend to be enhanced with acute doses of *d*-amphetamine up to about 50 mg (Jaffe, 1990). Paradoxically, a sizable minority of humans show the opposite effects, at least for the first hour or so, after taking amphetamine (Tecce & Cole, 1974). Somewhere in the 100 mg dose range, humans experience dysphoria, social withdrawal, and depression (Griffith et al., 1970). Continued exposure to these high doses can precipitate a psychosis with symptoms very similar to paranoid schizophrenia (Jonsson & Gunne, 1970; Lyon et al., 1986). Behavior often becomes very stereotyped and repetitive. Simple movements such as continuous chewing, rubbing of the tongue on the inside of the lips, and teeth grinding occur. The individual may engage in a repetitious thought or meaningless act for hours. Often users seem fascinated or preoccupied with their own thought processes and with philosophical concerns on a grand scale. The person may get very suspicious of others and become antisocial, and in some cases may become very prone to violence. Similar actions have been described with the other amphetamine-like substances—for example, methylphenidate (Franz, 1985) and cocaine.

Very similar behavioral effects have been noted to occur in all mammals, although in each case the specific type of stereotypic reaction is dependent on the species. Rats typically bob their heads back and forth and display gnawing behaviors. Monkeys have been observed to exhibit continuous grooming-like movements of body and limbs without actually grooming, and chimpanzees have been observed to rock and sway back and forth. Because of the similarities between the behavioral effects of high doses of amphetamines in humans and nonhumans, and because the human reactions are so similar to paranoid schizophrenia, the effects in nonhumans induced by higher doses of amphetamine are commonly viewed as a way of producing a model animal "psychosis."

One of the curious aspects of the amphetamine-induced psychosis in animals is that repeated exposure to amphetamine appears to sensitize, rather than reduce, the organism's susceptibility to it. This phenomenon can occur even if the exposures are several days apart (Kilbey &

Ellinwood, 1977). Exposure to similar-acting drugs such as cocaine, and severe stress also appear to sensitize the organism (Antelman et al., 1980; MacLennan & Maier, 1983). These findings have led to the speculation that humans who have been exposed to stress or drugs of this nature may also be predisposed to developing the psychotic reactions to amphetamine or cocaine. As yet, there has been no satisfactory explanation for this sensitization effect with these drugs. One possibility is that the prolonged depletion of catecholamines following heavy use (see "Dependence") induces increased receptor density/sensitivity (receptor up-regulation). At any rate, tolerance to some of amphetamine's effects, as well as sensitization (or reverse tolerance, as it is sometimes called) to others, may occur with chronic use (Sparber & Fossom, 1984).

In addition to their central effects, amphetamines and related compounds have a number of sympathomimetic effects. They increase blood pressure and heart rate, constrict the blood vessels to the viscera, increase body temperature and muscle tension, and induce intestinal relaxation and bronchial dilation.

Clinical Uses for Amphetamines

The acute effects of low to moderate doses of amphetamine in humans include increased energy, concentration, alertness, and self-confidence, and mood elevation. In some individuals these effects can occur almost to the point of elation and euphoria (Jaffe, 1990). Social interactions, such as increased talkativeness, friendliness, and activity, may be enhanced. Amphetamine also suppresses appetite (anorexia).

The clinical uses of amphetamine and related drugs reflect these effects. Following its use in the treatment of asthma, one of amphetamine's first clinical uses for its CNS effects was in the treatment of *narcolepsy,* a rare but serious disorder in which the person falls asleep repeatedly during the day, often without warning. Shortly thereafter, amphetamine was found to significantly reduce many of the symptoms of children whose cognitive functioning was impaired by the inability to concentrate and who were overly active (a disorder now called *attention deficit disorder*). At present, these are the only two disorders for which most experts agree amphetamines may be legitimately prescribed.

However, over the past 50 years, amphetamines have been used for a variety of purposes. During World War II, most of the armed forces on both sides of the war issued amphetamines to their men to counteract fatigue, elevate mood, and heighten endurance (Brecher, 1972). Whether this practice hurt or helped their cause in the long run is debatable, for as we shall see, escalating the dose of amphetamine is a tempting probability in such times of stress. It can lead to a psychotic state involving a severe case of perceptual and cognitive disorganization. Some historians have suggested that at the end of the war, Adolf Hitler's increasingly bizarre behavior may have been due to his use of amphetamines, along with a variety of other stimulants. As stated by one historian:

> No one who has read about his behavior during this time or about his pronouncements at the situation conferences on 23, 25 and 27 April 1945, then still being recorded, can fail to recognize what it was that made him conjure up in all good faith such patently harebrained schemes. The rapid alternation of depression and euphoria, exhaustion and artificially induced buoyancy clearly reflect Hitler's dependence on the stimulants prescribed by Morell. (Maser, 1971, pp. 228–229)

After the war, amphetamines were routinely prescribed for weight control and mood depression, now recognized as inappropriate because amphetamine can lead to a person becoming even more depressed and suicidal. To blunt the nervousness and sleep-disrupting properties of amphetamine, individuals often combined it with a sedative-hypnotic, or tranquilizer. In some of these combinations, the compound actually served as an amphetamine antagonist.

In the early 1970s, more than 30 amphetamine-containing preparations were on the market. Some government sources estimated that there were enough doses of amphetamine and related compounds being marketed in the United States to supply every man, woman, and child several times daily. Furthermore, there were plenty of unscrupulous and ignorant physicians around willing to prescribe it. In addition to its medically prescribed uses, it was being used by truck drivers who were doing long hauls without adequate rest, students who were cramming for exams, and "speed freaks" who were injecting it just to get high. With all of its use and potential misuse, something had to give. Since the mid-1970s, the use of amphetamines has gradually decreased, for many reasons. First, the government began to exert legal pressures on pharmaceutical companies to decrease their production. Second, the number of legitimate medical uses was drastically reduced. Third, the general population and physicians became more educated about the potential hazards and misuse. Fourth, compounds with less abuse potential and more specific actions with respect to major mood depression were developed—for example, antidepressants. Finally, cocaine, which users were led to believe was much less harmful than amphetamine, came on the scene to replace it as a drug for recreational use.

Dependence

Despite the dysphoric effects of high doses or chronic use, the dependence liability of amphetamine and similar-acting drugs is considered to be among the highest of all drugs (Jaffe, 1990). Although physical dependence may be a factor, unequivocal evidence for abstinence symptoms associated with these drugs is lacking. There is no question that when individuals stop taking amphetamines after a few days of moderate to heavy amphetamine exposure, they generally "crash"; that is, they experience exhaustion, depression, lethargy, and hunger. These are all symptoms opposite to the direct effects of the drug. However, rather than being signs of an abstinence syndrome, these symptoms may be due to lack of decent sleep, low blood sugar, or depletion of norepinephrine, among other things. One can speculate that because of the enhanced activity at catecholamine receptors, there may also be a short-lived decrease in the sensitivity of postsynaptic catecholamine receptors, an effect that would be consistent with a true abstinence syndrome. (However, note that this speculation contrasts with the possibility for up-regulation of receptors following catecholamine depletion.) Even if the postdrug symptoms associated with chronic psychostimulant use were due to a true abstinence syndrome, they clearly would be qualitatively and quantitatively very different from those symptoms associated with the sedative-hypnotics and the narcotics. Furthermore, it is questionable whether these symptoms are a major factor in the maintenance of drug-taking behavior with this class of drugs.

On the other hand, the psychological dependence associated with amphetamines and related drugs can be overwhelming. The euphoria, feelings of well-being, and enhanced self-confidence in both physical and mental ability serve as powerful primary reinforcers—even more powerful than food in a hungry animal (Aigner & Balster, 1978). Even animals find their effects very reinforcing. Recent self-administration studies with nonhumans have indicated that, if given free access to amphetamines or cocaine, they are highly likely to administer larger and larger amounts—in many cases to the point of administering lethal doses (which induce convulsions) (Aigner & Balster, 1978; Brady & Griffiths, 1977). This phenomenon rarely occurs with narcotics like heroin, where animals typically stabilize at a fairly constant daily dosage somewhat below lethal levels. Thus it appears that these drugs have very strong primary reinforcing properties, and it is these properties that potentially lead to the heavy psychological dependence on them.

As with all psychotropic drugs, there is considerable individual variability in vulnerability to dependence on amphetamines. Some users go for months or years before becoming daily users, whereas others report such an intense positive response with the first dose that addiction occurs almost immediately. Some of the factors leading to this variability are likely to be genetic (e.g., differential reactivity to novel stimulation), whereas others may be environmental (e.g., the result of differential exposure to stressful events during some critical period of life) (Piazza et al., 1989).

Effects of Chronic Amphetamine Exposure

Even in animals that do not administer lethal amounts, continued exposure to amphetamines and related drugs eventually leads to problems associated with malnutrition, nonhealing ulcers, high blood pressure, and brain damage resulting from restricted blood flow to the brain. These effects can also occur in humans. Repeated administration of high doses of amphetamines has also been found to induce irreversible neuronal damage in animals (Wagner et al., 1985). This includes long-lasting depletion of central monoamine concentrations, a decrease in the number of monoamine uptake sites, a decrease in monoamine synthesis, and nerve terminal degeneration. It has been speculated that these effects are due to amphetamine's ability to enhance the release of both dopamine and serotonin as well as inhibit MAO activity, which leads to the nonenzymatic oxidation of these monoamines into neurotoxins (Sonsalla et al., 1989). Consistent with this view are studies that have demonstrated that the neurotoxic actions of methamphetamine can be attenuated by pretreatment with vitamin C (an antioxidant) and alpha-methyl-p-tyrosine (a catecholamine synthesis inhibitor), and can be exacerbated by pretreatment with reserpine (a drug that enhances cytoplasmic pools of monoamines) and iprindole (an inhibitor of dopamine and serotonin reuptake). Whether these types of neurotoxic effects occur with the doses of amphetamines used by humans is not presently known.

Cocaine

South American Indians have been using cocaine for centuries to increase their endurance and reduce fatigue and hunger. The early European explorers of South America, who essentially enslaved the natives, soon found the natives' fondness of the coca leaf to be useful as an incentive for performing hard labor. Eventually, the coca leaf was introduced in Europe with little fanfare. In the mid-1800s cocaine was isolated from coca extracts, but its general use did not begin until the late 1800s. Sir Arthur Conan Doyle's famous detective, Sherlock Holmes, was reported to have injected cocaine (circa 1888) occasionally between cases. He said he found it "transcendentally stimulating and clarifying to the mind" (Grilly, 1980). (A recent novel revolving around Holmes's cocaine use—*The Seven-Per-Cent Solution* by Nicholas Meyer—is obviously not authentic, because it often confuses the effects of cocaine with those of opiates, and cocaine is clearly not an opiate.)

Perhaps the earliest leading proponent of cocaine's clinical use, for its antidepressant and antifatigue properties, was a young physician by the name of Sigmund Freud (Brecher, 1972). Between 1884 and 1887

Freud performed the functions of a psychopharmacologist by testing the various mood- and behavior-altering properties of cocaine, primarily on himself and a few friends. Freud initially concluded that cocaine had many beneficial characteristics. He found that it could be used to enhance mood, alleviate depression, reduce the effects of fatigue, and enhance sexual potency. He felt it could be a potential treatment for morphine and alcohol addiction, numerous psychological disorders (such as hysteria and hypochondria), and a variety of physical debilities (for example, diseases involving tissue degeneration, asthma, and digestive problems). Finally, he suggested that its local anesthetic properties might be of value.

Although Freud initially believed that cocaine was a wonder drug through which he could establish his medical reputation (as well as provide himself with recreation), he eventually became disillusioned with the drug (Jones, 1953). One reason may have been that his own work indicated that there was tremendous individual variability in the reaction to cocaine. He also attempted to wean a good friend off of his dependence on morphine, using cocaine as a substitute. Although the friend was successfully weaned from his morphine habit, he quickly developed a very strong cocaine dependence. After observing the effects of both kinds of dependence, Freud was perhaps the first to recognize that dependence on cocaine can have far more deleterious effects than morphine dependence. As will be discussed in Chapter 10, chronic morphine use has relatively benign effects on the person, whereas chronic cocaine use induces a psychotic state, extreme loss of appetite leading to nutritional deficiencies, impaired interpersonal relations, and a variety of other pathological effects.

Freud has long been recognized as a high achiever who wanted to become famous—something that was unattainable as long as he was associated with a drug with such a poor reputation. In recognizing his error in judgment regarding cocaine's therapeutic promise, Freud turned away from pursuing physical, organic approaches to the treatment of mental illness—perhaps leading him toward an approach emphasizing unconscious forces in its cause. However, his work with cocaine may have led to its use by an eye surgeon, Karl Koller, as a local anesthetic in the eye. It was the first drug physicians had for this purpose. Cocaine was later used as therapy for asthma and colic. Although Freud's work with cocaine ceased, he continued to use cocaine regularly until at least 1895, and probably quite a bit longer (but encouraged the widely held view that he stopped using the drug in 1887). Many have speculated that his cocaine use not only was a factor in his prodigious writings but may also have played a causal role in the early development of his psychoanalytic theories by facilitating his capacity for introspection and self-analysis (Fuller, 1992).

Pharmacokinetics of Cocaine

Despite the South American Indians' long-term use of cocaine, there are no reports of them suffering from any unpleasant side effects or toxicity. On the other hand, in the 1980s in the United States, we began to experience an epidemic of use and abuse of, and extreme dependence on, cocaine. Why is there such a difference in these two cultures' reactions to cocaine? Basically the difference lies in the way in which the drug is administered. The South American Indians generally chew the coca leaf, which contains very small amounts of cocaine. Since cocaine in the coca plant is an alkaloid that is slowly absorbed from the G.I. tract, very little cocaine accumulates in the brain. North American users administer a highly concentrated form of cocaine intranasally, intravenously, or, most recently, through inhalation—all of which result in a rapid and high concentration of the drug in the brain (American Society for Pharmacology, 1987).

South American Indians have traditionally administered cocaine in its untransformed alkaloid form by chewing the leaves with an alkaloid substance so that absorption through the oral mucous membranes is enhanced. Apparently, there are very few cases in which this practice results in acute overdosage, psychosis, neglect of one's responsibility, or extensive focus on cocaine use. More recently, though, some young South Americans in urban areas have begun to mix the cocaine paste, which is extracted from the leaves for subsequent synthesis into cocaine hydrochloride, with tobacco and smoke it. In these individuals, the same patterns of pathological states, neglect of work, and preoccupation with cocaine use seen in North American users are evidenced (Jaffe, 1990).

In North America and other developed countries, cocaine hydrochloride is commonly self-administered by sniffing it (referred to as "snorting") so that it is absorbed through the nasal membranes. This leads to a somewhat faster onset of action and higher brain concentrations than when it is ingested orally (Van Dyke & Byck, 1982). The local vasoconstrictive properties of cocaine result in slower absorption and longer effects when the drug is snorted as opposed to smoked. Cocaine's vasoconstrictive properties in the nose also lead to tissue degeneration (for example, a perforated septum) because of ischemia (localized tissue anemia). Although much higher brain concentrations of cocaine can be achieved when administered intravenously, this mode of administration is uncommon in the vast majority of users, perhaps because users recognize the hazards associated with this route of administration. On the other hand, the smoking of cocaine is becoming increasingly popular because it allows high concentrations of cocaine to accumulate in the brain in a fashion very similar to intravenous administration, but avoids the hazards of injections—particularly the development of the inevitably lethal disease AIDS. Also, since users generally have had experience with smoking marijuana, they do not have to learn a new drug administration procedure.

Because cocaine hydrochloride is volatilized at temperatures that degrade it, in order for it to be effective when smoked, it must be reconverted chemically to its alkaloid (base) state. This practice is generally called **free-basing**, and in its crystalline form the compound is commonly referred to as **crack** (Gawin, 1991). In this mode it is easily volatilized in active form at relatively low temperatures. Crack is relatively inexpensive—a day's use can be financed for $10 to $20—and produces a rapid-onset, intense high, which makes it extremely addictive. Unfortunately, the toxic and lethal effects of cocaine, as well as the profound dependency, are just as readily induced by smoking the drug as with intravenous administration (American Society for Pharmacology, 1987). The dependence liability of cocaine with either of these modes of administration may actually be greater than that of amphetamine, because the subjective "crash" following smoking or intravenous administration of cocaine is much more noticeable than with amphetamine (American Society for Pharmacology, 1987). This outcome is probably related to cocaine's very short duration of action.

Once in the body, cocaine is widely distributed throughout the body and is rapidly metabolized (American Society for Pharmacology, 1987). Minimal amounts of cocaine are excreted in an unmetabolized form. Although cocaine's plasma half-life is around 30 to 90 minutes, several metabolites can be detected by way of urinalysis for up to three days after administration. However, as yet, there is no way of determining precisely from such analysis how recently the person has used cocaine or how much was used.

Pharmacodynamics of Cocaine

Although, as indicated in Chapter 4, cocaine has local anesthetic properties because of its ability to block neural conduction, its CNS effects are mediated primarily by its potent ability to inhibit the reuptake of the catecholamines norepinephrine and dopamine from the synaptic cleft (Moore et al., 1977). It has now been fairly well established that the reinforcing properties of cocaine are predominantly due to its dopamine-reuptake-inhibiting properties (Ritz et al., 1987). Cocaine also appears to weakly facilitate the release of catecholamines from axon terminals.

The neurochemical effects of cocaine are similar to those of methylphenidate, amphetamine, and some antidepressants, although in many cases there are subtle, but potentially important, differences. Amphetamine, for example, has weaker catecholamine-reuptake-blocking properties than cocaine but more potent catecholamine-releasing actions

(Moore et al., 1977). Furthermore, cocaine appears to have considerably more dopaminergic activity, whereas amphetamine has considerably more noradrenergic activity. Because of the greater access of catecholamines to their receptors, one might expect chronic exposure to these drugs to lead to down-regulation of receptors. Apparently, however, it is not that simple; although initial doses of these substances lead to excessive receptor activity, they also lead to catecholamine depletion (Dackis & Gold, 1985; Short & Shuster, 1976). If the depletion were to last long enough, it would lead to lower than normal receptor activation and their up-regulation. Thus, depending upon when receptor binding is measured, one may find increased or decreased binding, or no change at all in binding. This may be why in a recent review it was concluded that amphetamine exposure leads to lower receptor dopamine binding, whereas chronic cocaine exposure induces the opposite effect—that is, it leads to increased dopamine receptor binding (Dackis & Gold, 1985). To confuse the issue further, dopamine and norepinephrine mediate different behavioral effects and increase and decrease at different times during and following psychostimulant exposure (Short & Shuster, 1976), leading to a myriad of effects regarding tolerance, sensitization, and receptor binding with these drugs. Further speculations on this issue with respect to cocaine will be discussed shortly.

Finally, although antidepressants such as imipramine (to be discussed in Chapter 13) share cocaine's monoamine-reuptake-inhibiting properties, they do not elevate mood until after several days of exposure, nor do they elevate mood in nondepressed individuals. Some of these differences may be due to these drugs having considerably weaker effects at the dopamine-uptake-binding site than cocaine; for instance, it would account for their lacking reinforcing effects in humans and animals. In order to achieve blood levels of imipramine that would induce dopamine-reuptake blockade comparable to that of cocaine, the imipramine blood levels would be in the range of human lethality (Ritz et al., 1987).

Psychological Effects of Cocaine

Because of the similarities of the neurochemical effects of cocaine and those induced by amphetamine, it is not surprising that their mood-altering and behavioral effects are also quite similar. With few exceptions, the characteristics noted earlier for amphetamine apply to cocaine. Although users of the two drugs will swear that the effects of the two drugs are different, there is little scientific research to support this belief. In fact, most studies have found that, when users of cocaine and amphetamine are administered these drugs intravenously, they are unable to distinguish between them, except for the duration of the drug effect (Van Dyke & Byck, 1982). The time course for amphetamine is approximately 2 to 3 hours, whereas cocaine's effects dissipate in about 30 minutes. In studies with animals, the behavioral effects of cocaine and amphetamine are quite similar in a variety of procedures. Also, after chronic exposure to either substance, those effects exhibiting tolerance to one will sometimes confer tolerance to the other (Fischman et al., 1985; Wood & Emmett-Oglesby, 1986). Similarly, when enhanced sensitivity is observed with one, sometimes it will also be evidenced with the other (Kilbey & Ellinwood, 1977; Short & Shuster, 1976). On the other hand, neither is cross-tolerant with opiates like morphine (Short & Shuster, 1976; Jaffe, 1990).

High doses of cocaine induce the same psychopathological effects noted earlier with respect to amphetamine: suicidal thoughts, irritability, anxiety, rebound depression, and paranoid ideation. (Robert Louis Stevenson gives us a glimpse of this behavior in his story "The Strange Case of Dr. Jekyll and Mr. Hyde," which he wrote in six days and nights under the influence of cocaine [Siegel, 1989]. Presumably, the drug that Dr. Jekyll took that turned him into the demonic murderer Mr. Hyde was modeled after cocaine.) The most common of the perceptual changes and pseudohallucinations induced by cocaine are tactile disturbances, in which there is a sensation of bugs running over the skin (referred to as *formication*), and visual disturbances (termed snow lights) (Jaffe, 1990).

There are some differences between cocaine and amphetamine in addition to those mentioned earlier. Although the potency of cocaine is about 60% that of amphetamine when the two drugs are administered intravenously, it is considerably less potent when they are administered orally (Jaffe, 1990). Oral cocaine, because of its alkaloid nature and the effects of G.I. secretions, is not well absorbed, whereas amphetamine is readily absorbed from the G.I. tract. There is also a difference between them when taken intranasally; cocaine has local anesthetic properties, whereas amphetamine does not. This local anesthetic action also appears to make it difficult for cocaine users to distinguish cocaine from other local anesthetics with minimal CNS actions, such as procaine (Novocain) (Van Dyke & Byck, 1982). Perhaps some of the subjective differences between amphetamine and cocaine are due to reputation, expectation, and setting, all of which are potent factors in many so-called drug-induced effects.

Cocaine Dependence

Although most reports prior to 1980 indicated that cocaine had relatively benign effects on most individuals, the majority of reports in the 1980s have indicated considerable concern over cocaine's dependence liability and toxicity. These reports have indicated that, particularly when administered intravenously or through smoking (popularly known as free-basing), cocaine can induce a very strong psychological dependence (Gawin, 1991). For example, cocaine addicts report that virtually all thoughts are focused on cocaine during binges (which can last up to several days); nourishment, sleep, money, loved ones, responsibility, and survival lose all significance. It is estimated that one out of 10 recreational users of intranasal cocaine becomes heavily dependent or experiences numerous severe consequences. However, cocaine abusers in treatment report that 2 to 4 years intervene between initial exposure to cocaine and the development of addiction—a delay that may have contributed to the lack of recognition of its addictive and toxic properties.

Although it has been known for several years that sensitization to some of cocaine's effects may occur with chronic use (Stripling & Ellinwood, 1977), until recently there has been some question whether tolerance occurs with cocaine use. There is now considerable evidence that tolerance does develop to many of the physiological and subjective effects of cocaine, and in some cases it develops very rapidly (American Society for Pharmacology, 1987; Fischman et al., 1985; Wood & Emmett-Oglesby, 1986). Whether tolerance or sensitization occurs with chronic cocaine use appears to depend on the complex interactions among dose, the behavior involved, and the species, as well as other, as yet unknown, factors (Grabowski & Dworkin, 1985).

It has been demonstrated that a major component of cocaine sensitization is attributable to the environmental context and Pavlovian conditioning (Post et al., 1987). However, with sufficiently high doses of cocaine, an environment context-independent sensitization effect can also appear. Panic attacks and seizures may be particularly prone to develop. It has been speculated that these are due to the biochemical properties of cocaine that produce its local anesthetic actions. Local anesthetics, when administered repetitively in high doses, produce an alteration in the threshold for seizures such that previously subconvulsive doses become capable of eliciting major motor seizures. (This phenomenon appears to be similar to that of electrophysiological "kindling," in which repeated electrical stimulation below the convulsive threshold eventually provokes full-blown seizures.) However, studies with animals have shown that, in contrast to seizures kindled by lidocaine (a local anesthetic with minimal euphoric properties), which are generally well tolerated for weeks or months of repetitions, cocaine-induced seizures are extremely lethal.

Recent studies have also strongly suggested that withdrawal after extensive cocaine use does occur. Furthermore, the withdrawal appears to involve several phases, with mixtures of different dependence-inducing processes being implicated (Gawin, 1991). During the first few hours after a binge (which generally ceases only when all the cocaine is gone), the user feels depressed and agitated, lacks appetite, and experiences high cocaine craving. In the next several hours or days, the user experiences extreme hunger, although cocaine craving is absent. In some individuals there is also a strong abhorrence for cocaine during this time period, and the need for sleep is overwhelming. During the next several days, the user's sleep patterns and mood return to normal, and there is little cocaine craving. However, subsequently the user experiences anxiety, a lack of energy, an inability to enjoy normal activities, and high cocaine craving that is exacerbated by environmental cues previously associated with cocaine use. After several weeks, the user's mood and pleasure response return to normal, and he or she experiences only episodic cocaine craving, which again is most common in the presence of specific environments. If the person begins taking cocaine again at any point, he or she generally returns to the first phase.

Cocaine addiction is a growing problem in American society and many others. Understanding how it develops and how it can be treated is very important. From the preceding description, it should be clear that environmental and internal stimuli (that is, mood states) trigger or exacerbate the craving for cocaine. In addition, there is abundant evidence that pharmacologically induced biochemical disruptions, particularly central dopamine neuronal systems, play a role in the craving for cocaine (Dackis & Gold, 1985; Gold & Dackis, 1984; Ritz et al., 1987).

There are at least four major biochemical phases which play a role in cocaine dependency (Dackis & Gold, 1985). (Actually there are more than four, but for simplicity, this discussion will be limited to four.) First, cocaine inhibits dopamine reuptake (while cocaine can alter norepinephrine and serotonin activity, its effects on dopamine appear central to its rewarding properties—that is, euphoria). Second, acute cocaine exposure abruptly elevates extraneuronal dopamine levels—that is, levels in the synaptic cleft. This increase is followed by a sharp reduction to normal within minutes. Presumably, the latter is due to the activation of a negative feedback system, such as autoreceptor activation. Third, chronic cocaine exposure depletes intraneuronal dopamine stores, either because of reduced synthesis via autoreceptor activity or enhanced catabolization via COMT or other enzymes. Fourth, chronic cocaine exposure increases the number of functional dopamine receptors, presumably because of dopamine depletion and underactivation of receptors; that is, dopamine receptor up-regulation occurs.

These biochemical phenomena can account for a number of behavioral phenomena that have been reported to occur with cocaine use. First, the subjective effects of cocaine are reported to be short-lived. Second, over a period of several hours, users report that repeated cocaine exposures induce the same effects. Third, following such an episode, users experience a crash. Fourth, following such episodes, chronic users often report mood depression for days or weeks. Fifth, the combination of reduced levels of dopamine with greater dopamine receptor sensitivity could explain a number of apparently paradoxical phenomena associated with cocaine use. For example, cocaine users or their acquaintances some-times report that the user is moody—happy one moment and sad the next. Sometimes cocaine tolerance is evident; sometimes it is not. At other times, the person is overly sensitive to cocaine's effects. One can specu-late that if the drug were not present, the lower than normal level of dopamine would be somewhat counterbalanced by hypersensitive dopa-mine receptors, such that if one's daily life experiences were stimulating, mood would be relatively normal. Under nonstimulating conditions, the person may feel depressed and crave cocaine. If the person were to admin-ister cocaine while dopamine stores were low, there would be little in-crease in dopamine levels in the cleft. Thus there would only be slight mood elevation; that is, tolerance would be evident. If the person were to administer cocaine after dopamine stores had been replenished some-what (but were still below normal), the increase in dopamine levels in the cleft, combined with hypersensitive receptors, would induce euphoria. Finally, if the person were to administer cocaine after dopamine stores had been replenished to normal levels, but while the dopamine receptors were still hypersensitive, the resulting arousal might be great enough to induce a psychotic-like reaction (Post, 1977). These are provocative specu-lations that future researchers can address in attempting to understand the varying aspects of cocaine addiction.

In terms of patterns of use, cocaine is one of the few controlled substances in which the chances of initiating its use persist or increase well into adulthood (Kozel & Adams, 1986). As noted in Chapter 6, its use generally follows exposure to more licit drugs, such as tobacco and alcohol, and marijuana. Epidemiological studies are needed to answer more specific questions about predictors for initiation and maintenance of cocaine use, what interventions might mitigate these, and how fre-quently cocaine use impacts other aspects of the user's life, such as use of other drugs, socioeconomic status, health, and driving.

Cocaine has a reputation of enhancing a person's subjective self-worth, competence, and performance, and we would expect this to be a factor in the maintenance of cocaine drug use. However, whether the enhanced performance and competence actually occur or are simply due to alterations in the user's perception is not clear.

Direct Adverse Consequences of Cocaine

Many of the problems attributed to cocaine, such as lower productivity, financial losses, family disruptions, legal difficulties, and so on, are indi-rectly related to its use. These problems come about because of the user's preoccupation with the drug or the U.S. legal system's views on its posses-sion and use. However, unlike opiates, where most of the problems with their use are due to these factors rather than to direct effects on the body, cocaine also has several potential direct adverse consequences. As noted previously, the adverse effects of heavy amphetamine use—for example, psychosis, profound irritability, misperception, paranoid thought, impaired interpersonal relations, and eating and sleeping disturbances—have also been well-documented to occur with heavy cocaine use (Post & Contel, 1983). Cocaine has also been shown to precipitate panic attacks, which may subsequently recur without further cocaine use (Aronson & Craig, 1986).

Cocaine can produce a variety of neurological problems, including seizures, headache, and transient symptoms such as sensory loss on one side of the body, visual impairment, and tremor (Rowbotham & Lowenstein, 1990). Other than seizure activity, which is dose related, there does not appear to be a correlation between these neurological problems and the dose, route of administration, or prior cocaine use patterns.

While news reports such as those discussing the deaths of well-known athletes like Maryland basketball player Len Bias and Cleveland Browns football player Don Rogers tend to emphasize cocaine's potential lethality, it is not clear how many deaths are directly due to cocaine overdoses. Statistics regarding fatalities attributable to cocaine use are not particularly reliable, but it does appear that only about one-quarter of the deaths are actually due directly to the recreational use of cocaine. The majority of cocaine-associated deaths can be attributed to suicide induced by or facilitated by cocaine; accidental overdoses (for example, the person swallowed cocaine for smuggling purposes or to elude detection when arrested); homicides; death from natural causes; or the combining of cocaine with other drugs (primarily opiates) (Finkle & McCloskey, 1977; Lichtenfeld et al., 1984). For most individuals, the lethal dose of cocaine—approximately 1 to 2 grams in an hour—would be quite expensive. Cocaine use may cause sudden death because of cerebral hemorrhaging (bleeding within the brain) (Lichtenfeld et al., 1984), convulsion induction (Ellinwood et al., 1977), or acute myocardial infarction (sudden insufficiency of blood to the heart muscles)—even in individuals with no preexisting arterial dysfunctions (Isner & Chokshi, 1991). The mechanism behind sudden deaths is still obscure, but recent evidence suggests that even low doses of cocaine can lead to inflammation of the muscular walls of the heart in certain individuals. Also, contrary to what is commonly believed, intranasal cocaine can lead to sudden death (Finkle & McCloskey, 1977).

As noted in Chapter 3, most psychoactive substances are likely to be teratogenic. Considering cocaine's lipid solubility, there is no reason to believe that cocaine is an exception. Although only a small fraction of babies exposed to cocaine in the womb develop medical problems, since 1985 a number of studies, with both humans and non-humans, have documented the potential teratogenic effects of cocaine (Slutsker, 1992). In humans cocaine abuse has been associated with an increased stillbirth rate and premature delivery. Physically, cocaine-exposed neonates exhibit lower average birth weights, body lengths, and head circumferences. There is also evidence that such infants exhibit retarded brain growth and skull defects. Behaviorally, these infants exhibit more jitteriness and irritability and appear less attentive than non-cocaine-exposed infants. After birth, there is evidence that cocaine-exposed neonates are more prone to sudden unexplained infant death syndrome. Many of these effects are likely to be the result of impaired fetal oxygenation caused by cocaine's tendency to constrict blood vessels. Cocaine also produces a number of biochemical disruptions that may be responsible for many of its observed neurobehavioral effects. Unfortunately, the true extent of the severity and incidence of the harmful effects of prenatal cocaine exposure in humans is simply not known, because of a number of methodological problems in the studies addressing this issue. Among many problems, for example, the women in these studies (1) are more likely to be poor and undereducated; (2) may differ considerably in the amount, frequency, and time of cocaine use; (3) commonly use other drugs, such as alcohol, nicotine, marijuana, and heroin, that may also compromise prenatal development; (4) may under- or overreport their drug use; and (5) may practice other poor health behaviors, such as inadequate nutrition and prenatal care (Mayes et al., 1992).

Treatment of Psychostimulant Abuse

The characteristics of psychostimulant dependence are essentially the same as those for alcoholism; thus treatment for cocaine or amphetamine dependence is usually similar to that for alcoholism. The important factor in drug dependence is the dynamics among the individual's environment, genetic predispositions, behavior, and drug exposure—not the drug. The key to treatment is getting compulsive drug users to acknowledge that they are out of control and should do whatever it takes to get well. Most therapists demand abstinence from all drugs. In addition, self-help peer groups, conducted in either inpatient or outpatient settings, are a primary form of therapy (Dackis & Gold, 1985).

There are some differences in the chemical interventions potentially used in the treatment of psychostimulant dependence, as opposed to sedative-hypnotic or narcotic dependence. In the case of the psychostimulants, physical withdrawal is neither life-threatening nor exceedingly uncomfortable. Thus there is no need to substitute a long-acting psychostimulant (if there were such a compound) and then gradually reduce the dosage because of concern over precipitating a convulsive episode or cardiovascular collapse.

Because of the linkage between the cravings for cocaine and the depletion of the catecholamines dopamine and norepinephrine (Dackis & Gold, 1985), one potential way of alleviating the overwhelming craving for cocaine (and amphetamine) is to use drugs that augment catecholamine activity without inducing euphoria or positive mood changes (Gawin, 1991). The use of tricyclic antidepressants (see Chapter 13), which, like cocaine, inhibit catecholamine reuptake but do not induce euphoria, has been attempted, and several reports have indicated that the tricyclics such as desipramine (Norpramin) are effective in the treatment of cocaine and amphetamine dependence. However, successful abstinence may occur only with long-term, but not short-term, tricyclic exposure (Gawin & Ellinwood, 1988).

Drugs that specifically enhance dopamine activity have been shown in double-blind studies to significantly reduce cocaine craving and other withdrawal symptoms (Dackis et al., 1985–86; Tennant & Sagherian, 1987). Amantadine (Symmetrel), a drug that releases dopamine and norepinephrine from neuronal storage sites and delays their synaptic vesicle reuptake, and bromocriptine (Parlodel), a direct dopamine agonist, have both been demonstrated to alleviate the symptoms of cocaine withdrawal without producing euphoria themselves. Why these drugs are not capable of inducing euphoria and other pleasant reactions is still a puzzle. In fact, patients in one study using bromocriptine reported that the effect of cocaine was considerably reduced when they used it while also taking bromocriptine (Tennant & Sagherian, 1987). This result would suggest that bromocriptine may be a mixed agonist-antagonist.

Bromocriptine may induce side effects, like headaches and vertigo, that may lead patients to discontinue treatment. Amantadine also has its problems. Because it releases dopamine and norepinephrine from storage sites, it could exacerbate the cocaine-induced depletion of these neurotransmitters. If this proves to be the case, the precursors tyrosine or L-dopa may be administered concomitantly with amantadine (Tennant & Sagherian, 1987). It is unclear whether adding precursors to a patient's diet without additional drug treatment is beneficial or not.

In order to prevent the euphoric effects of cocaine from being experienced (should the patient relapse), the antimanic drug lithium may be used prophylactically (that is, as a preventative measure) (Gawin, 1991). Lithium may also be useful indirectly in the treatment of psychostimulant abuse because it reduces the symptoms of an affective disorder (see Chapter 13) that may be underlying causal factors in the person's use of psychostimulants.

For cocaine addicts concurrently dependent on opiates, treatment with the mixed opioid agonist/antagonist buprenorphine (discussed in Chapter 10) has been examined in several studies (Kosten et al., 1992). Preclinical studies with primates and rodents have indicated that buprenorphine may significantly attenuate the euphoric properties of cocaine, and preliminary human studies have suggested that buprenorphine treatment may be associated with less cocaine abuse than occurs with methadone treatment (also discussed in Chapter 10). Other clinical studies have failed to support these findings, but they do suggest that the dose of buprenorphine used (higher doses being more effective than lower doses) may be a critical factor in the attenuation of cocaine effects.

Other Drugs with Psychostimulant Properties

Nicotine

Every year thousands of young people take up smoking tobacco. Over time their use changes from sporadic, occasional use to more continuous, daily use. On the other hand, thousands of people who have smoked for years try to stop; in most cases these attempts fail because the process is so aversive. In fact, the Surgeon General of the United States recently issued a report that states that the pharmacologic and behavioral processes that determine tobacco addiction are similar to those that determine addiction to drugs such as heroin and cocaine (Byrne, 1988). Most people—smokers and nonsmokers—recognize that there are costs for smoking. Although cheap in comparison to most other drug habits, smoking is not inexpensive. "Pack-a-day" smokers currently pay more than $700 a year for their habit. However, this expense is a drop in the bucket compared to the potential health costs of lung cancer, emphysema, cardiovascular dysfunction, and other diseases associated with cigarette smoking. The problems are compounded by the fact that cigarette smoking is prominant among most abusers of other drugs; for example, more than 90% of alcoholic inpatients are smokers (Bien & Burge, 1990). Smoking exacerbates their health risks and complicates their treatment. (For example, it is not clear whether treatment for alcohol, cocaine, or heroin dependence would be facilitated or worsened by concomitant cessation of smoking.)

Questions as to why people start smoking in the first place and what makes stopping smoking so difficult for the majority of heavy smokers have been addressed by researchers for years. So far only pieces of the puzzle exist. There do appear to be some factors that predispose one toward taking up smoking. Adolescents who take up smoking tend to exhibit lower self-esteem, perceive themselves as having less internal control over their lives, and have higher levels of trait anxiety than those who do not take up smoking (Penny & Robinson, 1986). In the majority of these individuals, the initial smoking experiences are unpleasant. Apparently, the psychosocial rewards, like peer acceptance and role-model identification, are sufficiently strong to maintain smoking behavior until the individuals learn to monitor the amount of smoke, and the unpleasant side effects subside.

Once smoking begins, it is likely that genetic factors play a role in developing nicotine dependency. It has long been recognized that nicotine dependency is strongly associated with alcohol dependency, which, as we have noted earlier, has an established linkage to genes. Recent studies have also noted that nicotine-dependent persons, at some point in their lives, are more than twice as likely as nondependent nicotine users (or nonusers) to have suffered from major depression, which has also been viewed as involving a genetic predisposition (Glassman et al., 1990). In addition, persons with histories of major depression or any anxiety disorder tend to report more severe nicotine withdrawal symptoms than persons with neither of these disorders (Breslau et al., 1992). Thus, as has been noted on previous occasions in this book, there is likely to be some common genetic background that predisposes individuals to exhibiting a variety of pathological characteristics—the particular type or types being generated by environmental factors that are not yet clearly delineated.

Despite a multitude of studies on nicotine and tobacco use, it is still not clear what is so reinforcing about the drug and the practice. It has been long presumed that nicotine is the most important, but not the only, reinforcing factor behind smoking tobacco (Henningfield & Goldberg, 1988). If it were, then chewing nicotine gum would induce effects identical to smoking tobacco, which it does not do, and the treatment for smoking using nicotine gum would be much more effective than it is (Pickworth et al., 1986). In fact, most tobacco smokers cannot describe any attractive effect except what they might describe as the "taste" of tobacco smoke in their mouth, lungs, and nasal passages (Schelling, 1992).

One can present a case for nicotine as the principal reinforcer for smoking behavior, but the theory has holes in it (Henningfield & Goldberg, 1988). One early study, in which smokers were given nicotine injections, reported that most subjects described the sensation as pleasant and that craving for cigarettes during abstinence could be relieved. Working on the hypothesis that chronic smokers maximize the reinforcing effects of nicotine by titrating their intake, several studies have attempted to determine whether or not cigarette smokers can effectively regulate the amount of nicotine in their blood when given high- and low-nicotine cigarettes to smoke. Most agree that while some regulation of nicotine plasma levels is often achieved—by increasing the number of low-nicotine cigarettes or reducing the number of high-nicotine cigarettes consumed—it is nowhere near perfect. In two of the studies that varied nicotine and tar content independently, the number of cigarettes smoked was inversely related to nicotine content, not tar content. Finally, studies in which the subjects were preloaded with nicotine (in gum or in capsules) found a decrease in cigarettes consumed, whereas when a nicotine antagonist was administered, cigarette smoking increased.

In self-administration studies with nonhumans, nicotine infusions appear to have very minimal reinforcing properties, unless a discrete signal accompanies the nicotine infusions. For example, in one study, monkeys self-administered nicotine at a relatively high rate if a discrete signal came on just as the nicotine infusions were delivered, but their rate of administering nicotine dropped sharply when the signal did not occur (Goldberg et al., 1981). Perhaps this relationship explains why nicotine by way of smoking is the most popular route of administration; that is, with this route, discrete stimuli (smoke upon exhalation) always accompany the nicotine just before it reaches the brain (Schelling, 1992).

In some individuals, nicotine has a mild psychostimulant effect, particularly with respect to enhanced vigilance (Jaffe, 1990). In fact, socially relevant doses of nicotine may be comparable to socially relevant doses of caffeine in facilitating choice reaction time, motor tracking, and short-term memory retrieval as well as antagonizing some of the debilitating effects of alcohol (Kerr et al., 1991). For example, cigarette smoking has been shown to increase speed and accuracy in a concentration-demanding, rapid-processing task (Wesnes & Warburton, 1984). In most cases nicotine shifts EEG patterns toward those often associated with increased psychological arousal—that is, higher-frequency, lower-amplitude waves—and are most pronounced when the individual is relaxed with eyes closed (Pickworth et al., 1986). On the other hand, smokers often report that a cigarette calms them down and reduces tension (Schelling, 1992)—perhaps because it relieves their craving for a cigarette or stops withdrawal.

The effects of nicotine on performance are subtle and variable. While it is commonly believed that nicotine in cigarettes improves mental performance, recent studies have suggested that this improvement may occur only for the simplest tasks, such as finding a particular letter in a mixed group of letters (Spilich, 1987). In more complex tasks, such as understanding articles or solving problems, the performance of smokers was found to be worse than that of nonsmokers. Also, while smokers tended to work faster on some psychomotor tasks, such as driving simulators, they also committed more errors. Whether these findings were due to the nicotine or to inherent characteristics of the smokers that led to their being more or less efficient, and perhaps predisposed them to smoke, is unknown.

Presumably these psychological effects occur because of nicotine's ability to stimulate nicotinic receptor sites normally activated by acetylcholine. Which of the particular receptors are most important is not clear, since nicotine acts on receptors found throughout the nervous system. Furthermore, nicotinic receptors outside the brain may be involved. In the peripheral nervous system, activation of nicotinic receptors produces sympathomimetic effects, primarily because the nicotinic receptors found in the adrenal gland trigger the release of adrenaline (epinephrine) from the adrenal gland into the bloodstream. Adrenaline, in turn, is transported to adrenergic receptors in the heart and blood vessels, leading to increases in heart rate and elevated blood pressure (through constriction of blood vessels). Although adrenaline may potentially affect CNS function, it is unlikely to have much effect because it does not cross the blood-brain barrier very well. (Since there are nicotinic receptors on postganglionic parasympathetic neurons, activation of nicotinic receptors would also be expected to enhance parasympathetic activity, but the sympathetic effects predominate over the parasympathetic effects.) Despite these multiple PNS effects, they are probably not of major importance in reinforcing smoking because they can be blocked without appreciably altering the psychological effects of nicotine in humans.

There are also numerous nicotinic receptors in the CNS, which could account for nicotine's ability to alter cortical neuron function. Nicotine may also affect neurotransmitter systems other than cholinergic. For example, animal studies have shown nicotine to release norepinephrine and dopamine from brain tissue (Jaffe, 1990). It is also possible that the light-headed feeling that one gets by depriving the brain of oxygen—because of the carbon monoxide in smoke—is perceived as pleasurable.

Following chronic tobacco exposure, nicotine may also be reinforcing because it immediately stops withdrawal symptoms indicative of the physical dependence on nicotine that many believe exists. The onset of withdrawal symptoms may occur within hours of the last cigarette. In addition to a craving for tobacco, these symptoms may consist of decreased heart rate, EEG slowing, irritability, increased hunger, sleep disturbances, gastrointestinal disturbances, drowsiness, headache, and impairment of concentration, judgment, and psychomotor performance (Hughes et al., 1987).

However, observations that none of these symptoms may occur, that they may be delayed for several days, or that they may wax and wane over a period of months suggest that many of these symptoms may be more psychological than pharmacodynamic in origin (Henningfield & Goldberg, 1988). In other words, if the symptoms were purely physiological in origin, they would be strongly and inversely related to how much the person had been smoking recently and how long it had been since the person's last cigarette. If this were the case, all heavy smokers (those smoking at least 20 cigarettes a day) would undergo withdrawal every morning, because nicotine plasma levels are essentially zero at this time; yet many do not start smoking until the afternoon. Others may forgo smoking altogether for proscribed periods of time without undue discomfort—for example, Orthodox Jews on the Sabbath.

Conversely, if abstinence symptoms were psychological in origin, they would be directly related to the type of environment, social setting, and mood states that regularly have accompanied cigarette smoking, as well as the person's expectations and attitudes about cigarette withdrawal. The fact that these vary considerably within and among individuals more easily accounts for the variability in the degree of discomfort and the times when it occurs. For example, one recent study found that smokers in a treatment program who believed they were getting nicotine gum, but actually were receiving a placebo, reported fewer withdrawal symptoms and smoked fewer cigarettes during the first week of quitting smoking than those smokers who thought they were getting a placebo (Gottlieb et al., 1987). Also, there was no relationship between the actual nicotine content of the gum and reported withdrawal symptoms or eventual relapse rates. Unfortunately, as stressed in Chapter 6, once the underlying conditioning factors take place and the expectations develop, their presence may be felt for the rest of the person's life.

Finally, smoking may be reinforcing because it gives one something to do with one's hands, it may affect one's public image (although lately the image of a smoker has become considerably more negative), or it may be associated with other social reinforcers, such as acceptance by one's peers.

Although concerns over cigarette smoking have probably been a factor in the significant decline of smoking in young men and women over the past several years, use of smokeless tobacco—namely, snuff and chewing tobacco—has recently increased at an alarming rate in young males (National Institutes of Health, 1986). This increase has been attributed to the perception that smokeless tobacco is safer and more socially acceptable than cigarette smoking, and that smokeless tobacco enhances athletic performance. Unfortunately, smokeless tobacco is not harmless, nor does it appear to facilitate performance. Its use has been associated with oral and pharyngeal cancer, numerous dental and gum problems, and cardiovascular abnormalities related to elevated blood pressure and heart rate. Also, differences between users and nonusers of smokeless tobacco have not been observed with respect to neuromuscular reactivity or perceptual-motor task performance (Edwards & Glover, 1986; Edwards et al., 1987).

Many people "mature out" of their drug habits because their drug use ceases to match a change in their life-style—for example, marriage, job, or parenthood. Hardly anybody matures out of cigarettes. Smokers quit, but not through loss of interest—it requires determination (Schelling, 1992). The most promising aids to quitting are medicines that contain nicotine, such as chewing gum (Nicorette) or nicotine-containing skin patches (ProStep, Habitrol, Nicoderm), which release a constant, small amount of nicotine into the bloodstream and presumably lessen the craving for cigarettes. After a few weeks patients can chew less gum or receive smaller patches that release less nicotine until they are weaned off the substance. It is too soon to determine the effectiveness of skin patches (the FDA approved their use in 1992), but a few studies with Nicorette have indicated a permanent success rate as high as one-third—about double what is generally estimated to occur without it (Schelling, 1992). It should be emphasized that, while using these aids, smoking tobacco is absolutely to be avoided, because of nicotine's potential cardiovascular toxicity at high doses.

Convulsants

Mention the word "strychnine" to most people, and their immediate impression is that it is a poison used to kill rodents. Its lethality is due to the induction of convulsions, which are followed by impaired respiration and hypoxia. However, in low doses, *convulsants* do have some properties of other psychostimulants (Franz, 1985). Convulsants, like strychnine, do increase arousal at low doses, primarily as a result of their antagonistic action at postsynaptic receptors for glycine, which serve an inhibitory function in numerous interneurons in the brain stem. In other words, these neurons are released from inhibition by these drugs. However, their therapeutic indexes are very low, and thus they are highly toxic and lethal in relatively small amounts. I am not aware of any self-administration studies with nonhumans that could assess whether these drugs have any primary reinforcing effects, but humans do not use these drugs, perhaps because they are so aware of their toxic qualities. Convulsants, like other types of drugs, seem to facilitate retention in the passive avoidance task (discussed later in this chapter), but studies with humans are obviously limited because of the toxicity of these drugs.

Antidepressants

Antidepressants, which will be discussed in Chapter 13, would seem to be the type of drugs that would be appropriately classified as psychostimulants, and vice versa. However, most drugs now used for the treatment of depression do not increase attention and vigilance and enhance mood in nondepressed individuals. In fact, the major type of antidepressant used actually may cause drowsiness and mental confusion. On the other hand, the potent psychostimulants are not generally used as antidepressants because tolerance to their mood-elevating effects develops rather rapidly, they have a high potential for abuse, and they tend to induce a rebound depression when drug administration is terminated.

Pemoline Magnesium

Pemoline magnesium (Cylert) increases attention and relieves fatigue somewhat as methylphenidate does (Franz, 1985). It does not appear to have any unique behavioral properties that distinguish it from other psychostimulants. However, there are no reports of its abuse, possibly because of its slow onset of action. Its present use seems limited to the occasional treatment of the attention deficit disorder in children, presumably in cases where the usual psychostimulants, like methylphenidate or amphetamine, do not work or have noticeable side effects. It may take two to four weeks of daily administration of pemoline before its behavioral effects become apparent, with a lag of six to eight weeks before the maximum effect. These lags are only partially explained by the drug's slow rate of accumulation. Pemoline's mechanism of action is still unknown, but based on studies of urinary excretion of catecholamines, serotonin, and their metabolites in humans, its mechanism appears to be different from that of traditional psychostimulants like amphetamine and methylphenidate (Zametkin et al., 1986).

Psychostimulants, Learning, and Memory

Because of the enhanced mood and alertness associated with low doses of amphetamines and similar drugs, one might expect this type of drug to enhance learning. Indeed, this has been a common assumption of many a college student for years. But do these drugs really enhance learning? The evidence on the issue is equivocal, primarily because learning is never observed directly and involves a variety of complex processes for it to take place. Therefore, before beginning a discussion of this issue, one must be familiar with the basic phases of learning and memory. These consist of an acquisition phase, a consolidation phase, a retention phase, and a retrieval phase (Heise, 1981).

Acquisition is the phase in which the behavior or information is practiced and encoded. *Retention* is the preservation of this behavior or information between the end of the training period and the period during which it is utilized. *Retrieval* is the phase during which the organism attempts to utilize the behavior or information acquired earlier. Note that the acquisition phase corresponds to what we commonly refer to as learning, and the retention and retrieval phases correspond to what we refer to as memory. Memory is commonly viewed as consisting of two different storage systems: short-term memory, lasting a few seconds or minutes, and long-term memory, which is relatively permanent. During the time that it takes to create the long-term changes (perhaps resulting from the creation of new proteins that modify the permanent responsiveness of neurons), the information is maintained in short-term memory. There is a time period during which only temporary (short-term) memory exists and the permanent memory has not yet been established. The establishment of permanent traces from temporary ones is called *consolidation,* and the time it takes to form the permanent traces is called the consolidation phase.

A schematic representation of these four phases is shown in Figure 9–2. In the figure, times A, B, C, and D indicate where a drug would be administered in order to assess its effects on different components of learning and memory. Differences in performance between drug-treated and non-drug-treated animals are assessed during retest procedures. Any differences would be due to the drug's effects on acquisition processes (for example, attention, motivation, and general arousal) if the drug were administered at time A, consolidation if administered at time B (or if the duration of action of the drug given at A was such that it was also present during time B), retention if administered at time C, and retrieval if administered at time D (modified from Heise, 1981). From this discussion, we can see that when we ask the question of whether a particular drug affects learning or memory, we must first clarify during which phase(s) the drug is present.

Under conditions in which the person is fatigued or has an attention deficit disorder (see Chapter 14), there do seem to be some beneficial effects of low doses of amphetamine in the acquisition of new information, presumably because of increased attention to the material (Jaffe, 1990; Wender et al., 1981). Under conditions in which the person is already alert and rested, or with higher doses of amphetamine, the evidence is not as clear. In some cases it facilitates and in some cases it interferes with acquisition. Perhaps these contradictory results occur because, although amphetamine may enhance attentional processes, it may also increase one's attention to irrelevant details or tangential material. Thus relevant information may not be acquired. Regardless of whether there are benefits to the acquisition process or not, there are questions as to whether the information will be efficiently retrieved at appropriate times later on. This issue will be dealt with shortly.

Once information has been acquired, there is some evidence that exposure to adrenaline-stimulating drugs, like amphetamine, immediately following a learning experience (that is, during consolidation) can affect subsequent retention—with retention being enhanced by low doses and impaired by high doses (McGaugh, 1990). Most of the evidence for these phenomena comes from studies with nonhumans learning a very particular type of behavior referred to as passive avoidance. Briefly, the task involves placing a rat or a mouse in an area that it generally will move away from, such as on a platform raised an inch or so off the ground. Normally, the animal will step down off the platform after a few seconds. It is then subjected to a brief aversive shock, and then transferred back to its home cage. Later, after about 24 hours, the animal is placed on the platform again, to see how long it takes to step down. Animals that were not shocked earlier will generally step down very quickly, whereas animals that had been shocked will generally stay on the platform for a consider-

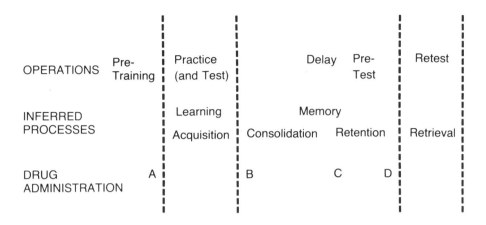

Figure 9–2

Schematic representation of operations over time and phases of inferred processes in the study of effects of drugs on learning and memory (modified from Heise, 1981).

ably longer period of time, presumably because they remember what happened the last time they stepped down. If the animal is administered an appropriate dose of amphetamine just after the initial shock, it generally will stay on the platform the next time even longer than saline-treated (undrugged) animals, presumably because it remembers even better what had happened to it the first time it stepped down.

Similar enhancements of retention in nonhumans with adrenaline-stimulating drugs have been obtained using positively motivated discrimination tasks (McGaugh, 1990). However, the tasks used to assess the effects of drugs on the consolidation phase of learning involve very special situations that may have no counterpart in the everyday learning experiences of humans. Thus we cannot really say that information acquired by humans will be similarly enhanced if it is immediately followed by amphetamine exposure.

Once information has been acquired and consolidated, there is little likelihood that amphetamine and similar-acting drugs will facilitate retrieval at a later time, unless the person is particularly fatigued to begin with. In fact, there is evidence of state-dependent learning with amphetamine. This means that if learning occurred without the drug, its presence during retention may actually interfere with the retrieval of the previously learned material. For example, in one study, hyperactive and normal children engaged in a paired-associate learning task (one in which the subjects are required to learn a set of stimulus-response pairs, such that when a stimulus item is presented the subjects are supposed to produce the appropriate response) after being administered a placebo or

Ritalin. They were then tested at a later time for their retention of the material, again after being given Ritalin or a placebo. Both groups showed greater retention when the drug state during retesting was the same as that during learning, as opposed to when the drug state was changed between the learning and testing phases (Swanson & Kinsbourne, 1976).

Bibliography

Aigner, T. G., & Balster, R. L. (1978). Choice behavior in rhesus monkeys: Cocaine versus food. *Science, 201,* 534–535.

American Society for Pharmacology and Experimental Therapeutics and Committee on Problems of Drug Dependence. (1987). Scientific perspectives on cocaine abuse. *The Pharmacologist, 29,* 20–27.

Anderson, K. J., & Revelle, W. (1983). The interactive effects of caffeine, impulsivity and task demands on a visual search task. *Personality and Individual Differences, 4,* 127–134.

Antelman, S. M., Eichler, A. J., Black, C. A., & Kocan, D. (1980). Interchangeability of stress and amphetamine in sensitization. *Science, 207,* 329–331.

Aronson, T. A., & Craig, T. J. (1986). Cocaine precipitation of panic disorder. *American Journal of Psychiatry, 143,* 643–645.

Battig, K. (1991). Coffee, cardiovascular and behavioral effects: Current research trends. *Reviews on Environmental Health, 9,* 53–84.

Benowitz, N. L. (1990). Clinical pharmacology of caffeine. *Annual Review of Medicine, 41,* 277–288.

Biel, J. H. (1970). Structure-activity relationships of amphetamine and derivatives. In E. Costa & S. Garattini (Eds.), *International symposium on amphetamines and related compounds* (pp. 3–19). New York: Raven Press.

Bien, T. H., & Burge, R. (1990). Smoking and drinking: A review of the literature. *International Journal of the Addictions, 25,* 1429–1454.

Brady, J. V., & Griffiths, R. R. (1977). Drug-maintained performance and the analysis of stimulant reinforcement effects. In E. E. Ellinwood & M. M. Kilbey (Eds.), *Cocaine and other stimulants* (pp. 599–614). New York: Plenum Press.

Brecher, E. M. (Ed.). (1972). *Licit and illicit drugs.* Boston: Little, Brown and Company.

Breslau, N., Kilbey, M. M., & Andreski, P. (1992). Nicotine withdrawal symptoms and psychiatric disorders: Findings from an epidemiologic study of young adults. *American Journal of Psychiatry, 149,* 464–469.

Byrne, G. (1988). Nicotine likened to cocaine, heroin. *Science, 240,* 1143.

Charney, D. S., Heninger, G. R., & Jatlow, P. I. (1985). Increased anxiogenic effects of caffeine in panic disorders. *Archives of General Psychiatry, 42,* 233–243.

Cho, A. K. (1990). Ice: A new dosage form of an old drug. *Science, 249,* 631–634.

Chu, B., & Kelley, A. E. (1992). Potentiation of reward-related responding by psychostimulant infusion into nucleus accumbens: Role of dopamine receptor subtypes. *Psychobiology, 20,* 153–162.

Cole, S. O. (1978). Brain mechanisms of amphetamine-induced anorexia, locomotion, and stereotypy: A review. *Neuroscience and Biobehavioral Reviews, 2*, 89–100.

Dackis, C. A., & Gold, M. S. (1985). New concepts in cocaine addiction: The dopamine depletion hypothesis. *Neuroscience and Biobehavioral Reviews, 9*, 469–477.

Dackis, C. A., Gold, M. S., Davies, R. K., & Sweeney, D. R. (1985–86). Bromocriptine treatment for cocaine abuse: The dopamine depletion hypothesis. *International Journal of Psychiatry in Medicine, 15*, 125–133.

Davidson, R. A., & Smith, B. D. (1991). Caffeine and novelty: Effects on electrodermal activity and performance. *Physiology Biochemistry and Behavior, 49*, 1169–1175.

Edwards, S., & Glover, E. (1986). Snuff and neuromuscular performance. *American Journal of Public Health, 76*, 45.

Edwards, S., Glover, E., & Schroeder, K. (1987). The effects of smokeless tobacco on heart rate and neuromuscular reactivity in athletes and nonathletes. *The Physician and Sportsmedicine, 15*, 141–147.

Ellinwood, E. H., Kilbey, M. M., Castellani, S., & Khoury, C. (1977). Amygdala hyperspindling and seizures induced by cocaine. In E. H. Ellinwood & M. M. Kilbey (Eds.), *Cocaine and other stimulants* (pp. 303–326). New York: Plenum Press.

Erikson G. C., Hager, L. B., Houseworth, C., Dungan, J., Petros, T., & Beckwith, B. E. (1985). The effects of caffeine on memory for word lists. *Physiology and Behavior, 35*, 47–51.

Eysenck, H. J. (1967). *Biological basis of personality.* Springfield, IL: Thomas Charles C.

Finkle, B. S., & McCloskey, K. L. (1977). The forensic toxicology of cocaine. In R. C. Peterson & R. C. Stillman (Eds.), *Cocaine: 1977.* National Institute of Drug Abuse-Research Monograph Series, *13*, pp. 153–179.

Fischman, M. W., Schuster, C. R., Javaid, J., Hatano, Y., & Davis, J. (1985). Acute tolerance development to the cardiovascular and subjective effects of cocaine. *Journal of Pharmacology and Experimental Therapeutics, 235*, 677–682.

Franz, D. N. (1985). Central nervous system stimulants. In A. G. Gilman, L. S. Goodman, T. W. Rall, & F. Murad (Eds.), *The pharmacological basis of therapeutics* (pp. 582–588). New York: Macmillan.

Fudin, R., & Nicastro, R. (1988). Can caffeine antagonize alcohol-induced performance decrements in humans? *Perceptual and Motor Skills, 67*, 375–391.

Fuller, R. C. (1992). Biographical origins of psychological ideas: Freud's cocaine studies. *Journal of Humanistic Psychology, 32*, 67–86.

Gawin, F. H. (1991). Cocaine addiction: Psychology and neurophysiology. *Science, 251*, 1580–1586.

Gawin, F. H., & Ellinwood, E. H. (1988). Cocaine and other stimulants: Actions, abuse, and treatment. *New England Journal of Medicine, 318*, 1173–1182.

Glassman, A. H., Helzer, J. E., Covey, L. S., et al. (1990). Smoking, smoking cessation, and major depression. *Journal of the American Medical Association, 264*, 1546–1549.

Gold, M. S., & Dackis, C. A. (1984). New insights and treatments: Opiate withdrawal and cocaine addiction. *Clinical Therapeutics, 7*, 6–21.

Goldberg, S. R., Spealman, R. D., & Goldberg, D. M. (1981). Persistent behavior at high rates maintained by intravenous self-administration of nicotine. *Science, 214,* 573–575.

Gottleib, A. M., Killen, J. D., Marlatt, G. A., & Taylor, C. B. (1987). Psychological and pharmacological influences in cigarette smoking withdrawal: Effects of nicotine gum and expectancy on smoking withdrawal symptoms and relapse. *Journal of Counseling and Clinical Psychology, 55,* 606–608.

Grabowski, J., & Dworkin, S. E. (1985). Cocaine: An overview of current issues. *International Journal of the Addictions, 20,* 1065–1088.

Griffith, J. D., Cavanaugh, J. H., Held, J., & Oates, J. A. (1970). Experimental psychosis induced by the administration of d-amphetamine. In E. Costa & S. Garattini (Eds.), *International symposium on amphetamines and related compounds* (pp. 897–904). New York: Raven Press.

Griffiths, R. R., Bigelow, G. E., & Liebson, I. A. (1986). Human coffee drinking: Reinforcing and physical dependence producing effects of caffeine. *Journal of Pharmacology and Experimental Therapeutics, 239,* 416–425.

Grilly, D. M. (1977). Rate dependent effects of amphetamine resulting from behavioral competition. *Biobehavioral Reviews, 1,* 87–93.

Grilly, D. M. (1980). Sherlock Holmes and cocaine: Fact and fiction. *Sherlock Holmes Journal, 15,* 11–13.

Gupta, U., & Gupta, B. S. (1990). Caffeine differentially affects kinesthetic aftereffect in high and low impulsives. *Psychopharmacology, 102,* 102–105.

Heise, G. A. (1981, June). Learning and memory facilitators: Experimental definition and current status. *Trends in the Pharmacological Sciences,* pp. 158–160.

Henningfield, J. E., & Goldberg, S. R. (1988). Pharmacologic determinants of tobacco self-administration by humans. *Pharmacology, Biochemistry, and Behavior, 30,* 221–226.

Holtzman, S. G. (1986). Discriminative stimulus properties of caffeine in the rat: Noradrenergic mediation. *Journal of Pharmacology and Experimental Therapeutics, 233,* 706–714.

Holtzman, S. G. (1987). Discriminative stimulus effects of caffeine: Tolerance and cross-tolerance with methylphenidate. *Life Sciences, 40,* 381–389.

Hughes, J. R., Gust, S. W., & Pechacek, T. F. (1987). Prevalence of tobacco dependence and withdrawal. *American Journal of Psychiatry, 144,* 205–208.

Isner, J. M., & Chokshi, S. K. (1991). Cardiac complications of cocaine abuse. *Annual Review of Medicine, 42,* 133–138.

Jaffe, J. H. (1990). Drug addiction and drug abuse. In A. G. Gilman, T. W. Rall, A. S. Nies, & P. Taylor (Eds.), *The pharmacological basis of therapeutics* (pp. 522–573). New York: Pergamon Press.

Johnson, L. D., Spinweber, C. L., & Gomez, S. A. (1990). Benzodiazepines and caffeine: Effect on daytime sleepiness, performance, and mood. *Psychopharmacology, 101,* 160–167.

Jones, E. (1953). *Life and work of Sigmund Freud, Volume I (1856–1900).* New York: Basic Books.

Jonsson, L. E., & Gunne, L. M. (1970). Clinical studies of amphetamine psychosis. In E. Costa & S. Garattini (Eds.), *International symposium on amphetamines and related compounds* (pp. 929–936). New York: Raven Press.

Kerr, J. S., Sherwood, N., & Hindmarch, I. (1991). Separate and combined effects of the social drugs on psychomotor performance. *Psychopharmacology, 104,* 113–119.

Kilbey, M. M., & Ellinwood, E. H. (1977). Reverse tolerance to stimulant-induced abnormal behavior. *Life Sciences, 20,* 1063–1076.

Kosten, T. R., Rosen, M. I., Schottenfeld, R., & Ziedonis, D. (1992). Buprenorphine for cocaine and opiate dependence. *Psychopharmacology Bulletin, 28,* 15–19.

Kozel, N. J., & Adams, E. H. (1986). Epidemiology of drug abuse: An overview. *Science, 234,* 970–974.

Lecos, C. (1984). The latest caffeine scorecard. *Consumer's Research, 67,* 35–36.

Lichtenfeld, P. J., Rubin, D. B., & Feldman, R. S. (1984). Subarachnoid hemorrhage precipitated by cocaine snorting. *Archives of Neurology, 41,* 223–224.

Lieberman, H. R., Wurtman, R. J., Emde, G. G., Roberts, C., & Coviella, I.L.G. (1987). The effects of low doses of caffeine on human performance and mood. *Psychopharmacology, 92,* 308–312.

Lombardo, J. A. (1986). Stimulants and athletic performance (part 1 of 2): Amphetamines and caffeine. *The Physician and Sportsmedicine, 14,* 128–139.

Lyon, N., Mejsholm, B., & Lyon, M. (1986). Stereotyped responding by schizophrenic outpatients: Cross-cultural confirmation of perseverative switching on a two-choice task. *Journal of Psychiatric Research, 20,* 137–150.

MacLennan, A. J., & Maier, S. F. (1983). Coping and the stress-induced potentiation of stimulant stereotypy in the rat. *Science, 219,* 1091–1092.

Maser, W. (1971). *Adolf Hitler: Legend, myth and reality.* New York: Harper & Row.

Mayes, L. C., Granger, R. H., Bornstein, M. H., & Zuckerman, B. (1992). The problem of prenatal cocaine exposure. *Journal of the American Medical Association, 267,* 406–408.

McGaugh, J. L. (1990). Significance and remembrance: The role of neuromodulatory systems. *Psychological Science, 1,* 15–25.

Moore, K. E., Chiueh, C. C., & Zeldes, G. (1977). Release of neurotransmitters from the brain in vivo by amphetamine, methylphenidate and cocaine. In E. H. Ellinwood & M. M. Kilbey (Eds.), *Cocaine and other stimulants* (pp. 143–160). New York: Plenum Press.

National Institutes of Health Consensus Development Conference Statement. (1986). Health implications of smokeless tobacco use. *Cancer Journal for Clinicians, 36,* 310–317.

Penny, G. N., & Robinson, J. O. (1986). Psychological resources and cigarette smoking in adolescents. *British Journal of Psychology, 77,* 351–357.

Piazza, P. V., Deminiere, J.-M., Le Moal, M., & Simon, H. (1989). Factors that predict individual vulnerability to amphetamine self-administration. *Science, 245,* 1511–1513.

Pickworth, W. B., Herning, R. I., & Henningfield, J. E. (1986). Electroencephalographic effects of nicotine chewing gum in humans. *Pharmacology, Biochemistry, and Behavior, 25,* 879–882.

Post, R. M. (1977). Progressive changes in behavior and seizures following chronic cocaine administration: Relationship to kindling and psychosis. In E. H. Ellinwood & M. M. Kilbey (Eds.), *Cocaine and other stimulants* (pp. 353–372). New York: Plenum Press.

Post, R. M., & Contel, N. R. (1983). Human and animal studies of cocaine: Implications for development of behavioral pathology. In I. Creese (Ed.), *Stimulants: Neurochemical, behavioral, and clinical perspectives* (pp. 169–202). New York: Raven Press.

Post, R. M., Weiss, S.R.B., & Pert, A. (1987). The role of context and conditioning in behavioral sensitization to cocaine. *Psychopharmacology Bulletin, 23,* 425–429.

Rall, T. W. (1985). Central nervous stimulants (continued). In A. G. Gilman, L. S. Goodman, T. W. Rall, & F. Murad (Eds.), *The pharmacological basis of therapeutics* (pp. 589–603). New York: Macmillan.

Rapoport, J. L., Buchsbaum, M. S., Weingartner, H., Zahn, T. P., Ludlow, C., & Mikkelsen, E. J. (1980). Dextroamphetamine: Its cognitive and behavioral effects in normal and hyperactive boys and normal men. *Archives of General Psychiatry, 37,* 933–943.

Rees, D. C., Wood, R. W., & Laties, V. G. (1987). Stimulus control and the development of behavioral tolerance to daily injections of d-amphetamine in the rat. *Journal of Pharmacology and Experimental Therapeutics, 240,* 65–73.

Ritz, M. C., Lamb, R. J., Goldberg, S. R., & Kuhar, M. J. (1987). Cocaine receptors on dopamine transporters are related to self-administration of cocaine. *Science, 237,* 1219–1223.

Rowbotham, M. C., & Lowenstein, D. H. (1990). Neurologic consequences of cocaine use. *Annual Review of Medicine, 41,* 417–422.

Sawyer, D. A., Julia, H. L., & Turin, A. C. (1982). Caffeine and human behavior: Arousal, anxiety, and performance effects. *Journal of Behavioral Medicine, 5,* 415–439.

Schelling, T. C. (1992). Addictive drugs: The cigarette experience. *Science, 255,* 430–433.

Segal, D. S. (1977). Differential effects of serotonin depletion on amphetamine-induced locomotion and stereotypy. In E. H. Ellinwood & M. M. Kilbey (Eds.), *Cocaine and other stimulants* (pp. 431–444). New York: Plenum Press.

Short, P. H., & Shuster, L. (1976). Changes in brain norepinephrine associated with sensitization to *d*-amphetamine. *Psychopharmacology, 48,* 59–67.

Siegel, R. K. (1989). *Intoxication.* New York: Pocket Books.

Slutsker, L., (1992). Risks associated with cocaine use during pregnancy. *Obstetrics and Gynecology, 79,* 778–789.

Sonsalla, P. K., Nicklas, W. J., & Heikkila, R. E. (1989). Role for excitatory amino acids in methamphetamine-induced nigrostriatal dopaminergic toxicity. *Science, 243,* 398–400.

Sparber, S. B., & Fossom, L. H. (1984). Amphetamine cumulation and tolerance development: Concurrent and opposing phenomena. *Pharmacology, Biochemistry, and Behavior, 20,* 415–424.

Spilich, G. J. (1987). Cigarette smoking and memory: Good news and bad news. Paper presented at the American Psychological Association Convention, New York.

Stripling, J. S., & Ellinwood, E. H. (1977). Sensitization to cocaine following chronic administration in the rat. In E. H. Ellinwood & M. M. Kilbey (Eds.), *Cocaine and other stimulants* (pp. 327–352). New York: Plenum Press.

Swanson, J. M., & Kinsbourne, M. (1976). Stimulant-related state-dependent learning in hyperactive children. *Science, 192,* 1354–1356.

Tecce, J. J., & Cole, J. O. (1974). Amphetamine effects in man: Paradoxical drowsiness and lowered electrical brain activity (CNV). *Science, 185,* 451–453.

Tennant, F. S., & Sagherian, A. A. (1987). Double-blind comparison of amantadine and bromocriptine for ambulatory withdrawal from cocaine dependence. *Archives of Internal Medicine, 147,* 109–112.

Van Dyke, C., & Byck, R. (1982). Cocaine. *Scientific American, 246,* 128–141.

Wagner, G. C., Carelli, R. M., & Jarvis, M. F. (1985). Pretreatment with ascorbic acid attenuates the neurotoxic effects of methamphetamine in rats. *Research Communications in Chemical Pathology and Pharmacology, 47,* 221–228.

Weidner, G., & Istvan, J. (1985). Dietary sources of caffeine. *New England Journal of Medicine, 313,* 1421.

Wender, P. H., Reimherr, F. W., & Wood, D. R. (1981). Attention deficit disorder ("minimal brain dysfunction") in adults. *Archives of General Psychiatry, 38,* 449–456.

Wesnes, K., & Warburton, D. M. (1984). Effects of scopolamine and nicotine on human rapid information processing performance. *Psychopharmacology, 82,* 147–150.

Wood, D. M., & Emmett-Oglesby, M. W. (1986). Characteristics of tolerance, recovery from tolerance and cross-tolerance for cocaine used as a discriminative stimulus. *Journal of Pharmacology and Experimental Therapeutics, 237,* 120–125.

Zahn, T. P., & Rapoport, J. L. (1987). Acute autonomic nervous system effects of caffeine in prepubertal boys. *Psychopharmacology, 91,* 40–44.

Zametkin, A. J., Linnoila, M., Karoum, F., & Salle, R. (1986). Pemoline and urinary excretion of catecholamines and indoleamines in children with attention deficit disorder. *American Journal of Psychiatry, 143,* 359–362.

Zwyghuizen-Doorenbos, A., Roehrs, T. A., Lipschutz, L., Timms, V., & Roth, T. (1990). Effects of caffeine on alertness. *Psychopharmacology, 100,* 36–39.

Chapter Ten

Opioids (Narcotics) and Their Antagonists

Some of the oldest psychotropic drugs used by humans are morphine and codeine; their use may go back 7,000 years. Originally these drugs were used in the form of extracts from the poppy plant, which contains opium, and in purified form they are still used extensively. They belong to a class of drugs that includes the most potent pain relievers available, so they are the most commonly used analgesic treatments for moderate to severe pain. Since users often experience euphoria, drowsiness, and mental clouding—perhaps resulting in the feeling that all their problems are trivial—these drugs are also used recreationally and are highly subject to abuse.

The most common term for morphine and similar-acting drugs is **narcotic**, which is a derivation of the Greek word for stupor (narkē). Unfortunately, the term "narcotic" has taken on many unwarranted connotations. It has been used primarily to refer to a class of drugs that promote sleep and induce analgesia, but many laypersons often think of narcotics as any highly abusable or addicting drug. From this perspective, drugs that bear little similarity to morphine in terms of their neurochemical actions or their psychological effects (like cocaine and marijuana) have been designated as narcotics for legal purposes. However, pharmacologically, only a drug with the following qualities can be appropriately classified as a narcotic: (1) It generally has sedative-hypnotic and analgesic properties; (2) it acts stereospecifically on endorphin/enkephalin receptors; and (3) its actions are antagonized by naloxone (Narcan). In essence, narcotics are restricted to extracts of opium (**opiates**), opiate derivatives, and synthetic drugs with opiate properties. Perhaps because of the confusion surrounding the term "narcotic," many authorities now refer to these substances as **opioids**. Routinely throughout this chapter, I will refer to these substances as narcotics, opiates, and opioids interchangeably. In this way, you will become familiar with all three terms.

Endogenous Opioid Peptides

The definition of a narcotic has become more confusing and complex since the discovery of a multitude of substances, endogenous to the brain and body, with opiate properties (researchers often refer to these as *endogenous opioid peptides*). Three distinct families have been identified thus far: the *enkephalins,* the *endorphins,* and the *dynorphins* (Akil et al., 1984). However, as mentioned previously, these are often categorized in a general sense as endorphins. Each family is derived from different precursor polypeptides, more than 200 amino acids long, with different anatomical distributions. Each precursor contains a number of biologically active opioid and nonopioid peptides, which are cleaved (split) at specific sites by specific enzymes (called *proteases*) to produce the active agents (Marx, 1987). For example, the precursor pro-opiomelanocortin contains three separate hormones, one of which contains the opioid peptide beta-endorphin, which in turn contains the opioid peptide met-enkephalin (a peptide of five amino acids with methionine at one end). The precursor proenkephalin contains several met-enkephalin segments and a leu-enkephalin segment (the same amino acid sequence as met-enkephalin except that leucine is substituted for methionine). The precursor prodynorphin contains two endorphin segments, three leu-enkephalin segments, and two types of the opioid peptide dynorphin.

Pro-opiomelanocortin peptides are found in the pituitary gland (indicating that they play a role in a variety of neuroendocrine functions) and in relatively limited areas of the CNS. Peptides from the other two precursors are distributed widely throughout the CNS, particularly on those regions related to the modulation of pain perception (such as the spinal cord and midbrain), affective behavior (for example, amygdala, hippocampus, locus coeruleus, and cerebral cortex), and the autonomic nervous system (for example, medulla). They are also found in other parts of the body, such as the stomach and intestines.

Though the endogenous opioid peptides are believed to function as neurotransmitters, neurohormones, or neuromodulators, their physiological role is not well understood. Furthermore, they frequently coexist with other hormones or neurotransmitters within a given neuron.

To confuse matters, at least three distinct opioid receptors have been identified, and there may well be subtypes of each of these (Collin & Cesselin, 1991). Those designated as *mu* receptors are localized in pain-modulating brain regions, are morphine- and naloxone-selective (that is, morphine and naloxone bind to them more readily than enkephalins do), and probably mediate the euphorigenic properties of mu agonists (such as morphine) as well as opioid withdrawal. *Delta* receptors are found in the emotion-modulating areas of the brain (the limbic system) and are enkephalin-selective. *Kappa* receptors are localized in deep layers of the cerebral cortex, have a high affinity for dynorphin, and may mediate sedating analgesia. These receptors also probably mediate aversive, psychosis-mimicking opiate effects, and this fact may explain why some narcotics that are primarily kappa agonists (for example, cyclazocine) do not produce drug-seeking behavior (Slifer & Dykstra, 1987). These three types of receptors may represent independent and structurally different entities, but they do not always act independently of one another; that is, stimulation of one type of opioid receptor can affect another opioid receptor. As opioid research progresses, it is likely that other putative opioid receptors will be discovered and their functions determined.

Typical Opiates

Considering the various types and subtypes of opioid receptors, it should not come as any surprise that not all drugs classified as narcotics have identical effects. In some cases, drugs with narcotic-like effects by themselves may actually block the effects of other narcotics.

In addition to the natural opiates (morphine and codeine), derivatives or semisynthetic opiates, like heroin, nalorphine, and hydromorphone (Dilaudid), have resulted from minor modifications in structure. A number of other drugs with very similar properties, but very dissimilar molecular structures, have been synthesized, including meperidine (Demerol), fentanyl (Innovar), propoxyphene (Darvon), and methadone (Dolophine).

In addition to having somewhat different pharmacological effects, these drugs differ with respect to potency, intensity, duration of action, and oral effectiveness, in many cases because of differences in pharmacokinetics (Oldendorf et al., 1972). For example, heroin is one of the most potent of the nonendogenous types of opiates. It is approximately two to four times more potent than morphine when injected (that is, one-third as much is needed to achieve the same degree of analgesia as morphine). Because of this difference in potency, many individuals have campaigned to make heroin, which is presently a Schedule I drug, a legally available medication in the United States for the treatment of severe pain for use in terminally ill patients (Holden, 1977). However, what most people do not realize is that the differential potency is due to pharmacokinetics and not to intrinsic activity at receptors. The heroin molecule is simply a slight modification of morphine. This modification allows heroin to penetrate the blood-brain barrier much more rapidly than morphine does. This characteristic allows it to accumulate in the brain much more quickly. Once in the brain, heroin is metabolized into morphine, but because it gets there so much more quickly, it exerts effects that are much more rapid and intense.

Administered subcutaneously for analgesia in humans, methadone has approximately the same potency as morphine and approximately half the potency of heroin (Jaffe & Martin, 1985). With respect to suppression of opiate withdrawal symptoms, methadone is about twice as potent as heroin and four times as potent as morphine. It is much more effective than either heroin or morphine when administered orally and has an action approximately three to four times longer than that of morphine. Codeine is approximately 12 times less potent than morphine when injected; however, it is more readily absorbed through oral administration than morphine. Neither heroin nor morphine, being weak alkaloids, are readily absorbed orally; heroin administered orally is about 100 times less potent than when it is administered intravenously. The endogenous opioid peptides are far more potent than heroin (Smith & Griffin, 1978), but they are rapidly inactivated by enzymes throughout the body (Schulties et al., 1989).

Pharmacodynamics and Behavioral Effects of Opiates

Because of the multiplicity of endorphin receptors in the brain and body, the neuropharmacological properties of narcotics have not been well defined. In addition to acting at endorphin receptors, dopamine receptors have been directly implicated in the action of narcotics. Narcotics depress the rate of neuronal firing in most areas of the brain, but some groups of neurons increase their rate of firing, possibly because they are released from the inhibitory control by other neurons whose rate of firing has been directly depressed by opiates (Jaffe & Martin, 1985). Although the predominant effect of narcotics is a sedative-hypnotic one, there may be a brief stimulant-like effect immediately after administration, particularly if administered intravenously. Some species, such as cats, and some people show only the stimulant type of effect (Jaffe & Martin, 1985).

The most prominent clinically useful effect of opiates is to reduce pain—a complex perceptual and emotional phenomenon dependent on several neurotransmitter systems located in the spinal cord and supraspinal structures (i.e., areas above the spinal cord such as the locus coeruleus and medulla). Opiates like morphine, which interact with opioid receptors and produce analgesia by the same mechanisms as enkephalins, hyperpolarize the pain-modulating interneurons in the spinal cord and depress the release of transmitters associated with the transmission of pain (Lipp, 1991). They also can interact with opioid receptors located in supraspinal structures to reduce pain.

Table 10–1

Effects of Opiate Administration and Opiate Withdrawal

Opiate Administration	Opiate Withdrawal
Hypothermia	Hyperthermia
Decrease in blood pressure	Increase in blood pressure
Peripheral vasodilation, skin flushed and warm	Piloerection (gooseflesh), chilliness
Miosis (pupillary constriction)	Mydriasis (pupillary dilation)
Drying of secretions	Lacrimation, rhinorrhea
Constipation	Diarrhea
Respiratory depression	Yawning, panting
Decreased urinary 17-ketosteroid levels	Increased urinary 17-ketosteroid levels
Antitussive	Sneezing
Decreased sex drive	Spontaneous ejaculations and orgasms
Relaxation	Restlessness, insomnia
Analgesia	Pain and irritability
Euphoria	Depression

Note. From Jaffe (1985) and Jaffe and Martin (1985).

The discovery of multiple pathways involved in pain perception should allow us to control chronic pain more effectively while reducing the tolerance and dependence that now limit the usefulness of most opiates. For example, when a patient shows signs of tolerance to morphine, which has a high affinity for mu receptors in supraspinal structures, he or she could be switched to a compound with a high affinity for delta receptors, which are more prominent in the spinal cord, in order to maintain analgesic activity (Pasternak, 1988).

Some of the most notable effects of narcotics are shown in Table 10–1 (from Jaffe, 1985; Jaffe & Martin, 1985). In addition to their analgesic properties, opiates, presumably because of activity in the limbic system, also relieve what some call psychological pain—that is, anxieties, feelings of inadequacy, and hostile or aggressive drives—as well as inducing extremely pleasant mood states or euphoria in the majority of users. Intravenous administration, or so-called "mainlining," results in what is subjectively referred to as a "whole-body orgasm" or "rush," an experience for which there is presently no explanation (primarily because only humans can verbalize such a subjective experience, and ethical constraints prevent researchers from administering narcotics intravenously just to assess the experience). However, in general, chronic narcotic use severely reduces the person's sex drive and leads to impotence.

Actions in the medulla decrease the rate and depth of breathing (respiratory depression—a primary cause of death associated with narcotic use), suppress the cough reflex, and induce vomiting (emesis) and nausea. This last effect generally occurs with the first administration, unless the person is in pain or is lying down, but shows relatively rapid tolerance.

Narcotics have a number of peripheral actions. Most notably, they induce a marked constriction of the pupil, called "pinpoint pupil" or miosis (primarily found with morphine, heroin, and hydromorphone, but not with meperidine), and they slow the movement of the contents of the G.I. tract, resulting in constipation.

There are drugs that are classified as narcotics but they have some unusual properties that distinguish them from the prototype narcotics like morphine and heroin. Some, like nalorphine and cyclazocine, have an analgesic effect, but they may induce a dysphoric reaction, cause anxiety, or have psychotomimetic effects. These are also capable of blocking the effects of the prototype narcotics. Because these drugs have agonist as well as antagonist properties, they are often referred to as **mixed agonist-antagonists**. Although these drugs have no psychological dependence liability (for example, there is an absence of craving for them), if taken chronically, discontinuing their use can precipitate an abstinence syndrome similar to that of other narcotics, indicating that they can induce physical dependence. However, as indicated in Chapter 6, because physical dependence plays a minimal role in motivating drug-seeking behavior, these drugs are viewed as having little or no potential for abuse. Other mixed agonist-antagonist drugs that have the more typical narcotic effects that make them prone to induce drug-seeking have been synthesized. Pentazocine (Talwin) is such a drug. Nevertheless, they are capable of blocking the effects of prototypic narcotics, and in fact, may provoke withdrawal if taken by someone physically dependent on morphine or heroin. As indicated previously, these various actions seem to be determined by their differential affinity for or activity at the different opioid receptors.

Although the chronic use of narcotics might be expected to lead to significant deterioration in the body, many studies have found no major damage to any organ of the body that is solely due to the presence of a narcotic—even heroin (Brecher, 1972). Most of the damage that is found is due to the poor nutritional practices of addicts, the use of adulterated drugs under nonsterile conditions, concomitant use of other drugs, and the general life-style of the addicts. Also their narcotic use decreases their ability to recognize pain that normally is present when something is pathologically wrong with them, and thus they fail to seek treatment. Their recognition that medical treatment may also reveal their addiction and lead to termination of their drug use may also be a factor in failing to seek treatment. If pure narcotics are taken under sterile conditions and proper nutritional practices are followed, there is little damage to the body. It is possible for chronic exposure to narcotics to permanently alter the body's synthesis or regulation of endorphins and their receptors, so that normal psychological processes that are believed to be associated with them, like pain perception, mood, and pleasure, may be affected for the remainder of the person's lifetime.

It has long been observed that opiate addicts have increased susceptibility to infections. Whether this is a result of the addict's life-style or a direct result of opioid exposure is not clear, since opiates have been shown to exert effects on immune functions of the body (Weber & Pert, 1989). For example, opiate agonists tend to suppress antibody production, alter the ability of white blood cells to respond to substances that stimulate white blood cell transformation, and decrease the toxicity of other types of natural killer cells. Recent studies have indicated that many of these effects are mediated through opiate receptors in the midbrain.

There may be significant damage to a fetus and neonate if a woman is chronically exposed to narcotics during pregnancy (Bauman & Levine, 1986). Newborns of narcotic-dependent women tend to have lower birth weights and be more excitable and irritable than normal babies. Some of these symptoms are probably due to their experiencing narcotic withdrawal at birth. Symptoms that persist for several weeks or months, or longer, may be due to any number of factors. Prior to birth, the developing nervous system of the fetus may be particularly sensitive to the periodic withdrawal that the mother (and the fetus) probably undergoes (Kuwahara & Sparber, 1981). Or there may be alterations in the endorphin systems of the fetus during development. After birth, the mother-infant bonding may be disrupted, inadequate maternal care or nutrition may be provided, and dependent mothers may perform less adaptively in areas of intelligence, personality, and parenting behaviors.

Tolerance and Dependence on Opiates

After continued use of an opiate, especially if it is taken often and in fairly high doses, the user becomes very tolerant to many of its effects, and cross-tolerance occurs to all of the narcotics, including the endorphins. After several months of heavy use, some users can administer 40 to 50 times the dose that would kill the nontolerant individual. Tolerance occurs to some but not all effects of narcotics. The rush and euphoria probably show the fastest tolerance, whereas there is little or no tolerance developed to the constipation and pupil constriction.

Many of the mechanisms for inducing tolerance discussed in Chapter

6 have been suggested to be involved in tolerance development to narcotics with chronic exposure (Collin & Cesselin, 1991; Jaffe & Martin, 1985). A slight elevation in the drug-metabolizing enzymes of the liver has been shown. This could lead to faster metabolic inactivation of opiates. Tolerance might also be due to the down-regulation of opioid receptors with chronic opioid exposure. However, numerous studies have attempted to demonstrate this phenomenon with mixed results; that is, in some cases down-regulation occurs, in others it does not, and in still others up-regulation of some opioid receptors appears to occur. Whatever the opioid receptor modifications observed, they are not likely, by themselves, to be responsible for the development of tolerance to opioids because they generally occur after tolerance develops (Collin & Cesselin, 1991). On the other hand, it appears that opioid tolerance is associated with a functional uncoupling of opioid receptors from their secondary messenger systems; that is, receptor desensitization occurs. This desensitization in turn may be responsible for the increase in activity of another secondary messenger system involving adenylate cyclase and cyclic AMP (which opiates normally inhibit) that follows chronic opiate exposure (Collin & Cesselin, 1991). This mechanism may also explain why unrelated agonists that also inhibit this secondary messenger system—for example, the alpha-2-adrenergic agonist clonidine—may be effective in reducing the symptoms of opiate withdrawal. In any case, opioid receptor desensitization appears to be partially responsible for both tolerance and physical dependence to opiates.

As opiates inhibit activity of several types of neurotransmitters—for example, they decrease norepinephrine and dopamine release—the receptors for these neurotransmitters may exhibit up-regulation (Martin & Takemori, 1987; Moises & Smith, 1987) and may be likely causes for some of the physical withdrawal symptoms that occur with narcotics.

NMDA receptors, a subtype of glutamate receptor important in mediating several forms of neural and behavioral modifiability, may also be a factor in the development of opiate tolerance and dependence, since an antagonist (MK-801) at this receptor has been shown to reduce morphine analgesia tolerance and withdrawal symptoms but does not affect morphine-induced analgesia (Trujillo & Akil, 1991). It is not clear whether pharmacodynamic or learning mechanisms are involved in these phenomena, but this finding does indicate that NMDA antagonists may prove valuable in extending the clinical usefulness of opiates.

Recently, both Pavlovian and instrumental conditioning processes have been proposed to account for some types of tolerance to opiates (see the discussion in Chapter 6). The Pavlovian model, which hypothesizes that environmental cues associated with the drug elicit compensatory CRs (i.e., CRs that oppose the drug-induced UCRs), is particularly controversial. Although some studies indicate that environmental cues associated with the drug effects can be a factor in tolerance to some of morphine's effects, others suggest that environmental cues can have an additive effect (Eikelboom & Stewart, 1982). Other researchers suggest that the context-specific tolerance is not due to a Pavlovian CR, because most attempts to demonstrate specifically the presence of a compensatory response with opiates have generally failed (Tiffany et al., 1983), but that the context-specific tolerance to opiates is actually due to simple stimulus habituation.

Clear signs of abstinence symptoms, indicative of physiological dependence, have been documented to occur with narcotics. The symptoms of withdrawal from opiates are essentially opposite to the direct effects of these drugs (see Table 10–1 for examples of some of the direct and withdrawal effects associated with opiates). The intensity and duration of the abstinence syndrome are directly correlated with the intensity and duration of the particular drug's effects (see Figure 10–1). For example, the withdrawal from heroin, which induces a rapid and intense effect of short duration, is relatively intense but dissipates within a few days. On the other hand, withdrawal from methadone, which induces a gradual and mild effect of long duration, is relatively mild, but the syndrome takes several days to weeks to subside (Jaffe & Martin, 1985). For this reason, many opiate addicts find methadone withdrawal to be more disruptive and disturbing than heroin withdrawal.

Whatever the case, many experts believe that, because of the poor quality of heroin available in the United States and its expense, most American addicts experience withdrawal that is no more severe than what is commonly experienced with a bad case of the flu (Hofmann, 1983). One might also note that opiate withdrawal is rarely life-threatening, unlike the withdrawal associated with the sedative-hypnotics, unless there are preexisting cardiovascular problems that could result in stroke or heart failure during the heightened sympathetic nervous system activity. Several investigators have further suggested that many of the physical complaints are really of psychological rather than physical origin, in which case they would be very context-specific (Childress et al., 1986a, 1986b; Jaffe, 1985). In fact, in one recent study, the psychological factors of neuroticism and the degree of distress expected were more related to the severity of withdrawal symptoms during methadone detoxification than either the methadone dose or the length of opiate use prior to methadone treatment (Phillips et al., 1986).

For a number of years, many experts believed that the physical dependence on opiates was the primary motivating factor in continued drug taking. However, study after study has noted that even after the abstinence syndrome has long since dissipated, the vast majority of addicts, if left without further treatment, eventually start taking opiates again. Addicts often report that the craving for opiates may be present even after several months of abstinence. This craving has been attributed to the development of a Pavlovian conditioned drive state.

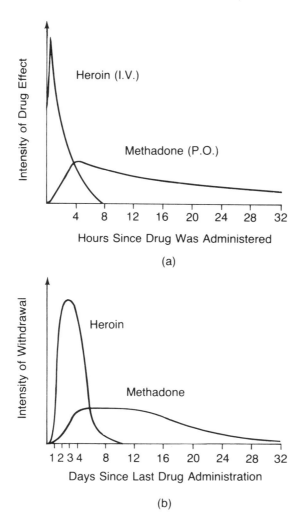

Figure 10–1

Intensity-duration relationships for the direct effects (a) and abstinence symptoms (b) of the narcotics heroin and methadone.

This type of CR is different from the compensatory CR discussed earlier, but functionally it does the same thing; that is, it creates an unpleasant state that can be effectively eliminated by administering a narcotic. Studies demonstrating how the context can trigger conditioned reactions that could subserve the craving subsequently supported these reports (Childress et al., 1986a, 1986b). Also, as noted in Chapter 6, conditioned abstinence symptoms have been shown to develop when organisms undergo physical withdrawal when opiate actions are terminated rapidly in specific contexts (which would occur with a short-acting opiate such as heroin, or if an opiate antagonist were administered). Thus the prevailing view now is that the psychological dependence on opiates is the far more powerful factor, in the long run, in maintaining opiate drug-taking behavior.

All forms of dependence—primary and secondary psychological, as well as physiological—have been documented to occur with narcotics. Other than these effects, heroin and other narcotics are not particularly damaging as far as the body is concerned (Brecher, 1972). However, they have such primary reinforcing value that people will engage in some very maladaptive behaviors (such as using dirty syringes and dirty water, exposing themselves to unknown adulterants, or engaging in criminal activities) to obtain them and experience their effects (Stephens, 1987). (As will be discussed shortly, many of these maladaptive behaviors are due to American culture's legal system regarding access to narcotics.) The high incentive value of narcotics may also decrease the person's desire for engaging in more socially acceptable activities. This outcome is not inevitable, as there are some very successful people who have been heavily dependent on narcotics for much of their adult careers. Two such individuals are the actor Bela Lugosi and William Halstead, one of the founders of Johns Hopkins Medical School, who is considered by some to be the father of modern surgery (Brecher, 1972). These people are probably the exception rather than the rule. However, we may never know how many such people there are because addiction has been so stigmatized in American society that few people volunteer information of this nature.

Contrary to popular belief, patients taking opiates solely to control pain generally do not become addicted. The common misconception, however, has resulted in their being undertreated and having to experience unnecessary agony. The traditional approach has been to administer morphine or other opiates at fixed intervals, with the expectation that the analgesia will last 4 to 6 hours. Unfortunately, the pain may then become so severe that a larger dose is needed, which then increases the likelihood of side effects, such as mental clouding and nausea. A more enlightened approach that has recently come into use allows patients to self-administer opiates, either orally or by pushing a button on an electronically controlled pump to give themselves small doses of morphine through an I.V. tube. Numerous studies have shown that patients generally maintain their doses at a reasonable level, often using lower amounts of morphine than when it is administered in the traditional fashion, experience more effective pain relief, and decrease their dosage when pain diminishes. Rarely do such patients develop rapid and marked tolerance to, and dependence on the narcotic; those that do usually are patients who have a history of psychological disturbance or substance abuse (Melzack, 1990).

Treatment for Opiate Dependence

Although some chronic compulsive opiate users eventually stop of their own accord, for the most part dependence on opiates is so strong that some type of intervention is required in order to overcome it. A variety of treatments have been tried, all with limited success. Many addicts go into therapeutic communities, like Synanon and Daytop, that have been established by addicts to support narcotic users through the most difficult periods of their dependence. One study of a Synanon group in West Berlin found that over a 10-year period approximately 15% of the individuals who stayed in the community were still abstaining from narcotic use and that only about 4% of those who left the community were still abstinent (Cohen, 1981).

The finding that abstinent opiate abusers (who completed a 30-day treatment program in a therapeutic community setting) experienced intense drug craving and withdrawal symptoms when exposed to drug-related stimuli has led to recent attempts to eliminate these responses through the process of extinction. This process basically involves exposing the person to the conditioned stimuli that provoke the craving without allowing the person to experience the drug (that is, the unconditioned stimulus). This has been found to virtually eliminate the conditioned craving and withdrawal symptoms within 20 hour-long treatment sessions (Childress et al., 1986a). How long these reductions last and how well they generalize to other drug-related stimuli after the patients' discharge remains to be determined.

Some of the more common treatments for narcotic addicts involve the use of drugs that either block narcotic effects or are substitute narcotics with less disruptive effects than those on which the person is dependent (Kosten, 1990). One of the first drug treatments for narcotic dependence involved the administration of **narcotic antagonists**. Initially, either nalorphine or cyclazocine was used. While these drugs did block the effects of heroin and morphine, thereby theoretically breaking up the relationship between the drug-taking behavior and the reinforcing effects of these drugs, they had a number of properties that prevented them from being practical tools in the treatment of narcotic dependence. First, as noted earlier, these drugs sometimes induced dysphoric side effects. Second, taken chronically, they were capable of inducing a mild physical dependence. The introduction of the pure narcotic antagonist naloxone (Narcan) eliminated these problems because it induced neither dysphoria nor physical dependence. One disadvantage of naloxone was its short duration of narcotic blockade. The subsequently developed narcotic antagonist naltrexone (Trexan), with a blocking action of up to three days, eliminated the need for several daily administrations. However, there has been concern that pure narcotic antagonists will never be very effective in the treatment of compulsive narcotic users because they do not deal with the major motivating factor behind the narcotic use; that is, they do not eliminate the psychological craving for narcotics. Therefore, without any further intervention, these individuals will probably stop taking the antagonist and go back to taking narcotics. It is argued that these drugs would only be useful in highly motivated individuals. These concerns have been supported by a recent study indicating that only 27% of naltrexone-maintained narcotic addicts remained in treatment for the 12-week observation period, whereas 87% of methadone-maintained addicts remained in treatment (Osborn et al., 1986).

Perhaps one of the most successful drug "treatments" for narcotic dependence is not really a treatment at all, in that it involves administering one narcotic in the place of another. However, the substitute narcotic has more socially acceptable qualities and fewer disruptive effects on the individual. The narcotic is methadone (Dolophine), a synthetic narcotic developed in Nazi Germany during World War II. Although it is a very effective analgesic, it did not come into use in the United States until the late 1960s.

The way in which methadone came into use for the treatment of narcotic dependence is an interesting story (Dole & Nyswander, 1976). It came about somewhat by accident through the combined efforts of Dr. Vincent Dole, a specialist in metabolic disorders, and Dr. Marie Nyswander, a psychiatrist who specialized in the treatment of narcotic addicts. Dole was interested in establishing whether narcotic addicts had a metabolic disorder that resulted in their craving for narcotics, and Nyswander was interested in pursuing alternatives to the multiple approaches to the treatment of addiction that were being used in the 1960s, and that almost always failed.

To pursue the metabolism research, a few heroin addicts were first maintained on morphine. This required several injections per day and kept the patients in a generally lethargic and inactive state. For detoxification purposes, the patients were given methadone, which was known to produce a more protracted, but less intense, withdrawal. However, rather than immediately beginning to decrease the dose of methadone, the patients were maintained on rather high doses so that the metabolic studies could be repeated with methadone. Although the metabolic research did not turn up anything notable, the researchers noticed a number of other developments in their patients. First, the patients' craving for narcotics was eliminated, and second, they began to engage in socially relevant activities. Follow-ups with more patients revealed other developments. There was a dramatic decrease in their heroin use and drug-related crimes, and an increase in their ability to function in the community. Patients began attending school, receiving passing grades, maintaining a family, and working at a job.

In summary, Dole and Nyswander (1976) concluded that, despite most of their patients' preexisting disadvantages of low socioeconomic levels, poor education, prison records, and years of addiction, the majority of those individuals maintained on methadone became self-supporting, law-abiding citizens. Furthermore, the longer they were maintained on methadone, the more probable this scenario became. More recent studies have supported these conclusions (Kosten et al., 1986).

The primary advantages of methadone over other narcotics are that it is readily and reliably absorbed orally and has a relatively long duration of action—approximately 24 hours. These characteristics eliminate the hazards of the injection method and, although it has some mood-elevating effects, methadone induces a more gradual and stable effect on the individual than heroin or morphine does. Tolerance develops to methadone, and through cross-tolerance, methadone blocks the effects of other narcotics unless they are taken in very high (and expensive) amounts. Because it is active at opiate receptors, it greatly reduces the craving for narcotics generally experienced by addicts and reduces their motivation for returning to their original drug-taking behavior. The side effects of methadone—namely, constipation and impotence—are qualitatively the same as those of other narcotics (Jaffe & Martin, 1985).

Methadone is used either as a maintenance drug, much as insulin is used by diabetics, or as a drug that can be administered in smaller and smaller doses to gradually reduce the addict's physical dependence on narcotics. Most studies indicate that the former approach is more satisfactory in decreasing illicit narcotic use (Kosten et al., 1986). Further decreases in illicit drug use can be obtained if the dose of methadone is made contingent on drug-free urinalysis; for example, when the urine is drug-free, the client receives a higher dose of methadone (Stitzer et al., 1986).

Studies have shown that methadone does decrease the use of illicit narcotics but does not eliminate their use in a large portion of addicts. They often get into methadone treatment, gradually reducing the dose until their tolerance to narcotics decreases, and then return to their original drug-taking activities. Addicts under methadone are also more likely to have higher employment rates than nontreated addicts and are less likely to engage in criminal activities. However, access to methadone does not eliminate criminal behavior entirely, since most American addicts have developed over the years a number of skills, such as selling drugs and stealing, that may still be useful to them, even though they may not be needed for obtaining narcotics any more.

Other drugs used in the treatment of narcotic dependence are LAAM (levo-alpha-acetyl-methadol), buprenorphine (Buprenex), and clonidine. LAAM is a narcotic agonist similar to methadone (Jaffe & Martin, 1985), and buprenorphine is a mixed agonist-antagonist (Richards & Sadee, 1985). Both of these have even longer durations of action than methadone. Thus they induce a much more stable effect on mood and psychological processes, necessitate far fewer drug administrations, and induce a very mild withdrawal when drug administration is terminated. It is too soon to tell whether either of these drugs will supplant methadone as the drug of choice in the treatment of narcotic dependence. One potential problem with the use of very long-acting narcotics is that, after a history of taking other narcotics daily or several times daily, addicts may not feel subjectively that the longer-acting substance is actually working. Therefore, they may feel some psychological discomfort with a compound that only needs to be taken once or twice a week. On the other hand, many opiate addicts prefer LAAM over methadone because they need to attend a clinic less frequently, experience fewer side effects, and feel that LAAM has a better maintenance effect (Tennant et al., 1986).

Preliminary studies with buprenorphine have found it to be acceptable to heroin addicts who will not accept methadone maintenance treatment, either because they view methadone as "just another addicting drug" with less desirable effects than heroin or have experienced methadone effects as aversive (Resnick et al., 1992). It has also been shown to suppress their use of heroin, be effective in detoxification, block the effects of other opiates, and satisfy their opiate craving. However, before it receives FDA approval for the treatment of opiate addiction, discussion is needed about how best to integrate buprenorphine into public policy—for example, who will be permitted to prescribe it for addicts and where it will be dispensed.

With the discovery of the endogenous opioid peptides, there was hope that one or more of these might be usefully employed as a nonaddicting substitute for opiates. Unfortunately, the duration of effect of these peptides proved to be short because they are rapidly inactivated in the body by enzymes. Furthermore, tolerance occurs with chronic endorphin or enkephalin exposure, and withdrawal may occur when administration ceases (Cooper et al., 1991).

Clonidine, a nonopiate alpha-2-adrenoceptor agonist, has been found to significantly alleviate opiate withdrawal without inducing euphoria (Svensson, 1986). Detoxification with clonidine is generally faster, and may be more effective, than with methadone. Its efficacy appears to be due to its ability to reduce noradrenergic activity within the locus coeruleus, a part of the reticular-activating system. It projects extensively to limbic regions and autonomic centers. Firing rates and norepinephrine release from locus coeruleus neurons tend to be inhibited by opiates initially, but these effects show tolerance with repeated opiate use. When opiate use ceases, locus coeruleus cells become hyperactive. Clonidine significantly reduces this hyperactivity via its actions at these cells' autoreceptors; that is, it activates the inhibitory feedback system regulating norepinephrine synthesis and release. While facilitating opiate detoxification, clonidine is not a drug likely to be beneficial in reducing the psychological cravings for opiates, perhaps because these feelings are more directly tied to opiate receptor activity. Furthermore, clonidine is only effective in suppressing withdrawal symptoms specifically associated with heightened activity in the locus coeruleus of the CNS and the sympathetic nervous system (both are heavily noradrenergic) (Jaffe, 1985). Anxiety, restlessness, insomnia, and muscular aching are suppressed only minimally.

Many users of narcotics never seek treatment. Those who do not are less likely to have severe non-drug-related problems (for example, employment, legal, or psychiatric problems) than those who do (Corty & Ball, 1986). Many of those who do not seek treatment may eventually become abstinent on their own—a process called "maturing out." While maturing out tends to be a time-related phenomenon, it is less likely to occur in addicts who are deeply involved in crime and drug dealing (Brecht et al., 1987).

The "Overdose" Phenomenon

Perhaps one of the more notable properties of narcotics in the eyes of the general public is their lethality. Reports occur periodically in the mass media describing what appears to be a death induced by an overdose of a narcotic. However, there is little scientific evidence that the vast majority of these deaths are actually due to narcotic overdose. An excellent discussion of this phenomenon was presented in 1972 (Brecher, 1972), but remarkably little has been done to advance our knowledge of it since then. First of all, although respiratory depression and death do occur at high doses of narcotics, such doses are much higher than those obtainable by most addicts. It takes approximately 50 mg/kg of morphine to kill a nontolerant rat and approximately 7 mg/kg to kill a nontolerant baboon. Assuming that humans are physiologically similar to baboons and that heroin is three times more potent than morphine, it would take somewhere in the vicinity of 150 mg of heroin administered intravenously to kill the average nontolerant human. To the vast majority of addicts, that is a lot of heroin to be administered. A gram (1,000 mg) of illicitly obtained heroin, which may cost around $100, may actually contain 5 to 30% heroin (50 to 300 mg), and injecting that amount all at once is highly unlikely. Furthermore, addicts generally have developed tolerance to narcotics. Second, there is little evidence from autopsies of addicts who supposedly have died from narcotics that an excessive amount of narcotic was in the body. Nor is there clear evidence that the concentration of heroin found in the syringe or supplies used by the person was particularly high. Third, addicts often share a supply of heroin, but only one may die from the injection. Finally, in some cases, death is so rapid that the needle is still in the arm of the deceased, whereas sufficient respiratory depression to cause death with narcotics generally occurs after several minutes or hours.

If the majority of deaths associated with illicit narcotics are not due to excessive amounts of narcotics, then to what can these deaths be attributed? One possibility is that they are due to an interaction between an opiate and another drug (a phenomenon common to a wide variety of drug-related deaths). The fact is, it is a rare narcotic user who uses only narcotics. Alcohol use is quite abundant. Mixing a narcotic with cocaine (commonly called a speedball) or with a drug that has sedative-hypnotic properties (like Valium) is also common. Such drug mixtures can have synergistic effects or interact in ways still not understood. The deaths of Janis Joplin, Jimi Hendrix, and Elvis Presley, as well as many other well-known celebrity narcotic-related deaths, probably occurred in this fashion. Although Elvis's autopsy did not reveal large concentrations of any particular drug, traces of a dozen or so psychoactive substances were found in his body. John Belushi died following an injection of heroin and cocaine, administered after a heavy night's drinking.

The adulterants mixed with illicit narcotics may also be a factor. There is an interesting direct correlation between death rates associated with heroin use and the percentage of quinine mixed with heroin. Adding quinine to heroin was first done in the 1930s as a way of preventing malaria, but it was soon discovered to be an effective way of disguising the actual purity of heroin because of its taste and because it acted synergistically with heroin. Since the 1930s, as adding quinine to heroin has become more common, the death rates associated with heroin use have risen dramatically. It is also possible that many narcotic-related deaths are due to *anaphylactic shock*—an immediate, transient kind of extreme allergic reaction characterized by contraction of smooth muscle and dilation of capillaries resulting from the release of histamine and other pharmacologically active substances. Such a reaction could result in rapid pulmonary edema (a filling of the lungs with fluid) and asphyxiation, which are not uncommon among narcotic-related deaths. The Pavlovian conditioning model of tolerance has even been proposed as a factor (Hinson & Siegel, 1982). That is, an addict may inject a narcotic—perhaps one that is more pure than usual—in a novel environment. In such an environment, compensatory CRs normally elicited by the environment associated with the drug would not be present to counteract the drug UCRs. In effect, much of the tolerance to the drug would be lost, and the person could die.

Whatever the case, there are a multitude of factors, other than simply an overdose of narcotics, that may contribute to deaths associated with their use. For example, of the almost 2,000 narcotic-related deaths in New York City in 1986, approximately 12% were regarded as general overdose deaths. The remainder were attributed to AIDS (45%) and other diseases resulting from the addicts' life-styles (e.g., pneumonia, liver damage, cardiovascular complications, tuberculosis) (Stoneburner et al., 1988).

Legal Factors in the Narcotics Problem

It seems appropriate at this point to discuss briefly the legal system's contribution to the present problem with narcotics in the United States (Brecher, 1972; Stephens, 1987). Up until the early 1900s, it was possible to obtain any drug available over the counter for a relatively small price. A wide variety of tonics and medicines contained unknown mixtures of alcohol, opium, cocaine, and other psychoactive substances. We can assume that, with such easy access to these mixtures, dependence was widespread. But we can also assume that the dependence was rather mild, because the common route of administration was oral. With the recognition of increasing dependence associated with these drugs, a number of governments around the world became concerned about the ramifications of this problem. In 1914 the United States legislated the Harrison Act to deal with it. In essence, it classified a number of drugs as narcotics (curiously, cocaine was among these) and made it illegal for them to be sold except by prescription obtained from a physician, who could only prescribe them during the course of professional practice. Initially, this restriction presented no problem to those dependent on opium or heroin, because they simply went to their local doctor for a prescription. However, before long, some law officials began prosecuting physicians for prescribing narcotics to dependent persons, because addiction was not viewed as a disease and, therefore, prescribing narcotics solely to alleviate the symptoms of withdrawal was not an acceptable medical practice. Physicians soon stopped prescribing narcotics to their addicted patients.

Immediately, some enterprising individuals, recognizing the ready market for narcotics, set up shop and started dispensing narcotic drugs—at somewhat inflated prices. The law's attempts to prosecute these individuals, as well as to legislate more severe penalties for the sale and possession of narcotics, started a vicious cycle that escalated for more than a half century.

With higher and higher prices for narcotics, individuals turned to crime to support their habits. Little money went for proper nutrients, and the physical health of the average addict began to decline. More and more misrepresentation of drugs, in terms of quantity, quality, and type of drug, and the addition of adulterants led to increased toxicity and lethality in the addicted population.

Recently the danger of adulteration was well illustrated by the discovery that the sloppy laboratory practices of a man attempting to synthesize analogues of the narcotic meperidine for street sale in northern

California resulted in the chemical l-methyl-4-phenyl-1,2,5,6-tetrahydro-pyridine (MPTP) (Lewin, 1984). The substance has been found to metabolize in the brain into a compound that kills midbrain dopaminergic cells whose axons project to neurons in the basal ganglia. This effect produces clinical symptoms essentially identical to those of Parkinson's disease. This phenomenon was first described in 1979 in the case of a 23-year-old graduate student who had developed a parkinsonian-like condition after using a meperidine-like drug that he had synthesized in his own laboratory. In taking shortcuts in his manufacturing process, the student contaminated his chosen product with MPTP. Unfortunately, the student was not the only one who used the adulterated substance, and several dozen young users of this new synthetic heroin have now succumbed to a similar fate—a lifetime (which could be quite short) of tremors, partial or complete paralysis, and abnormal posture. Unfortunately, these symptoms can only be temporarily reversed with the drug most commonly used in the treatment of Parkinson's disease (L-dopa), and they get worse with time.

Low availability of narcotics also eventually led to the more dangerous intravenous method of administration. Problems with the injection procedure were compounded by the failure to protect against infectious diseases, in part because of lack of education. Finally, vigorous enforcement of narcotics laws in the United States allowed organized crime to strengthen itself with the immense profits associated with narcotic sales. That is, the greater the penalties for sale, the higher the price and the greater the profit from selling. This phenomenon persists to this day. The basic problem is that the majority of the money spent to buy illicit drugs like heroin or cocaine goes to the bottom level of the market—to the street and near-street sellers. Only a small portion of the final price goes to the production and smuggling sector. As a result, seizures of big drug shipments, which may cost the government on the order of $1 million per drug seizure, have almost no impact on buyers and thus no impact on demand or on the huge profits to be made (Marshall, 1988).

In essence, what started out as an effort to protect consumers from becoming mildly dependent on relatively nontoxic substances resulted in their becoming strongly dependent on very toxic and lethal substances. The question many of us ask is: Would we have been better off to have left well enough alone? Although there is no way of knowing the answer to this question as far as the United States is concerned, another "experiment," conducted in Great Britain at about the same time, leads many to answer yes to the question, or at least suggests that an alternative route might have been more productive.

Around the time the United States legislated the Harrison Act, Great Britain was instituting its own similar legislation. However, it viewed dependence from a less moralistic perspective, as something to be treated. Thus, narcotic addicts in Great Britain were able to obtain heroin and other narcotics by prescription from their family physicians, while the law attempted to keep illicit narcotics out of the hands of nonaddicts. Thus illicit trade in narcotics was minimized and the population of addicts was maintained at a fairly constant level until the 1960s. Unfortunately, some physicians were rather lackadaisical in their prescription practices, and more narcotics were being prescribed than was necessary to maintain just the addicted population. This excessive prescribing led to a change in policy whereby addicts were required by law to be registered and only physicians connected with specific clinics could prescribe narcotics, a policy that basically is still in effect today.

Great Britain's policy with respect to narcotic addiction is not a panacea (Leech, 1985). Addicts still die from narcotic-related deaths and suffer infectious diseases because of nonsterile injection procedures. There is still a black market trade in narcotics, and the rate of addiction in Great Britain is still growing. In the late 1960s there was an apparent tripling of known narcotic addicts; however, this may have been due more to the duplication in registered addicts than to a significant increase in the addiction rate (Brecher, 1972). In any event, the problems with narcotics in Great Britain appear to be of a lower magnitude than those in the United States, and the lower incidence of criminal activities by addicts who do not need much money to obtain clean supplies of narcotics definitely benefits the general population.

Opiate Antagonists: Potential Uses

As discussed earlier, the CNS has a variety of pain-reducing systems, many of them involving opioid peptides. It appears that the CNS also has natural antianalgesic transmitters that do not act at opioid receptors but induce actions opposite to those of opiates—for example, the neuropeptide cholecystokinin (Wiertelak et al., 1992). To date no clinically useful drugs have been developed that act as agonists at these receptors, but several drugs that act as antagonists at opioid receptors have been developed that do have clinical value. These opiate antagonists are currently being used primarily for their ability to reverse the effects of narcotics in acute overdose and as a diagnostic tool for assessing the degree of opiate physical dependence. The long-acting and orally effective antagonist naltrexone is also being used as a prophylactic measure in opiate addicts who have terminated their opiate use but who are concerned that they may relapse. Should they do so and administer a narcotic such as heroin, they are aware that they would not experience any of the effects and that it would be a waste of money.

Opiate antagonists may also be used to reduce the abuse potential of opiates. Some opiates that are normally taken orally for their analgesic effects often are converted for illicit use into injectable form for intravenous administration. This enhances the opiate's euphoric properties as well as its dependence liability. However, if an opiate antagonist like naloxone is added to the tablet, injection no longer works. That is, naloxone, which in small amounts is ineffective orally, does not reduce an opiate's effectiveness if taken orally. But when the combination is injected, sufficient amounts of naloxone get into the brain to effectively block the opiate's action. In essence, the combination eliminates the opiate's effects if injected, and significantly reduces its likelihood of being channeled into illicit use. Such an approach has recently been taken with the opiate analgesic pentazocine (Talwin Nx). Unfortunately, if the combination is injected, it can cause severe, potentially lethal, reactions. Again, it appears that our attempts to reduce illicit opiate use can lead to worse consequences for the user than the opiate itself.

Opioid antagonists may have a variety of other potential uses outside the scope of narcotic dependence (Jaffe & Martin, 1985). With the discovery of a variety of endogenous opioid peptides in the body, there has been much speculation as to their function. Obviously, one of these is in the area of pain regulation, but there are many other areas. It has been speculated that endogenous opioids are involved in a variety of psychopathological conditions, including schizophrenia, obsessive-compulsive disorders, eating disorders such as bulimia, sleep apnea syndrome (disruptions in breathing possibly associated with sudden infant death syndrome), and attention deficit disorders. These disorders and their potential involvement with endorphins will be discussed in later chapters.

Numerous studies have explored the potential value of opioid antagonists in reducing the symptoms of these disorders, unfortunately with very limited success. While positive reports have frequently been made, failures to replicate are quite common (see studies by Hatsukami et al., 1986; Mitchell et al., 1986; Serby et al., 1986; Tariot et al., 1986). In many cases, this may be due to initial investigations being done without appropriate controls (for example, use of the double-blind procedure in which neither the person receiving the drug nor the person measuring the effects is aware of the actual drug given), or small sample sizes. In some studies noting positive effects, the test procedures themselves may have been stressful. It has now been established that acute stressors may activate endorphin systems. If the test procedures were sufficiently stressful to activate endorphin activity and exacerbate the pathological symptoms being measured, then it would appear that the symptoms would be reduced if an opiate antagonist were administered. In other cases, the heterogeneity of the factors causing similar symptoms may lead to discrepant findings. Finally, the degree to which opioid antagonists have therapeutic effects may depend on whether endogenous opioids are active all the time in a particular disorder or only under specific conditions, if indeed they are involved at all. It is clear that much work remains to be done in this area before we will have any definitive answers regarding the efficacy of opiate antagonists in these disorders.

Bibliography

Akil, H., Watson, S. J., Young, E., Lewis, M. E., Khachaturian, H., & Walker, J. M. (1984). Endogenous opioids: Biology and function. *Annual Review of Neuroscience, 7*, 223–225.

Bauman, P. S., & Levine, S. A. (1986). The development of children of drug addicts. *International Journal of the Addictions, 21*, 849–863.

Brecher, E. M. (Ed.). (1972). *Licit and illicit drugs.* Boston: Little, Brown.

Brecht, M. L., Anglin, M. D., Woodward, J. A., & Bonett, D. G. (1987). Conditional factors of maturing out: Personal resources and preaddiction sociopathy. *International Journal of the Addictions, 22*, 55–69.

Childress, A. R., McLellan, A. T., & O'Brien, C. P. (1986a). Abstinent opiate abusers exhibit conditioned craving, conditioned withdrawal and reductions in both through extinction. *British Journal of Addiction, 81*, 655–660.

Childress, A. R., McLellan, A. T., & O'Brien, C. P. (1986b). Conditioned responses in a methadone population. *Journal of Substance Abuse Treatment, 3*, 173–179.

Cohen, S. (1981). *The substance abuse problems.* New York: Haworth Press.

Collin, E., & Cesselin, F. (1991). Neurobiological mechanisms of opioid tolerance and dependence. *Clinical Neuropharmacology, 14*, 465–488.

Cooper, J. R., Bloom, F. E., & Roth, R. H. (1991). *The biochemical basis of neuropharmacology,* 6th ed. New York: Oxford University Press.

Corty, E., & Ball, J. C. (1986). What can we know about addiction from the addicts we treat? *International Journal of the Addictions, 21*, 1139–1144.

Dole, V. P., & Nyswander, M. E. (1976). Methadone maintenance treatment. *Journal of the American Medical Association, 235*, 2117–2119.

Eikelboom, R., & Stewart, J. (1982). Conditioning of drug-induced physiological responses. *Psychological Review, 89*, 507–528.

Hatsukami, D. K., Mitchell, J. E., Morley, J. E., Morgan, S. F., & Levine, A. S. (1986). Effect of naltrexone on mood and cognitive functioning among overweight men. *Society of Biological Psychiatry, 21*, 293–300.

Hinson, R. E., & Siegel, S. (1982). Nonpharmacological bases of drug tolerance and dependence. *Journal of Psychosomatic Research, 26*, 495–503.

Holden, C. (1977). New look at heroin could spur better medical use of narcotics. *Science, 198*, 807–809.

Hofmann, F. G. (1983). *A handbook on drug and alcohol abuse.* New York: Oxford University Press.

Jaffe, J. H. (1985). Drug addiction and drug abuse. In A. G. Gilman, L. S. Goodman, T. W. Rall, & F. Murad (Eds.), *The pharmacological basis of therapeutics* (pp. 532–581). New York: Macmillan.

Jaffe, J. H., & Martin, W. R. (1985). Opioid analgesics and antagonists. In A. G. Gilman, L. S. Goodman, T. W. Rall, & F. Murad (Eds.), *The pharmacological basis of therapeutics* (pp. 491–531). New York: Macmillan.

Kosten, T. R. (1990). Current pharmacotherapies for opioid dependence. *Psychopharmacology Bulletin, 26*, 69–74.

Kosten, T. R., Rounsaville, B. J., & Kleber, H. D. (1986). A 2.5 year follow-up of treatment retention and reentry among opioid addicts. *Journal of Substance Abuse Treatment, 3*, 181–189.

Kuwahara, M. D., & Sparber, S. B. (1981). Opiate withdrawal in utero increases neonatal morbidity in the rat. *Science, 212*, 943–947.

Leech, K. (1985, January). Leaving it to the market. *New Statesman*, pp. 8–9.

Lewin, R. (1984). Trail of ironies to Parkinson's disease. *Science, 224*, 1083–1085.

Lipp, J. (1991). Possible mechanisms of morphine analgesia. *Clinical Neuropharmacology, 14*, 131–147.

Marshall, E. (1988). A war on drugs with real troops? *Science, 241*, 13–15.

Martin, J. R., & Takemori, A. E. (1987). Further evidence that a single dose of an opiate can increase dopamine receptor sensitivity in mice. *European Journal of Pharmacology, 135*, 203–209.

Marx, J. L. (1987). A new wave of enzymes for cleaving prohormones. *Science, 235*, 285–286.

Melzack, R. (1990). The tragedy of needless pain. *Scientific American, 262*, 27–33.

Mitchell, J. E., Laine, D. E., Morley, J. E., & Levine, A. S. (1986). Naloxone but not CCK-8 may attenuate binge-eating behavior in patients with the bulimia syndrome. *Biological Psychiatry, 21*, 1399–1406.

Moises, H. C., & Smith, C. B. (1987). Changes in cortical beta-adrenergic receptor density and neuronal sensitivity to norepinephrine accompany morphine dependence and withdrawal. *Brain Research, 400*, 110–126.

Oldendorf, W. H., Hyman, S., Braun, L., & Oldendorf, S. Z. (1972). Blood-brain barrier: Penetration of morphine, codeine, heroin and methadone after carotid injection. *Science, 178*, 984–986.

Osborn, E., Grey, C., & Reznikoff, M. (1986). Psychosocial adjustment, modality choice, and outcome in naltrexone versus methadone treatment. *American Journal of Drug and Alcohol Abuse, 12*, 383–388.

Pasternak, G. W. (1988). Multiple morphine and enkephalin receptors and the relief of pain. *Journal of the American Medical Association, 259*, 1362–1367.

Phillips, G. T., Gossop, M., & Bradley, B. (1986). The influence of psychological factors on the opiate withdrawal syndrome. *British Journal of Psychiatry, 149*, 235–238.

Resnick, R. B., Galanter, M., Pycha, C., Cohen, A., Grandison, P., & Flood, N. (1992). Buprenorphine: An alternative to methadone for heroin dependence treatment. *Psychopharmacology Bulletin, 28*, 109–113.

Richards, M. L., & Sadee, W. (1985). Buprenorphine is an antagonist at the k opioid receptor. *Pharmaceutical Research, 25*, 178–181.

Schulties, G., Weinberger, S. B., & Martinez, J. L., Jr. (1989). Plasma uptake and in vivo metabolism of (leu)enkephalin following its intraperitoneal administration to rats. *Peptides, 10*, 913–919.

Serby, M., Resnick, R., Jordan, B., Adler, J., Corwin, J., & Rotrosen, J. P. (1986). Naltrexone and Alzheimer's disease. *Progress in Neuro-Psychopharmacological and Biological Psychiatry, 10*, 587–590.

Slifer, B. L., & Dykstra, L. A. (1987). Discriminative stimulus effects of N-Allylnormetazocine in rats trained to discriminate a kappa from a sigma agonist. *Life Sciences, 40*, 343–349.

Smith, G. D., & Griffin J. F. (1978). Conformation of (leu5) enkephalin from x-ray diffraction: Features important for recognition at opiate receptor. *Science, 199*, 1214–1216.

Stephens, R. C. (1987). *Mind-altering drugs.* Newbury Park, CA: Sage.

Stitzer, M. L., Bickel, W. K., Bigelow, G. E., & Liebson, I. A. (1986). Effect of methadone dose contingencies on urinalysis test results of polydrug-abusing methadone-maintenance patients. *Drug and Alcohol Dependence, 18*, 341–348.

Stoneburner, R. L., Des Jarlais, D. C., Benezra, D., et al. (1988). A larger spectrum of severe HIV-1-related disease in intravenous drug users in New York City. *Science, 242*, 916–919.

Svensson, T. H. (1986). Clonidine in abstinence reactions: Basic mechanisms. *Acta Psychiatrica Scandivanica, 73*, 19–42.

Tariot, P. N., Sunderland, T., Weingarten, H., Murphy, D. L., Cohen, M. R., & Cohen, R. M. (1986). Naloxone and Alzheimer's disease. *Archives of General Psychiatry, 43*, 727–732.

Tennant, F. S., Rawson, R. A., Pumphrey, E., & Seecof, R. (1986). Clinical experiences with 959 opioid-dependent patients treated with levo-alpha-acetylmethadol (LAAM). *Journal of Substance Abuse Treatment, 3*, 195–202.

Tiffany, S. T., Petrie, E. C., Baker, T. B., & Dahl, J. L. (1983). Conditioned morphine tolerance in the rat: Absence of a compensatory response and cross-tolerance with stress. *Behavioral Neuroscience, 97*, 335–353.

Trujillo, K. A., & Akil, H. (1991). Opiate tolerance and dependence: Recent findings and synthesis. *The New Biologist, 3*, 915–923.

Weber, R. J., & Pert, A. (1989). The periaqueductal gray matter mediates opiate-induced immunosuppression. *Science, 245*, 188–190.

Wiertelak, E. P., Maier, S. F., & Watkins, L. R. (1992). Cholecystokinin anti-analgesia: Safety cues abolish morphine analgesia. *Science, 256*, 830–833.

Chapter Eleven

Psychotomimetics, Psychedelics, and Hallucinogens

What does one call a class of drugs taken primarily because of their ability to elicit in normal individuals such alterations as visual or auditory hallucinations, depersonalization, perceptual disturbances, and disturbances of thought processes at doses that exert minimal changes in other bodily functions? Before we answer this question, note that both the quantitative and the qualitative effects of these drugs are heavily dependent on the dose. Lower doses may alter mood and thought content with miminal sensory disturbances; somewhat higher doses may induce clear perceptual distortions without inducing true hallucinations (strongly experienced false perceptions that have a compulsive sense of the reality of the object but that have no relevant or adequate stimuli for their induction); and higher doses may actually induce true hallucinations. Common examples of such drugs with which you may be familiar are LSD, mescaline, and marijuana.

Since hallucinations are one of the more striking symptoms associated with such drugs, many authors commonly refer to this class of drugs as **hallucinogens**. Others prefer to use the term **psychotomimetic** (literally psychosis-mimicking) or **psychotogenic** (for psychosis-generating) because these drugs induce actual hallucinations only at the higher doses, whereas with the lower doses some of the fundamental characteristics of psychosis are still evidenced (such as gross distortion or disorganization of a person's mental capacity, affective response, and capacity to recognize reality, communicate, and relate to others). However, these two terms are also somewhat inappropriate. First, drugs referred to in this fashion rarely induce a condition that mimics the types of psychoses naturally found in humans—namely, schizophrenia and mania. Second, doses of some drugs that do mimic natural psychotic states, such as large doses of cocaine and amphetamine, are not voluntarily taken for this expressed purpose. The term **psychedelic** (for mind-expanding, -manifesting, -clarifying, or -revealing) has also been applied to these drugs, but the functional meaning of this term is also unclear. Philosophers and psychologists have grappled for years with the question of what the mind is or what it means. So what do we mean when we say it is expanded? Perhaps a new term should be coined for these drugs, but I will not be coining a new one here. For the purposes of this chapter, I will refer to them as psychotomimetic/psychedelic/hallucinogenic substances, or simply P/P/Hs. (See Jaffe, 1985, for further discussion of this issue.)

Some General Characteristics of P/P/Hs

Although P/P/Hs are used occasionally in a clinical context, the preponderant use of these substances is recreational. There are four major classes of P/P/Hs:

1. The **monoamine-related substances**, whose molecular structures and biochemical activity suggest that their effects are mediated by alterations in the activity of serotonin, dopamine, and norepinephrine in the CNS.

2. The **cannabinoids**, derivatives of the *Cannabis sativa* (marijuana) plant or synthetic analogues.

3. **Anticholinergics**, which block acetylcholine activity in the brain.

4. **Dissociative anesthetics**, which are analgesic-anesthetic drugs with P/P/H effects.

Most of these drugs gain their reinforcing value for humans because of their ability to alter consciousness and perceptual processes, rather than because they exert their effects on the primary reward centers of the brain, as do some of the drugs described earlier. I say this for several reasons. First, the subjective reports of humans consistently contain references to the perceptual and cognitive aspects of the drug-induced experience, while comments on the mood and emotions evoked appear secondary to these (Feeney, 1976; Wallace & Fisher, 1991). Second, although euphoria is commonly expressed as an effect of these drugs, it is highly context-specific. In some cases, an extreme dysphoric reaction, described as a panic or paranoid feeling, may occur without warning and may persist for several minutes to hours (Jaffe, 1985).

A third line of evidence that the reward value of most P/P/Hs is not directly related to their effects on the primary reward centers of the brain comes from research with nonhumans. In most instances, nonhumans will not self-administer P/P/Hs in their pure form (Jaffe, 1985), whereas they will do so with psychostimulants, sedative-hypnotics, and narcotics. There are reports of animals ingesting plants that contain P/P/H substances, but because they have nutritional value, it is not clear whether they are eating them for their P/P/H properties or for the nutrients (Siegel, 1979).

When pure LSD, mescaline, or delta-9-tetrahydrocannabinol (a major active ingredient in marijuana) is used with the catheter infusion method, animals avoid administering them. There are exceptions to this general rule, though. For example, in one report of monkeys self-administering a P/P/H substance under experimental conditions, the monkeys were completely isolated from all visual and auditory stimulation (Siegel & Jarvik, 1980). They were then allowed to self-administer the very short-acting P/P/H dimethyltryptamine (DMT) by way of a smoking response. Under these conditions, two of the three monkeys did so. Unfortunately, the interpretation of these observations is unclear because of the well-documented stress that occurs with isolation. Under such conditions, any perceptual experience, drug-induced or not, can have reinforcing properties. Furthermore, when the monkeys were returned to their normal test environment with visual and auditory stimulation, they refused to administer the DMT, even when the monkeys were water-deprived and water reward was made contingent on DMT smoking. Two types of P/P/Hs that are readily administered by nonhumans are phencyclidine (PCP) and derivatives of amphetamine with P/P/H properties (such as MDMA). However, this finding is still not unambiguous evidence that nonhumans will administer P/P/Hs for their consciousness-altering or perceptual effects, because PCP also has opiate-like properties, and the amphetamine derivatives have effects very similar to amphetamine.

Before beginning a discussion on P/P/Hs, it should be pointed out that research on most P/P/Hs over the last 15 years, particularly with humans, has been very limited, primarily because of governmental restraints and a lack of funding for this type of research (Neill, 1987). Furthermore, since many of these substances are classified as Schedule I drugs, researchers have to apply for a special DEA license to conduct research with them. Some of the restraints have come about because of public wariness over the potent consciousness-altering properties of these drugs (Holden, 1980). In some cases the early research was conducted without proper controls, with subjects who were not sufficiently informed of the type of research being conducted (or were not informed at all that they were involved in a drug experiment). Some subjects experienced very dysphoric, and occasionally long-lasting, reactions. During the 1960s, literally thousands of people experienced the effects of P/P/Hs, either in clinical settings as a potential therapeutic tool or in recreational settings. Unfortunately, information from these individuals consists mostly of self-reports of a highly variable nature.

Because present ethical concerns limit the type of research conducted with P/P/Hs in humans, much of the research with these substances is done with animals. Many of the questions we would like to address concerning P/P/Hs are somewhat limited by the nature of the primary properties of P/P/Hs. That is, animals cannot communicate about the highly subjective drug-induced experience, so their role is primarily one of determining what the neuropharmacological and biochemical actions of these drugs are. Unfortunately, trying to relate these actions to the cognitive and perceptual effects of P/P/Hs in humans is exceedingly difficult.

One very powerful tool for assessing subjective effects of P/P/H drugs (or any other psychoactive drugs) in animals is a technique known as the **drug discrimination paradigm** (Appel et al., 1982). Essentially, animals are trained to tell the difference (discriminate) between the effects of a placebo injection (saline) and those produced by a particular drug. For example, a rat may be reinforced occasionally for pressing a left lever if it was injected with water a few minutes earlier and reinforced for pressing a right lever if injected with a small dose of LSD. Rats can learn to do this fairly quickly. After the rat learns to respond on the appropriate lever more than 90% of the time, it is injected with a test compound. If the test compound induces subjective effects similar to LSD, the rat will press the right lever; if the effects are not LSD-like, the left lever will be pressed. This procedure can also be used to see which neurotransmitter systems are involved in a particular drug's subjective effects. After an animal has learned to discriminate between the presence and absence of a particular drug, the animal can be injected with a drug whose properties at specific receptors are known, prior to being injected with the placebo or the particular drug being tested. If, for example, we want to know if a particular drug works by activating 5-HT receptors, we could inject the drug after injecting a known 5-HT antagonist and test the animal to see whether it will press the lever that has been associated with the placebo. Thus the drug discrimination paradigm is a useful way in which to use animals to compare and contrast drugs with unknown CNS effects with those whose CNS effects have been established with humans, as well as to determine the specific sites at which a drug acts.

Monoamine-Related P/P/Hs

Monoamine-related drugs are so named because they share a basic similarity with the molecular structures of the monoamine neurotransmitters serotonin, dopamine, and norepinephrine (see Figure 11–1 for representative P/P/Hs of this type) (Glennon & Rosecrans, 1982). Examples of the serotonin-type P/P/H are lysergic acid diethylamide (LSD), psilocybin,

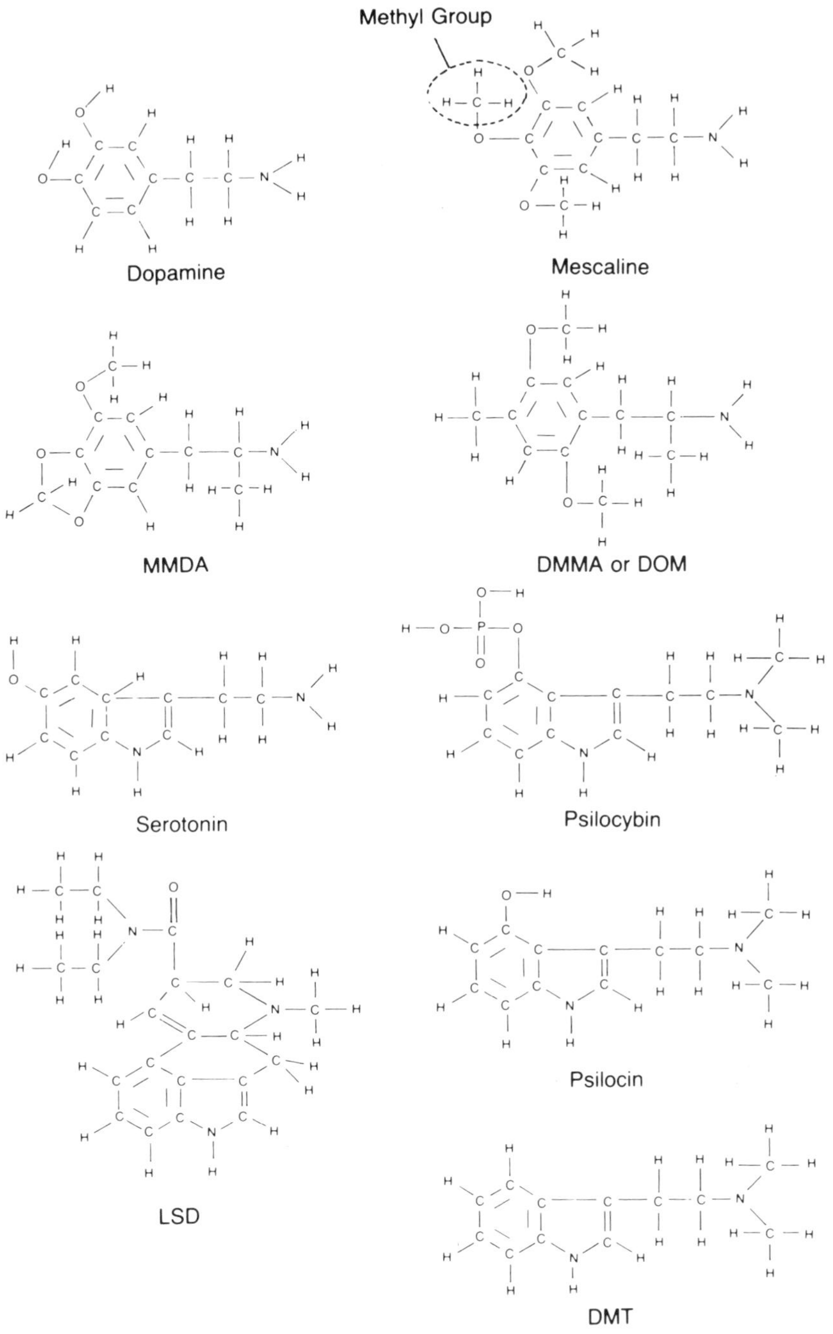

Figure 11-1

Examples of molecular structures of some drugs with psychotomimetic properties and two of the monoamine neurotransmitters in the brain. Note that all the psychotomimetic molecules have a number of methyl (CH_3) groups attached to them.

psilocin, dimethyltryptamine (DMT), and diethyltryptamine (DET). Examples of the catecholamine-type P/P/H are mescaline; dimethoxymethylamphetamine (DMMA, the main ingredient in the street drug known as STP); 3,4-methylenedioxyamphetamine (MDA); and methoxymethylenedioxyamphetamine (MMDA). Most of the discussion of this group of drugs will center on LSD, because the majority of work has been done with this compound.

The subjective effects of the monoamine-related P/P/Hs in the dose ranges that are effective are quite similar and often indistinguishable in both humans and animals. For example, in animal drug discrimination procedures, the serotonin- and catecholamine-type P/P/Hs generalize to each other (Appel et al., 1982). However, their potency may vary tremendously; for example, LSD is approximately 100 times more potent than psilocybin and approximately 4,000 times more potent than mescaline in humans (Jaffe, 1985). They may also differ in terms of their durations of action; for instance, the effects of LSD may last for several hours whereas the effects of DMT may dissipate within one hour. The durations of action of mescaline, psilocin, and psilocybin are in between these two.

The effects of monoamine P/P/Hs range from those very similar to amphetamine (strongly psychostimulant-like and weakly hallucinogenic, such as MDA), to those very similar to LSD (weakly psychostimulant-like and strongly hallucinogenic, such as mescaline and psilocybin) (Jaffe, 1985; Nichols, 1986). In some cases, the type of effect is largely dependent on which isomer of the compound is administered. For example, the dextro isomer of MDA induces amphetamine-like effects, whereas the levo isomer induces LSD-like effects (Nichols, 1986).

Most drugs in this category induce fairly rapid tolerance to both their mental and sympathomimetic effects; tolerance appears to be complete after three or four daily exposures (Freedman & Halaris, 1978). They are also cross-tolerant with each other, but do not appear to exhibit cross-tolerance with drugs in the other three P/P/H classes. The one exception seems to be DMT, in which tolerance (in cats) has not been shown to develop; nor does tolerance development to LSD transfer to DMT (Jaffe, 1985). However, the lack of tolerance to DMT may be due to the fact that DMT has a very short duration of action (perhaps tolerance would develop if an organism were exposed to DMT on an hourly basis for several days). In most cases, tolerance is lost after a few days of no drug exposure. As far as we know, there are no signs of an abstinence syndrome following chronic exposure to any of the monoamine-related P/P/Hs.

In addition to the similarity of the subjective effects of the monoamine-related P/P/Hs, as one might expect of drugs with some of the properties of the psychostimulants, they share the tendency to produce bodily effects largely sympathomimetic in nature. These may consist of pupillary dilation, increases in blood pressure and heart rate, exaggeration of deep tendon reflexes, tremor, nausea, piloerection (hair erection), and increased body temperature. As will be discussed later in this chapter, the other classes of P/P/Hs share these characteristics in some respects but differ greatly in other respects. For example, anticholinergics may increase heart rate and blood pressure and produce pupillary dilation, but unlike the monoamine-related P/P/Hs, the pupillary dilation is not responsive to light. While the monoamine-related P/P/Hs induce signs of heightened arousal, anticholinergics and cannabinoids tend to induce sedative-like effects, drowsiness, and fatigue. You should note other fundamental differences in the effects of the other P/P/Hs discussed in this chapter as we go along.

LSD's Historical Significance

Although the effects of LSD have only been experienced over the past 50 years or so, it has been hypothesized that its naturally occurring cousin, a form of ergot fungus, may have been the cause of the abnormal sensations and hallucinations reported by victims of the Salem witch trials in the 1700s (Caporael, 1976). In 1938 a pharmacologist for Sandoz, Albert Hofmann, synthesized LSD while working with several derivatives of ergot. Five years later, Hofmann was the first to describe its profound effects on consciousness, after he accidently ingested the compound while working on it in the laboratory. As Hofmann also found out rather quickly (after purposely taking what he considered to be a trivial amount—one-quarter of a milligram—and experiencing a psychotic reaction), it is one of the most potent pharmacological agents known. It can exert subjectively detectable effects in most people with doses as low as 50 micrograms (about the weight of a grain of table salt). It is up to 10 times more potent than our own hormones at its sites of action.

Following Hofmann's discovery of LSD, interest in it went through three distinct phases (Neill, 1987). The first was an interest in LSD's potential use for revealing the biochemical basis of psychosis, a phase that began to wane in the mid-1950s—primarily because it was determined that its effects did not mimic the symptoms of any "natural" psychosis. The second phase began in 1953 when it was proposed to be a potentially useful adjunct to various psychotherapeutic techniques, principally Freudian and Jungian psychoanalysis. Therapists, who often took LSD themselves so that they could better understand the therapeutic process in their clients, felt the drug could facilitate regression to obtain early childhood memories, shorten therapy, and, in particular, open up heretofore difficult patients, such as obsessive-compulsives and alcoholics. This phase came to an end in the mid-1960s—for two primary reasons. First, the psychiatric community was unable to decide how LSD should be used in the therapeutic process or to document its efficacy scientifically. Second, by the mid-1960s, nonmedical use of LSD, especially by young people comprising a counterculture that was opposed to traditional values, led to the belief that LSD had become a public health problem. As a result the U.S. government passed a law that banned the use and sale of LSD, as well as peyote, mescaline, and several similar drugs, by the public. At that point legitimate research on its effects on humans and on its potential therapeutic uses declined precipitously. In this third phase, LSD and similar drugs became just another class of abusable drugs that mainstream culture attempted to suppress. Psychedelic drug therapy still goes on unofficially—practitioners would not continue using it under difficult conditions unless they believed that they were accomplishing something. Whether it will ever return to mainstream use remains to be seen.

Pharmacodynamics of LSD and Related Compounds

LSD is absorbed within 30 to 60 minutes after oral administration, and its high lipid-solubility allows it to rapidly penetrate the blood-brain barrier and stay in the body for up to 15 hours. The potency of LSD is even more emphasized by the fact that there is general distribution of the drug throughout the body with relatively low levels found in the brain, where there is widespread regional distribution of LSD binding sites (Freedman & Halaris, 1978). Thus its mechanism and precise sites of action are difficult to determine because of the very small doses needed to induce its effects. Despite its potency with respect to perceptual, emotional, and cognitive alterations, there is only a single documented case of fatal poisoning by LSD in the literature (Fysh et al., 1985).

The mechanism through which LSD and other monoamine P/P/Hs induce their subjective effects is unknown but is most likely linked to serotonergic systems in the brain. Because of structural similarities between the LSD and 5-HT molecule and because LSD causes a cessation of spontaneous firing of serotonergic neurons of the reticular activating system, it was initially proposed that LSD acted as a presynaptic agonist on these neurons (Rech & Rosecrans, 1982). This hypothesis fit nicely with the observation that during normal REM sleep, when dreams are most vivid, these neurons also cease firing. Thus LSD could be viewed as inducing the intense emotions and vivid imagery of the dream state while the person was awake (Jacobs, 1976).

However, several subsequent lines of evidence were incompatible with this theory—the most important being that behavioral tolerance occurred with chronic LSD exposure while tolerance to its inhibiting effects on the serotonergic neurons did not. This discovery led to the theory that LSD and other P/P/Hs with its subjective effects acted as agonists postsynaptically—specifically via postsynaptic 5-HT$_2$ receptors

(Jacobs, 1987). This theory was supported by two major observations. First, the affinity of LSD-like P/P/Hs for 5-HT$_2$ receptors correlated highly with their potencies for causing hallucinations in humans. Second, 5-HT$_2$ antagonists were found to block the discriminative cue properties of LSD-like P/P/Hs in animals (Cunningham & Appel, 1987). But, again, subsequent research failed to support the theory—the most notable observation being that some highly specific 5-HT$_2$ antagonists did not block the discriminative cue properties of LSD (Pierce & Peroutka, 1990).

The most recent research on this issue still points to alterations in serotonergic functions, but the picture is much more complicated than previous theories assumed. It is now apparent that (1) LSD-like P/P/Hs bind to a variety of 5-HT receptors; (2) the hallucinogenic potencies of LSD-like P/P/Hs correlate well with their binding affinity at many of these receptors; (3) some of these 5-HT receptors are autoreceptors and some are postsynaptic receptors; and (4) depending on the type of receptor, LSD-like P/P/Hs may act as agonists, partial agonists, or antagonists (Frazer et al., 1990; Pierce & Peroutka, 1990; Sanders-Bush & Breeding, 1991). As the foregoing discussion should indicate, LSD-like drugs would be expected to exert a mixture of excitatory and inhibitory actions on serotonergic functioning; thus, even if alterations in serotonergic systems were solely responsible for the psychological effects these drugs produce, it is not at all clear how the combination of actions is related to the effects.

In addition to altering serotonergic function directly, monoamine-related P/P/Hs also affect noradrenergic and dopaminergic function, blocking reuptake (Nichols, 1986) in several areas of the brain. One area of the reticular-activating system that has been shown to be affected similarly by many monoamine-related P/P/Hs is the *locus coeruleus*, a noradrenergic system that distributes axon terminals directly to wide regions and most layers of the cerebral cortex, as well as to the cerebellar cortex (Rasmussen & Aghajanian, 1986). This nucleus has been implicated in modulating global brain functions such as emotion and vigilance. Both LSD and mescaline have been shown to depress the spontaneous activity of locus coeruleus neurons while simultaneously facilitating the activation of the locus coeruleus by external stimuli. These actions are most likely mediated by 5-HT$_2$ receptors located outside the locus coeruleus itself (Rasmussen & Aghajanian, 1986). Although it is tempting to speculate that these actions of monoamine-related P/P/Hs on the locus coeruleus may be important for their perceptual and emotional effects (such as enhancing the organism's responsiveness to both externally and internally produced stimuli), their general behavioral relevance remains to be established. From the preceding discussion, it is clear that much work remains to be done before we can gain an understanding of the mechanisms involved in P/P/H drug effects.

Psychological Effects of Monoamine P/P/Hs

The psychological effects of LSD and other P/P/Hs are very difficult to describe because they are almost entirely subjective and depend on self-reports. Furthermore, the effects are very dependent on the context and on the expectations of the person. The person may express deep religious feelings one moment, sexual feelings another, and extreme sadness, anxiety, and paranoia at another. Bizarre thoughts and feelings may represent a major break with reality and may lead the person to believe that he or she can fly, stop automobiles by stepping in front of them, or perform some other amazing feat. Occasionally, these feelings can lead to self-destructive behavior, such as attempting suicide or jumping out of windows.

In many instances, users report that they develop insights that never occurred to them before or that they see things regarding themselves or others that they have never seen before—much like looking into a mirror that strips away all preconceived notions about how they look, who they are, and the meaning of their existence. In some cases, this transcendental experience can leave them feeling quite at peace with themselves and their world; in others, it can be very disturbing.

Perceptual alterations are usually visual, auditory, or tactile and may involve extreme distortions of the physical environment or, with higher doses, actual hallucinations. With the eyes closed, the person experiences a virtual kaleidoscope of changing patterns and intense colors. Synesthesia, the transposition of sensations such as sounds into visual images, may occur.

Dysphoric reactions, often referred to as bad trips, generally occur if users take a larger than usual dose of these substances and suddenly get the feeling that they are completely losing control over the experience and that they may never return to normal. People and objects in the environment, as well as the person's own body image, may become so distorted that they are grotesque and threatening. Anxiety, panic, and paranoia (the belief that people are out to get you) are very common. Although these feelings may lead to assaultive behavior, the person is generally so paralyzed with fear that this is unlikely.

Although these acute effects dissipate within 6 to 12 hours after ingesting LSD-like P/P/Hs, a very small minority of individuals continue to experience mental confusion, perceptual distortions, and poor concentration beyond this time—in some cases for days or weeks. In very rare cases, individuals have complained about mental and emotional disturbances several years after being exposed to LSD (Jaffe, 1985). (Several individuals have tried to sue the United States government because of mental or emotional problems they allegedly suffered from involuntarily being administered LSD in experimental projects funded by or carried out by governmental agencies between 1953 and 1973. Although governmental officials have generally conceded that these projects were unethical, because of complicated circumstances these suits have not been successful. In one case—U.S. v. Stanley, 107 S. Ct. 3054 [1987]—the Supreme Court held that a former Army serviceman who was secretly administered LSD four times as part of an Army experiment could not seek redress through a suit for violations of his constitutional rights on the ground that the suit was barred by a doctrine that precludes governmental liability for injuries to servicemen resulting from activity incident to service. In another suit—Orlikow v. U.S., 682 F. Supp. 77 [D.D.C. 1988]—nine individuals claimed that they suffered mental or emotional problems resulting from their psychiatric treatment in a CIA-subsidized experimental program that included being administered LSD without their knowledge. The case dragged through the courts for a number of years until an out of court settlement was reached in Oct. 1988.) One of the key questions is whether the occasional prolonged psychotic reaction to LSD-like P/P/Hs constitutes a distinct syndrome or is a nonspecific reaction in personalities vulnerable to stress. Although this issue has not been resolved, most of the findings support the position that it is a drug-induced schizophrenia-like reaction in persons vulnerable to both substance abuse and psychosis (Vardy & Kay, 1983).

Antipsychotic drugs like chlorpromazine and haloperidol are effective in blocking most of the effects of LSD-like P/P/Hs, but these treatments are generally not needed in cases of dysphoric reactions. In most cases, placing the person in a quiet environment and talking him or her "down"—that is, talking to the person and offering continual reassurances that the effects will dissipate soon—are sufficient to calm the person (Jaffe, 1985).

Some users of LSD (and other P/P/Hs) may experience what they report as brief episodes similar to the LSD-induced state—commonly termed **flashbacks**—several weeks or months after they have ingested LSD. These are often, but not always, in the form of altered visual perceptions: geometric pseudohallucinations (patterns or figures that are clearly recognized by the observer as not being real), illusionary movements in the peripheral visual field, images that trail moving objects, flashes of color, intensified color for brief periods of time, and prolonged afterimages. Emergence into a dark environment is one of the most common precipitants of the disturbances (Abraham, 1983). Flashbacks may be very upsetting to some individuals, or they may be viewed as novel, curious phenomena by others.

Explanations for these phenomena are hard to come by because of confounding factors in the individuals who experience them (for example, multiple drug use or the presence of eccentric personality characteristics). Also, there is no way of determining when they might occur or of experimentally validating them. A pharmacological mechanism is an exceedingly remote possibility; these drugs simply do not stay in the body long enough (Cohen, 1981). Furthermore, the tendency to experience LSD flashbacks does not appear to be related to the time since the drug was last used, nor is there a clear relationship between the percentage of users who experience flashbacks and the number of times they have used LSD (Abraham, 1983). As noted previously, since the incidence of psychotic episodes (schizophrenia type) in the general population is not uncommon (approximately 1–2%), it is possible that the prolonged reactions to LSD occur in those individuals predisposed to psychosis and that the intense psychological disturbances of the LSD state then trigger the endogenous psychosis-like symptoms.

It has been suggested that flashbacks represent some type of learning phenomenon that occurs in predisposed individuals during acute stress (Cohen, 1981). Studies of individuals who have experienced flashbacks suggest that these individuals had strong tendencies to fantasize and were highly suggestible prior to their LSD use (Silling, 1980). Therefore, it is possible that after an LSD experience they may encounter a situation that reminds them of the experience (for example, a stressful situation that induces sympathetic arousal) and elicits a small conditioned response that they are able to elaborate on and interpret as a druglike experience. Others have hypothesized that some flashbacks represent episodes of visual seizures (Abraham, 1983). This theory would be consistent with reports that antipsychotics, which may reduce the seizure threshold (see Chapter 12), may actually enhance flashback episodes in some individuals.

Ever since the effects of LSD were first expressed, there has been much speculation about the similarity between these effects and those that occur during endogenous psychoses like schizophrenia. A number of authors have noted that there is a considerable difference between the two conditions (Jacobsen, 1968). With LSD, the hallucinations are mostly visual, generally consist of extreme distortions of the existing environment, and are viewed predominantly as pleasant or neutral in content. The LSD-induced psychotic state is highly responsive to suggestions from others. Finally, persons under the influence of LSD tend to be greatly concerned about their interpersonal relations. With schizophrenia, the hallucinations are almost entirely auditory, are generally superimposed on the environment, and are almost universally viewed as threatening and unpleasant. Schizophrenics are exceedingly resistant to suggestion (which makes psychotherapy difficult), and there is an almost total lack of concern over interpersonal relations. Finally, reports from schizophrenics in remission who have taken LSD indicate that they can distinguish between the two kinds of psychotic states.

Although the preceding accounts of both LSD and schizophrenia are highly simplified, they do suggest that different mechanisms are involved in the two conditions. However, it is important to point out that to some extent we may be comparing apples to oranges; with LSD, the psychosis is generally known by the person to be drug-induced and is short-lived, whereas, with schizophrenia, the psychotic episodes have no explainable cause and may be chronic or recurrent. These factors may contribute to some of the differences between the two kinds of psychoses. For example, if one's ability to communicate effectively with others is severely disrupted for a length of time, one might very well withdraw from contact with others and avoid any attempt to have normal interpersonal relations.

The latest controversy over monoamine-related P/P/Hs is centered on a chemical relative of methamphetamine known as ecstasy or MDMA (3,4-methylenedioxymethamphetamine). It is commonly referred to as a designer drug, but it was synthesized by a legitimate pharmaceutical company long before the concept of designer drugs came into being. It has been suggested that MDMA possesses both amphetamine-like and LSD-like effects, although it is relatively free of the hallucinations produced by the LSD-related compounds (Greer & Tolbert, 1986; Nichols, 1986). Users claim that it leaves them feeling more empathetic, insightful, and aware. Some psychotherapists who have used MDMA in their practice claim that it is useful in facilitating more direct communication between people involved in a significant emotional relationship. Others claim that it induces a state of reduced anxiety and lowered defensiveness, which makes it attractive to therapists wishing to speed up the therapeutic process (Greer & Tolbert, 1986).

MDMA is a derivative of MDA (a P/P/H of the 1960s that had a reputation as a "love drug"), and the effects of the two are quite similar. MDMA was originally synthesized more than 70 years ago, but until recently it received very little attention. Neuroscientists are just beginning to explore its potential mechanisms of action and its behavioral effects. As is the case with other monoamine P/P/Hs, serotonin seems to be heavily involved in the effects of both MDMA and MDA. However, rather than reducing serotonin release, as is the case with LSD, both have been found to be potent serotonin-releasing agents (Schmidt, 1987). As is the case with amphetamine, MDMA and MDA have some dopamine-releasing action. Studies with MDMA and animals have shown that following the serotonin-releasing action there is an acute depletion of cortical serotonin between 3 and 6 hours after administration, with recovery of normal serotonin levels within 24 hours. However, a second phase of depletion may occur several days later, which is suggestive of a neurotoxic reaction (Schmidt, 1987). Apparently, both the *d* and *l* isomers are involved in the first phase, whereas only the *d* isomer (or one of its metabolites) is involved in the second phase.

Because low doses appear to produce experiences characterized by consciousness-altering effects unaccompanied by intense hallucinations, users have often argued that MDMA is a unique drug that is distinctively different from mescaline and LSD. Tests with animals, using the drug discrimination procedure, support these assertions. MDA, but not MDMA, has been found to induce LSD-like stimulus properties, whereas MDMA has been found to induce amphetamine-like stimulus properties (Kamien et al., 1986).

With higher doses, which the frequent user is more likely to progress to, the perceptual effects of MDMA intoxication are typical of those induced by the classic monoamine-type P/P/Hs (Siegel, 1986). Users commonly report an orderly progression of visual imagery from simple geometric forms to complex scenes, a characteristic of these and other P/P/Hs. Auditory and body-image changes are also reported frequently.

As with other P/P/H drugs, MDMA intoxication is neither uniformly predictable nor uniformly controllable. Most users view the MDMA experience as positive and pleasant. The most common subjective positive effects include, in declining order of incidence, changes in feelings and emotions; enhanced communication, empathy, and understanding; cognitive insight or mental association changes; euphoria; perceptual distortions or hallucinations; and transcendental or religious experiences. Common negative effects are mostly of physiological origin and include, in declining order of incidence, elevation of blood pressure and pulse; muscle tension and jaw clenching; fatigue; insomnia; sweating; blurred vision; loss of motor coordination; and anxiety (Siegel, 1986). It appears that with subsequent use of MDMA, the positive effects often decrease, and the negative ones often increase (Barnes, 1988a).

The pattern of MDMA use is also typical of other P/P/H use, in that it is primarily social and experimental. Adverse reactions depend on the set and setting of the user or occur when higher than usual doses are taken. Most users adopt patterns of use and take doses that generally do not lead to dependence or significant psychopathology, although use of high doses can lead to prolonged physical and psychological reactions, such as anxiety. As is the case with other P/P/Hs, MDMA may predispose people to a recurrence of previous psychological disturbance.

Recent animal studies with MDMA have suggested that even short-term use of doses about two or three times greater than the average street dose may cause long-term, and possibly irreversible, effects on serotonergic systems of the brain (Ricuarte et al., 1985; Schmidt, 1987). Also, MDMA's potential dependence liability was revealed by studies showing that animals will self-administer MDMA by way of the catheter method (not true with the LSD-type P/P/Hs) (Lamb & Griffiths, 1987). These findings led to the DEA's classification of MDMA as a Schedule I drug. However, after several psychiatrists contested this classification in court, saying that they should be allowed to explore the use of mind-altering drugs in psychotherapy, the DEA was forced to remove the Schedule I classification (Barnes, 1988a). Six months later, the DEA reclassified MDMA as a Schedule I compound (Barnes, 1988b) because it had no proven medical value. In any event, other designer drugs of this type will probably be developed in the near future.

Cannabinoids

The leaves and buds of the *Cannabis sativa* plant have been used as a medicinal herb for centuries, perhaps as far back as 2737 B.C. Only for the last 100 years or so have the recreational uses of this plant been emphasized. Its medicinal use gradually declined, partially because other drugs for which it was used came into being with more selective action and partially because the shelf life of the active ingredients was short. About the same time, its recreational use began to increase gradually. Perhaps reflecting this shift in use, the term "marijuana" (also spelled "marihuana") was coined after the Mexican-Spanish word *mariguana*, which means "intoxicant."

Because its use changed from a medicinal one to a recreational one, certain public officials, particularly a zealous commissioner of the Federal Bureau of Narcotics by the name of Harry Anslinger, became concerned about its use. In the 1930s, Anslinger and other officials began to circulate stories about marijuana causing permanent brain damage and insanity, enhancing criminal and aggressive tendencies, and inducing sexual perversion. (These effects were duly noted in a 1936 film called "Reefer Madness," a completely serious movie that became a cult movie in the 1970s, when it came to be viewed by the audience as outrageously humorous.) In reaction to these allegations, the Marijuana Tax Act of 1937 made possession of marijuana without having paid a special tax on it a federal crime (Brecher, 1972).

A number of people were still skeptical of the potential damaging effects of marijuana. One of these was New York City's Mayor Fiorello La Guardia. In the early 1940s, he set up a special commission of experts to determine the actual consequences of marijuana use on people. The final report of La Guardia's panel suggested that marijuana was a fairly mild intoxicant with few side effects, even when used to excess. The panel's findings essentially concurred with those noted in the 1890s by the Indian Hemp Commission. Despite the findings of these presumably objective and unbiased observers, the report had little impact on the opinions of the majority of people in the United States. In most cases the report was ridiculed and criticized for its lack of rigor and its methodology (Brecher, 1972).

In the 1950s the beliefs about marijuana's effects changed somewhat. Its use supposedly resulted in a strong psychological dependence, led users to escalate their use to more potent and dangerous drugs (such as the dreaded heroin), induced a so-called *amotivational syndrome*, and was a cause of permanent brain damage. A plethora of empirical research on the effects of marijuana in the late 1960s and early 1970s dispelled some of these beliefs but led to speculation over some new potential detrimental effects (Harris, 1978; Hollister, 1986). There was a report that substantiated the view that irreversible brain damage was associated with its use—a report that was quickly and severely criticized for its methodological deficiencies. Other researchers suggested that heavy marijuana use was the cause of severe personality changes. The amotivational syndrome was still being discussed. However, contrary to the notions that marijuana caused one to become a sex maniac, studies indicated that marijuana actually caused sexual impotence and sterility in males due to reductions in the male sex hormone testosterone. Chromosomal aberrations, decreases in certain kinds of white blood cells and immunity, and alterations in DNA potentially leading to cancer were suggested by studies to be associated with cannabis use. The reliability and potential ramifications of these findings are still being debated.

Marijuana is not a drug itself; the word actually refers to the plant material, which contains over 400 different chemicals, more than 60 of which are specific to cannabis. These chemicals are referred to as *cannabinoids*. Most of these are probably not psychoactive even in high doses (Dewey, 1986; Hollister, 1986). The molecular structures of cannabinoids, which have no nitrogen atom and are not alkaloids, are very different from those of other classes of P/P/Hs and known neurotransmitters. It appears that cannabinoids possess complex and particularly unique properties, even though they induce effects similar to numerous other drugs.

The major psychoactive chemical in marijuana is delta-9-tetrahydrocannabinol, or THC for short. (Due to differences in numbering systems in describing chemical structures, the molecule may also be referred to as delta-1-THC.) Two other cannabinoids, cannabinol and cannabidiol, may be active at high doses. Although these two drugs may have minimal effects in the amounts found in street marijuana, research has indicated that they interact with THC to modify its effects (Karniol & Carlini, 1972). This finding is consistent with the common belief that varieties of marijuana grown in different localities have different effects not wholly related to their THC content. The actual THC concentration in marijuana has varied over the years (Stephens, 1987). Prior to 1974, few samples contained more than 1% THC. Between 1974 and 1979, samples averaged nearly 2% THC, and recently some samples with 4–5% THC have been observed. Hash oil, a concentrated liquid marijuana extract, has been found to have THC levels ranging from 11 to 28%.

Cannabinoid Pharmacokinetics

Marijuana is most commonly administered by smoking a "joint," but most cannabinoids are highly lipid-soluble and are also readily absorbed orally (Agurell et al., 1986). However, because of stomach acid degradation, enzyme alterations, and slow absorption, oral THC is about one-third as potent as THC that is smoked. However, if one takes sufficient amounts of THC orally in order to achieve the same peak intensity effects of smoked THC, the effects last considerably longer than when the THC is smoked. Initial metabolism of cannabinoids in marijuana smoke occurs in the lungs, whereas orally administered cannabinoids are metabolized in the G.I. tract and by the liver. There are more than 30 metabolites of THC, and over 20 each of cannabinol and cannabidiol. Many of these metabolites are also psychoactive. One of the principal psychoactive metabolites of THC is 11-hydroxy-delta-9-THC, which crosses the blood-brain barrier more readily than THC, and therefore may be more active than THC. However, because of the multitude of biotransformation pathways and metabolites and the complex interaction of the cannabinoids, no practical method has been developed for determining levels of intoxication based on detectable cannabinoids and metabolites.

What is quite apparent about cannabinoids is that their extremely high lipid-solubility results in their persisting in the body for long periods of time. Studies have shown that after a single administration of THC, detectable levels of THC are found in the body for weeks or longer, depending on how much was administered and the sensitivity of the assessment method. A number of investigators have suggested that this is an important factor in marijuana's effects, perhaps because cannabinoids may accumulate in the body, particularly in the lipid membranes of neurons. However, the actual consequences of such an accumulation, as well as the sites of accumulation, can only be speculated upon at this time. It is most likely that the major site of accumulation is adipose tissue (comprising some 10–20% of the human body), which would mean that these drugs would have no significant psychological consequences (Hollister, 1986).

Pharmacodynamics of Delta-9-THC

Little is known about the mechanisms of action of THC at the neuronal level. Our lack of understanding of these mechanisms is certainly not due to lack of interest or too little research in the area; rather, it is due to some unique characteristics of THC (Martin, 1986). First, THC has such high lipid-solubility that it is absorbed in high concentrations in practically all tissues. Second, THC alters just about every biological system in which it is examined. Unfortunately, establishing the significance of these effects with respect to THC's psychoactive properties is difficult.

THC exerts nonspecific "fluidizing" effects on lipid membranes—similar to those of general anesthetics and alcohol, but not to the same degree (Martin, 1986). This "fluidizing" could partially explain why THC has sedative-like effects without having anesthetic properties, but evidence for this possibility is still weak. Until recently, evidence for specific receptors for THC was circumstantial. As would be expected for a specific receptor interaction, modest structural modifications of the THC molecule can result in profound changes in its behavioral effects. Also, there is a definite stereospecificity of the THC molecule, with the levo isomer being from 6 to 100 times more active than the dextro isomer, depending on the species and the behavioral tests used.

Although receptor binding studies, which are normally used to assess the presence of specific receptors for ligands, have been hampered by THC's extreme lipid solubility and its large degree of nonspecific binding to membranes, researchers have now confirmed the existence of a cannabinoid receptor in the brain (Matsuda et al., 1990). Cannabinoids appear to alter mood and cognition by binding to this receptor (a G protein–coupled receptor) and inhibiting a secondary messenger system (adenylate cyclase) in a dose-dependent stereospecific manner. These receptors are widely distributed in the brain, but the pattern is uneven. The highest levels are found in the cerebral cortex, hippocampus, hypothalamus, and amygdala. These areas are critically important for higher mental processes, memory formation, primary drive regulation, and emotional expression—all of which are altered to some degree by cannabinoids.

At least one endogenous ligand for cannabinoid receptors has been isolated from brain tissue (Barinaga, 1992). Like THC, the ligand is fat-soluble, but it is a simpler molecule that is derived from arachidonic acid, a fatty acid common to cell membranes. The ligand has been christened "anandamide," from a Sanskrit word meaning internal bliss. What functions the cannabinoid receptor and its ligand actually serve in the CNS have yet to be determined, but these discoveries are likely to infuse new energy into the search for drugs with the therapeutic effects of marijuana (discussed later) without causing intoxication.

Depending on the concentration, THC has been shown to either enhance or inhibit release of various neurotransmitters (Campbell et al., 1986). Similarly, electrical recordings of CNS neuronal activity have suggested both excitatory and inhibitory effects of THC. Despite these inconsistencies, electrical recordings in the hippocampus of rats have been shown to change dramatically when behaviorally effective doses of THC are administered. Thus it is probable that THC-mediated changes in hippocampal operations are partly responsible for the distortions in memory and cognitive performance that commonly occur during marijuana intoxication (Campbell et al., 1986).

These speculations are supported by findings that suggest that THC disrupts cholinergic functioning because the hippocampus contains high concentrations of cholinergic neurons (Miller & Branconnier, 1983). The effects of cannabinoids on memory processes are similar to those found following administration of anticholinergics (such as scopolamine) and those found in neurological patients suffering from deficits in hippocampal (limbic) cholinergic functioning. Physiologically, cannabinoids exhibit some similarities to anticholinergics, including dry mouth, increased heart rate, decreased sweating, and bronchodilation (one notable exception is that whereas cannabinoids decrease pressure within the eyeball, anticholinergics increase it). It does not appear that THC operates at postsynaptic cholinergic receptors, since drugs that normally reverse the effects of competitive acetylcholine antagonists (such as physostigmine, a drug that reduces the enzymatic breakdown of acetylcholine in the synapse) do not change the subjective effects of THC. However, because THC (but not the weakly psychoactive cannabidiol) decreases acetylcholine turnover in the hippocampus, one mode of action of THC may involve a selective reduction of acetylcholine synthesis or its release from axon terminals, perhaps by acting through presynaptic cholinergic mechanisms.

There is now fairly good evidence that many of marijuana's rewarding effects are mediated by the same brain reward system (discussed in Chapter 6) through which other recreational and abuse-prone drugs act (Gardner & Lowinson, 1991). For example, THC has been found to enhance electrical brain stimulation reward and to enhance both basal and stimulated dopamine release in reward-relevant loci; both of these actions are reduced with opiate antagonists. However, it has not been established whether animals will work for microinjections of cannabinoids delivered into these regions. If future studies do find such a phenomenon, it will be difficult to reconcile with the fact that animals do not readily self-administer cannabinoids through inhalation or intravenous routes. It may be that cannabinoids exert actions in other brain areas that are aversive and counteract their rewarding properties (e.g., see comments at the end of this chapter).

Psychological Effects of Marijuana

Interpreting the effects of marijuana on behavioral variables is complicated by the fact that set and setting variables—for example, context, the user's personality, previous marijuana experiences, and expectations—have been shown to play a critical role in changes in mood and behavior that occur following marijuana use (Ferraro, 1980), and may even influence the rate of THC metabolism (Cami et al., 1991). Thus all the effects noted in this discussion of marijuana are likely to be due to the interaction between these factors and the actions of the drug on the nervous system.

The acute effects of marijuana (i.e., being "stoned") generally consist of an increasingly dose-dependent impairment of memory and cognitive functions, such as attending, speaking, problem solving, and concept formation (Azorlosa et al., 1992; Dewey, 1986; Ferraro, 1980). The person's speech is fragmented, suggestive of disjointed thought patterns, and the speaker often forgets what (s)he or others have recently said. Ideas extraneous to the focus of an individual's attention appear to enter consciousness, producing a loosening of associations. Phenomena that are not usually associated with each other in normal waking life tend to appear connected under the influence of marijuana, and phenomena or ideas that are commonly associated in normal waking life may seem irrelevant or unconnected. Sometimes the person under the influence of marijuana gains insights of great importance. Unfortunately, while under the influence, the person's ability to reflect on or analyze the quality of these insights is greatly impaired, and when the intoxication phase is over, the great insights often turn out to be mundane or unworkable ideas.

A multitude of studies using a wide variety of cognitive tasks strongly suggest that many of the cognitive deficits produced by marijuana can be attributed to alterations in memory functions (Hooker & Jones, 1987). There is a great deal of variability in the degree to which marijuana disrupts cognitive functions, some of which is dependent upon differences in the drug dose used and the specific task (Azorlosa et al., 1992). It is also well established that the level of motivation to perform well may affect the degree to which marijuana impairs performance (Cami et al., 1991). Cognitive and behavioral tolerance to marijuana's effects can also occur, such that cognitive deficits noted in infrequent users may not be observed in individuals who use it frequently.

One of the primary effects of marijuana is interference with short-term memory (the ability to maintain access to newly acquired information for several seconds or minutes). This is found to occur with both verbal and graphic material. Marijuana also disrupts long-term memory retrieval (the ability to gain access to information acquired several hours, or longer, prior to marijuana intoxication). This effect is more predominant with recall (the ability to reproduce the previously learned material) than with recognition (the ability to choose from a number of items which of those the person has previously learned). Much of the memory disruption appears to be due to increased imagery and thought flow coming out of the intrusion of irrelevant associations (Hooker & Jones, 1987). However, there is little evidence that, once the person returns from the intoxicated state, retrieval of information learned prior to the intoxicated state is affected.

There is also evidence for weak state-dependent retrieval effects with marijuana, in which information acquired under the influence of marijuana is retrieved better under marijuana than under nondrug conditions. But these effects are more likely to occur under recall conditions that provide minimal external cues to the person (Eich et al., 1975).

Although there are no studies directly assessing the effects of marijuana on classroom learning experiences, the similarity between the types of activities relevant to such settings and those observed in the laboratory is so close as to strongly suggest that marijuana interferes with classroom functioning and knowledge acquisition. This is an important factor considering the extent of marijuana use among high school students today.

The detrimental effects of marijuana on complex psychomotor skills in the laboratory have also been observed in real-life situations of driving and flying (Hollister, 1986). While marijuana may be less detrimental to driving performance than alcohol is, it nevertheless is a potential causal factor in accidents that occur while driving or engaging in similar activities. Some of the detrimental effects on performance may persist for some time, possibly up to 24 hours, beyond the period of subjective intoxication (Hieshman et al., 1990; Leirer et al., 1991). It is interesting to note that over the last decade there has been a significant change in the recognition of these effects by the general population and marijuana users in particular. Prior to 1975, the majority of marijuana users denied that marijuana impaired driving skills, whereas since 1975, there has been a growing recognition by these individuals that driving skills are impaired by the substance (Grilly, 1981). Whether this influences their actual drug use while driving is unknown.

As with most P/P/Hs, the euphoriant properties of marijuana seem restricted to humans and appear to be secondary to the alterations in consciousness. Psychoactive cannabinoids have a sedative-like action in most people, as opposed to the sympathomimetic-like effects of the monoamine-related compounds. There is no cross-tolerance between these two classes, and the monoamine-related compounds are more potent in their perceptual and hallucinatory actions (Jaffe, 1985). While many people find the marijuana experience pleasurable, others do not. Those who do experience pleasurable effects may find them to wax and wane during the period of intoxication, and in some cases they may develop a dysphoric reaction. This generally occurs if the person ingests an amount that is considerably higher than he or she is used to. Such cases are more common with oral administration, because the absorption of THC from the G.I. tract is considerably slower than absorption through smoking, and because the person has difficulty in regulating the amount of marijuana ingested.

Other effects of marijuana that may be viewed positively by the user are its effects on appetite (Foltin et al., 1986) and sexual experiences, although these appear to be heavily dependent on cultural expectations (Meyer, 1978). For example, North Americans commonly report and, in some cases, exhibit increases in appetite (particularly sweets) and weight gain (Foltin et al., 1986). They also report that they experience enhanced sexual stimulation under the influence of marijuana (Meyer, 1978). In other countries, cannabis is used as a sexual depressant (in India, for example) or to suppress feelings of hunger (in Jamaica). While acute use of marijuana in low doses may enhance the sexual experience, high doses or prolonged use may lead to a depression of sexual desire and even impotence (Hollister, 1986).

What makes the marijuana experience rewarding? We really do not know. The transient cognitive and memory disruptions associated with marijuana may account for both its popularity in some, but by no means all, humans, and its universal unpopularity in nonhumans (Feeney, 1976). That is, the new and unrelated intrusions into thought, the loosening of traditional or learned associations among stimuli and responses, the encoding of new information subject to associative links that normally would be inhibited, the ambiguity and variability in the perceptual experience, and so forth, result in novel experiences, feelings of creativity, and insightfulness (Feeney, 1976; Hooker & Jones, 1987). Those individuals who are not particularly anxious about the unfamiliar or the unconventional or about loss of control and the unpredictability of their world may find such effects pleasurable, as long as they can retain control over the time and degree of these effects. Those who are anxious about these may find such effects unpleasurable. (I suspect that all nonhumans fall into the latter category.) Millions of years of evolution have led to animals seeking the predictable and adaptively responding to the prevailing stimulus conditions. They had no time for reflecting, lowering their level of vigilance, or misinterpreting the potential dangers of a situation, because there was always another animal waiting around the corner ready to eat them if they did. In most cases, humans have transcended such evolutionary constraints. Thus we find ourselves in a world where the effects of drugs such as those contained in marijuana may in fact be viewed as pleasurable. Other drugs described in this chapter may have similar qualities, but marijuana's effects are relatively short-lasting and are easier to control, tolerance to them develops relatively slowly, and the immediate side effects associated with marijuana are less troublesome.

Psychopathological Effects of Marijuana

The acute panic anxiety reaction, noted particularly when unexpectedly strong marijuana is used, is the most common adverse psychological effect. More serious cannabis-related psychoses and other intellectual deficiencies have been reported in countries in which cannabis use is extensive. (Some of the individuals diagnosed as having cannabis psychosis had used cannabis for five years or more in amounts up to several grams per day; Imade & Ebie, 1991.) However, such reactions do not appear common in North America (Hollister, 1986). Interestingly, in a recent study evaluating the effect of cannabis on positive and negative symptoms in schizophrenics (described in Chapter 12), it was observed that negative symptoms were lower in schizophrenic cannabis abusers than nonabusers, supporting a self-medication hypothesis of cannabis abuse (Peralta & Cuesta, 1992).

The few studies that have investigated the effects of prolonged and heavy use of cannabinoids have not shown any systematic decrements in mental activities suggestive of impairments of brain or cerebral function and cognition—other than the previously noted transient cognitive impairments resulting from acute cannabinoid exposure (Ferraro, 1980; Hollister, 1986). For example, in one study of long-term cannabis use in 10 subjects born, raised, and educated in the United States, no cognitive deficits could be determined in any of the subjects, most of whom had engaged in extremely heavy use for over seven years (the subjects used a cannabis-tobacco mixture daily as a sacrament of communion in the context of their particular religion) (Schaeffer et al., 1981). In fact, the intellectual functioning among the adults tested was above average, and in two of the subjects where similar tests had been conducted 15 and 20 years previously, the I.Q. scores were virtually unchanged. It should be stressed that these adults were well educated prior to their cannabis use, did not use other psychoactive substances, observed a good diet consisting of vegetables, fruit, and small amounts of meat, and adhered to a strict religious doctrine. Obviously, such individuals are not particularly representative of a very broad spectrum of people.

Several studies conducted in the 1970s in Jamaica, Greece, and Costa Rica did not find any notable cognitive or physical differences between heavy users of cannabis (who had smoked in the vicinity of 10 "joints" a day for several years) and suitably matched nonusers (Hollister, 1986). Follow-up studies conducted on similar samples in Costa Rica and India also found no significant differences between users and nonusers on most tests of a variety of intellectual functions (Page et al., 1988; Varma et al., 1988). These later studies did find that users evidenced small, but reliable, deficits in some perceptual-motor tasks and sustained attention and short-term memory tests requiring considerable mental effort. A more recent study, which assessed brain wave patterns during a complex auditory selective attention task, indicated that chronic marijuana users had more difficulty than nonusers in setting up an accurate focus of attention and in filtering out irrelevant information (Solowij et al., 1991). Unfortunately from a methodological standpoint, the users in all three studies were only asked to abstain from cannabis use 12–24 hours prior to testing; considering the amount of cannabis normally consumed by the users in these studies, it is quite possible they were still somewhat "stoned" during these tests.

The one common adverse effect noted in some of these studies was related to lung damage; however, in most cases, cannabis was mixed with tobacco, so it is difficult to assess how much of the damage was due solely to the cannabis. Again, it must be stressed that the user samples studied were small (a total of just over 125 users were observed). In epidemiological studies it may be necessary to follow thousands of people over a period of years before we can definitively determine the true consequences of long-term cannabis use.

It should be pointed out that the quality of the studies in this area is variable, and their results often conflict. Some of the variability no doubt can be attributed to the variability in the users' personality and emotional dispositions, so that marijuana use may have either positive, negative, or benign effects on mental health and adjustment depending on the user's disposition (Zablocki et al., 1991). Also, it is difficult to distinguish between drug-induced psychological problems and preexisting determinants. It is often the case that extensive drug users are those who have had emotional problems prior to use (Hollister, 1986). Furthermore, use in North America is a relatively recent phenomenon, and the studies done with American users have involved relatively small samples of highly motivated college populations using smaller amounts of marijuana with lower amounts of THC. Whatever the case, most clinicians caution against the use of marijuana by persons with a history of serious psychological problems. This caution also applies to adolescents, who are generally going through a lot of turmoil regarding the psychosocial development of their identity, their role in the adult world ahead, and their cognitive and interpersonal skills.

While violence and aggression have sometimes been associated with marijuana use, there is little evidence to support such an association (Dewey, 1986; Hollister, 1986). In fact, the predominant finding is that low doses of marijuana have little effect on aggression, and moderate to high doses tend to inhibit aggression in humans. There may be some individuals with poor impulse control or a proneness to violence, or who are under stress, for whom marijuana use may trigger an aggressive episode.

Rarely, the *flashback* phenomenon may also occur with cannabis use (Fischer & Taschner, 1991). However, there does not appear to be a correlation between the amount of cannabis consumed and the occurrence of a flashback. On the other hand, the probability of the occurrence of a flashback in a cannabis user seems to increase with the amount of LSD-like P/P/Hs the person has used (Abraham, 1983). Therefore, these individuals' cannabis use may simply be coincidental with their experiencing flashbacks, or it may be a precipitating factor in inducing LSD flashbacks. Although a flashback may range from a mild to a quite vivid recreation of the drug-induced experience, most clinicians feel that it requires little or no treatment.

As is the case with cognitive deficits, brain damage associated with cannabis use has often been suspected. Again, however, there is little evidence for it (Hollister, 1986). One of the earliest studies—a British study in 1971—used air encephalography to assess the size of the ventricles in the brains of a small sample of marijuana users (the ventricles are spaces inside the brain containing cerebrospinal fluid). The researchers reported ventricular enlargements indicative of brain atrophy. However, the methodology of this study was heavily criticized because the subjects had used other illicit drugs and because the comparison group and diagnostic technique may have been inappropriate. Subsequent studies using echo encephalography and computerized transaxial tomography with heavy cannabis users failed to find any evidence of cerebral atrophy. (However, one's interpretation of these findings must be tempered by the fact that many individuals diagnosed with endogenous psychosis have no gross brain abnormalties that can be detected with present neurological techniques.) With respect to neuropsychological test performance, virtually all studies have failed to reveal irrefutable evidence of long-term impairments in humans following chronic marijuana exposure.

Tolerance and Dependence on Cannabis

Many users of marijuana report that continued use of it results in their becoming more sensitive to its effects (a so-called reverse tolerance). As suggested in Chapter 6, this phenomenon may be due to the novice user—exposed to low doses of THC—becoming more aware of marijuana's subjective effects, or to drug accumulation, since cannabinoids are stored in fat. However, the vast majority of studies indicate that tolerance can develop to most of the psychological effects (Dewey, 1986), but as is the case with most drugs, tolerance development to THC is dose dependent. Apparently, the usual patterns of marijuana smoking by North Americans—on the order of a joint or less a day (about 10 mg THC)—is such that tolerance to marijuana's effects does not develop (Perez-Reyes et al., 1991). However, with sufficiently high dosages, tolerance to most of THC's effects is likely to occur. Although some unknown pharmacodynamic mechanisms may be involved in the tolerance developed to cannabinoids, most of the evidence suggests that it is due to behavioral or perceptual adaptations to their disruptive effects (Ferraro, 1976).

Dependence on marijuana is primarily psychological—that is, it is due to its mood- and cognitive-altering properties. Although in some ways it is like comparing apples to oranges, most experts would probably agree that psychological dependence associated with cannabinoids (that is, the compulsive need to experience the effects) is of a considerably lower degree than that associated with alcohol and other sedative-hypnotics, opiates, or the psychostimulants (Dewey, 1986; Hollister, 1986; Jaffe, 1985). Physical dependence as a result of social use of marijuana is even more atypical; until the mid-1970s most experts even denied its existence. However, studies have determined that cessation of extremely high-dosage (e.g., 210 mg THC per day) chronic marijuana use by humans can precipitate an abstinence syndrome that may include one or more of the following: irritability, restlessness, decreased appetite, sleep disturbance, sweating, tremor, nausea, vomiting, and diarrhea. Similar symptoms have been observed in animals withdrawn from THC after chronic exposure (Beardsley et al., 1986). Although naloxone has been reported to precipitate narcotic-like withdrawal signs in rats administered THC chronically, these have not been found in monkeys. Thus it is not likely that chronic THC exposure induces dependence of the opiate type. (If it did, narcotic addicts would probably have figured it out a long time ago because they would attempt to use marijuana to alleviate opiate withdrawal.)

Non-CNS-Related Effects of Marijuana

Although they are outside the scope of the present text, there are a number of other potential consequences of marijuana use that the reader should be aware of, so these will briefly be discussed (see Dewey, 1986, and Hollister, 1986, for a more complete description). The peripheral manifestations of acute marijuana intoxication are minimal and consist predominantly of tachycardia (rapid heart rate) and conjunctival reddening of the eyes. There may be a slight increase in blood pressure with low doses and a slight decrease with high doses. Some individuals may experience blurred vision or headaches. Following acute intoxication there are generally no residual physiological effects analogous to the alcohol hangover, unless particularly large quantities are used. As an illustration of how high the dosage of THC must be to induce such effects, some of the studies cited earlier in this chapter reported no discomfort in the marijuana users who had smoked 10–15 joints a day for years (on the order of 150 mg THC a day) when they were asked to abstain from smoking for 12–24 hours.

With chronic marijuana use, there is considerable evidence that pulmonary function is impaired, perhaps more so than with cigarette smoking, because marijuana joints are not filtered. A number of studies have indicated that marijuana "tars" can be tumor-producing. Some studies have suggested that reproductive functioning may be impaired with marijuana, which may be reflected in lower testosterone levels (although generally within normal levels), reduced sex drive, and less vigorous sperm motility in males and interference with fertility in females. Most studies, however, have failed to show any significant effects of chronic marijuana use on the reproductive hormones of either men or women (Block et al., 1991). Given the potential alterations in hormonal functions, and the importance of these in the developing fetus, marijuana use (or any other drug use) during pregnancy is strongly discouraged. Although some studies have suggested that marijuana may interfere with the immune response and affect chromosomes, the clinical significance of those studies is questionable. Furthermore, many other studies have found no effects of marijuana in these areas.

On the other side of the coin, cannabinoids have been suggested to have some therapeutic value (Jaffe, 1985). Some of these are effective in significantly reducing the pressure in the eye associated with glaucoma. Others are effective in treating the nausea and vomiting associated with chemotherapy for cancer and AIDS. Although cannabinoids are not invariably superior to other medications used in these problems, they may prove useful in certain patients for whom these drugs are ineffective. However, because of the development of synthetic cannabinoid compounds with fewer intoxicating qualities and concerns over the potential harmfulness of marijuana, in 1992 the U.S. government stopped accepting new participants in its medicinal marijuana program, which, for some 15 years, had been supplying government-grown marijuana to patients suffering from cancer, glaucoma, and AIDS (Bowersox, 1992).

Dissociative Anesthetics: Phencyclidine and Ketamine

One of the most predominant effects of phencyclidine (or PCP, which stands for its chemical name phencyclohexyl piperidine) and its analog ketamine is profound anesthesia. Because patients anesthetized with these drugs are awake but appear disconnected from their environment, perhaps the simplest term to be used to describe these drugs is **dissociative anesthetic** (Jaffe, 1985). PCP is frequently misrepresented as LSD, mescaline, or THC. As is almost universally the case, PCP was discovered serendipitously. In the 1950s, while searching for new psychoactive drugs with therapeutic properties, chemists synthesized the drug, which psychopharmacologists immediately recognized as having some very unique effects in animals (Domino, 1980). In rats it had an amphetamine-like action, but, as with sedative-hypnotics, it induced a lack of muscular coordination. In dogs it induced convulsions, and in monkeys low doses had a calming effect (the monkeys appeared so serene that the drug was later marketed as Sernylyn), while higher doses eliminated sensitivity to touch or pain. It was this anesthetic action that was most promising for therapeutics, since most drugs with general anesthetic activity also have a strong lethal potential—due to the depression of the body's vital functions—at doses approximately double the anesthetic dose. With PCP the lethal dose was approximately 10 times the anesthetic dose. At appropriate doses, PCP induced insensitivity to pain while increasing blood pressure and heart rate. Also unlike any other general anesthetic, the organism remained awake with the eyes open.

When PCP was tested in human volunteers, it soon became apparent that it shared the properties of another class of drugs, the P/P/Hs.

However, unlike LSD with its definitive visual distorting properties, PCP prompted distortions in body image, feelings of depersonalization, and a sense of timelessness—a transient feeling of being in outer space or dead or not having any arms or legs. In approximately a third of the individuals, the drug also prompted symptoms that mimicked very closely those of schizophrenia (apathy, ambivalence, autism, and an inability to associate thoughts or ideas) and that, in some cases, persisted for several days or weeks. For this reason, the pharmaceutical company that developed Sernylyn withdrew it from the market except for veterinary purposes. Until it was totally withdrawn from the market, Sernylyn was used primarily as an anesthetic in primates and not, as it is commonly assumed, as an animal tranquilizer.

For some of the same reasons that clinical use of PCP with humans was discontinued, illicit drug manufacturers in the 1960s started synthesizing the drug (a relatively easy process) and selling it as a substitute for LSD, THC, mescaline, and amphetamine. Until the 1970s it was rarely purchased intentionally as PCP (in which case it was most commonly referred to as angel dust). Although still used by a very small minority of illicit drug users, PCP presents a very severe drug abuse problem in that it has been reliably linked to suicides (as a result of severe depression) and drownings, self-inflicted wounds, and violence (as a result of the dissociation from reality, incoordination, and hallucinations).

Pharmacodynamics and Psychological Effects of PCP

The CNS actions of PCP are quite complex and probably involve a wide variety of neurotransmitter systems. Stereospecific binding sites for PCP have been noted. Almost all of these sites appear to be located deep within an ion channel regulated by the NMDA receptor for the excitatory amino acids glutamate and aspartate; by binding to this site, PCP prevents Ca^{++} and Na^+ flow through the channel and into the neuron (Johnson & Jones, 1990). In fact, it is this action that has renewed neuroscientist's interest in PCP because PCP-like drugs can be especially useful in blocking neurotoxicity that can accompany excessive excitatory amino activity resulting from acute brain trauma or stroke. Although this action at NMDA receptors also accounts for some of PCP's behavioral effects, its ability to induce a psychosis resembling paranoid schizophrenia is more likely because of its action at a different site that enhances dopamine activity by inhibiting dopamine reuptake and facilitating its release (i.e., somewhat like the actions of amphetamine). Similar actions or norepinephrine and serotonin neurons may also be involved in PCP's behavioral effects.

Studies have also suggested that some of the properties of PCP are similar to those of the mixed agonist-antagonist narcotics like cyclazocine, which are generally viewed as kappa opioid receptor agonists (Pfeiffer et al., 1986). Adenosine receptors may be involved since agonists at these receptors block the CNS properties of PCP (Browne & Welch, 1982).

Despite the similarities of their neuropharmacological actions, the CNS effects of PCP are distinct from those of other drugs exhibiting these properties, including amphetamine, THC, LSD, methaqualone, scopolamine, and morphine (Jaffe, 1985). PCP's CNS effects are also clearly different from those of the monoamine-related P/P/Hs. In the drug discrimination procedure, animals show no generalization between PCP and any monoamine P/P/H (Appel et al., 1982) or for that matter between PCP and any cholinergic, dopaminergic, serotonergic, GABAergic, or opioid drugs (Johnson & Jones, 1990). Finally, whereas chlorpromazine (the antipsychotic) blocks the effects of LSD, it tends to potentiate PCP's depressant actions (Balster & Chait, 1976).

Electrophysiologically, sensory impulses to the cortex appear to be grossly distorted by PCP, particularly those involved in proprioception (the perceptual processing of stimuli originating in muscles, tendons, and other internal tissues) (Domino, 1980). Peripherally, PCP has the sympathomimetic effects of increasing heart rate and blood pressure. The persistence of the PCP-induced effects can be traced to the fact that PCP has a relatively long plasma half-life, in some cases as long as three days (Jaffe, 1985). In addition to the confusing array of effects possessed by PCP, there are dozens of its metabolites, with potential psychoactive properties, that also persist in the body for several days.

Behaviorally in humans, low doses of PCP (1–5 mg) produce a drunken state, or "floaty" euphoria, with numbness in the hands and feet. Persons often describe their experience as involving grotesquely distorted body shape, unreal size of body parts, a sensation of floating or hovering in a weightless condition in space, or a leaving of the body. Radiantly colorful visions that include images of moving from one room to another and moving, glowing geometrical patterns and figures are also reported, and the user may experience a complete absence of time sense (Domino, 1980).

Moderate doses (5–15 mg) induce analgesia and anesthesia, and an excited, confused intoxication can develop. Communication is definitely impaired. A body position may be rigidly maintained over extended periods of time (catalepsy). Larger doses of PCP induce a very definite psychosis and, in rare cases, convulsions (although low doses of PCP generally have anticonvulsant properties due to NMDA-mediated response blockade). Death is rarely directly caused by PCP because of its moderately high therapeutic index. There are distinct species differences in terms of reaction to PCP; some animals become very excited, and others become very sedated. The anesthetic dose is dependent on the complexity of the organism; as one progresses up the phylogenetic scale, lower doses are needed to induce anesthesia (Domino, 1980).

Tolerance develops to many of the effects of PCP, but much of it appears to be due to behavioral adaptations. For example, monkeys administered PCP (1.0 mg/kg) daily for four months were less affected by 1.0 mg/kg PCP than nondrug-treated monkeys in terms of their ability to stand on their hind limbs to reach for a food pellet, their ability to track a food pellet moved laterally across the field of vision, and their ability to reach out and take an offered pellet. However, in terms of nystagmus (rhythmical oscillation of the eyeballs), both groups of monkeys were affected to the same degree (Balster & Chait, 1976). Notice that the dependent variables to which tolerance developed were the ones in which you would expect behavioral adjustments to occur. Other studies with animals have confirmed these findings. For example, studies have demonstrated that tolerance occurs to some behavioral effects with both PCP and ketamine while the anticonvulsant action (with low doses) of these drugs remains unaffected after chronic drug exposure (Leccese et al., 1986).

PCP may also produce mild physical dependence because abrupt withdrawal from PCP after chronic use may be followed by fearfulness, tremors, and facial twitches (Jaffe, 1985). Some craving after stopping PCP use may also be experienced by chronic users.

With such a confusing array of pharmacological actions, it is not clear what accounts for PCP's popularity. Unlike other P/P/Hs, animals have been shown (using the catheter/infusion method) to self-administer PCP (Balster & Chait, 1976). The majority of PCP users report that they enjoy the intoxication state, viewing it as a novel experience that provides an escape from anxieties, depression, and other external pressures (Domino, 1980). To this outside observer, these effects seem a little like the effects from a combination of a sedative-hypnotic, a monoamine-related P/P/H, and an opiate.

PCP-Induced Psychosis

Although it has euphoriant effects in the majority of users, PCP can induce a distinct psychotic reaction in a significant minority of people (Erard et al., 1980). These people can generally be placed in one of three categories: (1) normal individuals who experience a schizophrenic-like syndrome lasting for several hours; (2) individuals with no previous history of psychotic episodes or other psychiatric problems, whose PCP-induced psychosis lasts an average of two weeks; and (3) those previously diagnosed with schizophrenia, in whom PCP triggers or exacerbates their original psychosis, a condition that may last for several weeks. Whether these three types of reactions are qualitatively different or are simply variations along a continuum involving persons with varying degrees of predisposition toward the development of schizophrenic symptoms is unclear.

The symptoms of PCP psychosis are indistinguishable from the core symptoms of schizophrenia (Erard et al., 1980). Most patients treated for it present global paranoia, persecutory and grandiose delusions, and auditory hallucinations, with periods of suspiciousness alternating with extreme anger or terror. As is common with schizophrenia, affect is blunted, and patients are ambivalent toward close friends and relatives. In some cases they profess superhuman strength and invulnerability, and they may become violent without provocation (it should be mentioned that this is rarely the case with schizophrenia). Other clinical signs are negativism, hostility, disorientation, repetitive motor behavior, and rigidity. In very rare cases, the psychosis is more similar to mania, with symptoms including elation, grandiose and paranoid delusions, and widely fluctuating affect, but no thought disorder or disorientation. Generally, the patients are amnesic for the events occurring during the PCP-induced state.

Schizophrenics are particularly sensitive to PCP and show profound disorganization in reaction to it (Erard et al., 1980). This is considerably different from their reaction to other P/P/Hs like LSD or mescaline. Intelligent schizophrenics can distinguish the effects of these latter drugs from their psychosis, and, as with normal individuals, they experience the kaleidoscopic visual effects (Jacobsen, 1968).

Treatment for PCP Psychosis

The treatment of PCP toxic reactions is somewhat different from treatments for other P/P/Hs (Aronow et al., 1980), which for the most part simply require time passage and reassurance. Some of the psychotomimetic effects of PCP can be antagonized by the nonsedating antipsychotics like haloperidol (Haldol), although some clinicians feel that these drugs may exacerbate the behavioral dyscontrol of PCP. Diazepam may be used to help control muscle spasms and restlessness, and the anticonvulsant Dilantin may be used prophylactically against convulsions. Nondrug treatment generally involves lavage (washing out the G.I. tract with large amounts of fluid) or gastric suctioning if the psychosis is treated shortly after the drug has been administered. Since PCP is a weak alkaloid administered as a salt (phencyclidine hydrochloride), a technique called *ion trapping*, where the urine is acidified to insure ionization of the PCP base, is used to facilitate PCP's removal from the body. Unlike the "talking down" strategy suggested for dealing with LSD-like or cannabinoid psychoses, it is suggested that the person experiencing a PCP psychosis be placed in as quiet and nonstimulating an environment as possible, because he or she may exhibit unexpected violence or aggression.

Ketamine

After noting the many side effects of PCP, chemists synthesized a number of analogues of PCP. Ketamine (Ketalar) was found to have the most therapeutic value as an anesthetic. While possessing the desirable characteristics of PCP (that is, high therapeutic index, minimal effect on respiration, and elevation of blood pressure and cardiac output), it did not induce convulsions and was shorter-acting than PCP (recovery occurs in less than two hours) (Domino, 1980).

Ketamine's pharmacodynamic actions are very similar to those of PCP, and essentially the same psychotic symptoms and perceptual distortions in vision, audition, body image, sense of time, and the like noted with PCP can occur during the recovery period following ketamine anesthesia, but to a lesser degree (Hansen et al., 1988). It is best used for short diagnostic procedures that require good analgesia and minimal relaxation, in cases in which the airway can be left undisturbed—that is, where the patient can continue to breath under his or her own power. Because reflexes are intact, there is no danger of vomiting or asphyxiation. Ketamine is especially useful in children for minor surgical or diagnostic procedures and in burn victims (Marshall & Wollman, 1985).

Anticholinergics

One of the oldest known groups of P/P/Hs is called the **anticholinergics** because of their specific blockade at acetylcholine receptors. The early writings of Homer describe potent agents with properties similar to those of the anticholinergics. These drugs are often called belladonna alkaloids because at one time women used one of these compounds (*Atropa belladonna*) to dilate their pupils and enhance their beauty (belladonna means beautiful lady). Throughout the Middle Ages, many witchcraft potions contained mushrooms and herbs with anticholinergic properties. The four deadly nightshades—*Atropa belladonna* (death's herb), *Datura stramonium* (Jamestown weed, jimson weed, thornapple, stinkweed), *Hyoscyamus niger* (henbane), and *Mandragora officinarum* (mandrake)—were also well known to oracles, assassins, seducers, and physicians. Jamestown weed was commonly used as an intoxicant by the early settlers of Jamestown, Virginia (circa 1676).

In addition to their CNS effects, anticholinergic drugs exert a number of peripheral effects that led to their being included in a variety of over-the-counter (OTC) medications. In the 1970s more than 100 OTC medications contained anticholinergics. These included a variety of sleep aids (Sominex, Compoz, Serene), cold remedies (Contac), antacids (Trangest), cough syrups (Endotussin), antidiarrhea compounds (Donnagel), analgesics (Femicin), antimotion sickness compounds (Travel-eze), and antiasthmatics (Asthmador). However, in the late 1970s and early 1980s, concerns over the effectiveness of OTC medications led the federal government to require that OTC medications be proven not only safe (a requirement established in the 1960s) but also effective in order for them to be marketed. These requirements led to the reformulation of most OTC medications containing anticholinergic drugs and, for the most part, the replacement of anticholinergics with more effective compounds (most of which are antihistamines).

At the present time, anticholinergics are not Schedule-controlled substances, even though they can only be purchased through prescription, nor is there any law preventing the cultivation of plants containing these alkaloids, primarily because the recreational use and the abuse potential for these drugs is currently very minimal. They have a number of side effects that reduce their reward value, and there are other drugs available with similar euphoriant properties that do not have these side effects.

Pharmacodynamics of Anticholinergics

The three most common anticholinergic compounds are atropine, scopolamine, and *l*-hyoscyamine. These drugs are pharmacological, competitive antagonists of acetylcholine (ACH) at muscarinic receptors (so named because the drug muscarine acts like acetylcholine at these receptors). Thus they are often, and more appropriately, termed **antimuscarinics**. Their blocking action at ACH receptors activated by nicotine (nicotinic receptors) is very weak. The fact that they compete with ACH means that their effects can be overcome by increasing the amount of ACH released or reducing its inactivation in the synaptic cleft. The latter technique is the most often used antidote to anticholinergic poisoning, carried out by administering physostigmine, a drug that inhibits the action of acetylcholinesterase (the enzyme that metabolizes ACH in the synaptic cleft). On the other hand, the use of antipsychotic drugs like chlorpromazine (Thorazine) in the treatment of anticholinergic-induced psychosis would only intensify the psychosis because these drugs also have anticholinergic properties.

Since muscarinic receptors for ACH are found in both the peripheral and central nervous systems, antimuscarinics have profound effects on both bodily and psychological functions. Atropine has a greater effect on the G.I. tract, heart, and bronchi, while scopolamine has a greater effect on the eyes, glands, and brain.

Psychological Effects of Antimuscarinics

The effects of antimuscarinics are heavily dose-dependent (Weiner, 1985). In small doses scopolamine causes quiet sedation with euphoria, amnesia, and dreamless sleep (probably associated with reduced REM activity). Sometimes, however, especially when the person is in pain, scopolamine causes excitement, hallucinations, or delirium in small doses. In general, the effects of antimuscarinics resulting from their CNS activity include the following: (1) confusion, slurred speech, disorientation similar to alcohol intoxication; (2) psychotic behavior similar to hebephrenia (a state in which the person acts very childish and silly); (3) hallucinations, primarily consisting of brightly colored objects and pleasant sounds; (4) drowsiness and fatigue; and (5) amnesia, where the person may forget the entire episode of intoxication. (At one time antimuscarinics, in combination with morphine, were given to women in labor to induce a "twilight sleep" so that they would forget the pain of childbirth.) At extremely high doses, coma can result. Although these drugs can be lethal and have been used as poisons in the past, their margin of safety is actually rather large. Deaths attributed to them nowadays generally involve abusers who might wander off into heavy traffic or fall into swimming pools, and children who ingest berries or seeds containing belladonna alkaloids.

Antimuscarinics generally shift the EEG rhythm to slower frequencies, an effect commonly found with sedative-hypnotic compounds (Weiner, 1985). As noted earlier, several cognitive and peripheral effects of marijuana resemble those of antimuscarinics. In therapeutic doses they also reduce abnormal EEG waves in approximately half of those individuals with grand mal seizures and may be useful in some cases of petit mal seizure activity. These drugs also have antitremor activity and have been used for many years in the treatment of parkinsonism.

Peripherally, antimuscarinics block activity of the parasympathetic nervous system (the system that regulates vegetative processes and that is most active when the organism is calm and relaxed). The reduction of parasympathetic input to the organs of the body results in effects that resemble those of drugs that amplify sympathetic nervous system activity (such as amphetamine), with respect to increased heart rate, blood pressure, and pupillary dilation. With antimuscarinics, pupillary dilation is not responsive to light, and testing this response is a good way to diagnose poisoning with these substances. Many other peripheral effects generally result in fluid retention in all areas of the body; for example, the mouth and nose dry up, sweating is absent, urination becomes difficult, and there is intraocular (inside the eye) fluid buildup. The person becomes very thirsty, hot, and flushed. Other effects include poor eye accommodation (blurred vision), decreased G.I. activity (constipation), and bronchodilation. It was because of several of these properties that small amounts of antimuscarinics were, until recently, often found in many over-the-counter medications for the treatment of cold symptoms, excess stomach acid, cough, diarrhea, motion sickness, and asthma.

Tolerance and Dependence

Tolerance to the belladonna alkaloids occurs in humans to a limited extent. Psychological dependence at the present time is extremely rare. Physical dependence is minimal, although vomiting, malaise, excessive sweating, and salivation have been recorded in parkinsonism patients treated with large doses (required for therapeutic benefit) of these compounds upon sudden withdrawal.

P/P/Hs: The Human Experience

We are built to process stimuli, and an important aspect of our living is our seeking out of stimuli to process. The popularity of P/P/Hs is a function of this general characteristic of stimulus seeking. The central property of any of the P/P/Hs is the enhancement of experience (Aaronson & Osmond, 1970). They seem to increase the capacity of the human brain to respond to fine gradations of stimulus input, to enhance our responses to stimulation at both the upper and lower levels of perceptual processing, and to remove the constraints imposed by the different sensory pathways through which stimulation is received. They produce new perceptions, alter our ways of looking at the world, and in some cases induce hallucinations. The experience can be very exhilarating or very frightening. In contrast, the sedative-hypnotics and narcotics reduce our attention to sensory input, although these substances may induce hypnagogic and dreamlike states. Psychostimulants may enhance endurance, improve mood, and increase alertness, but they do not alter our attention to the fine nuances of sensory experience to the degree that P/P/Hs do.

However, in order for the enhanced capacity for experience to occur with P/P/Hs, an adequate range of stimuli must be available, because exposure to them under conditions of sensory deprivation seems to reduce their effects considerably (Aaronson & Osmond, 1970). On the other hand, as the complexity of the stimulus situation increases, the variability of the experiences and perceptual reactions increases. Furthermore, in addition to the setting, the person's attitudes, motivations, cognitive set, and expectations play such a large role in the experience that it is impossible to predict in advance the type of experience one may have with these substances. This unpredictability may, in fact, be another reason why humans use them.

Bibliography

Aaronson, B., & Osmond, H. (1970). Introduction: Psychedelics, technology, psychedelics. In B. Aaronson & H. Osmond (Eds.), *Psychedelics* (pp. 3–18). Garden City: Anchor Books.

Abraham, H. D. (1983). Visual phenomenology of the LSD flashback. *Archives of General Psychiatry, 40,* 884–889.

Agurell, S., Halldin, M., Lindgren, J.-E., Ohlsson, A., Widman, M., Gillespie, H., & Hollister, L. (1986). Pharmacokinetics and metabolism of delta-1-tetrahydrocannabinol and other cannabinoids with emphasis on man. *Pharmacological Reviews, 38,* 21–43.

Appel, J. B., White, F. J., & Holohean, A. M. (1982). Analyzing mechanisms of hallucinogenic drug action with drug discrimination procedures. *Neuroscience and Biobehavioral Reviews, 6,* 529–536.

Aronow, R., Miceli, J. N., & Done, A. K. (1980). A therapeutic approach to the acutely overdosed PCP patient. *Journal of Psychedelic Drugs, 12,* 259–266.

Azorlosa, J. L., Heishman, S. J., Stitzer, M. L., & Mahaffey, J. M. (1992). Marijuana smoking: Effect of varying delta-9-tetrahydrocannabinol content and number of puffs. *Journal of Pharmacology and Experimental Therapeutics, 261,* 114–122.

Balster, R. L., & Chait, L. D. (1976). The biobehavioral pharmacology of phencyclidine. *Clinical Toxicology, 9,* 513–529.

Barinaga, M. (1992). Pot, heroin unlock new areas for neuroscience. *Science, 258,* 1882–1884.

Barnes, D. M. (1988a). New data intensify the agony over ecstasy. *Science, 239,* 864–866.

Barnes, D. M. (1988b). Ecstasy returns to Schedule I. *Science, 240,* 24.

Beardsley, P. M., Balster, R. L., & Harris, L. S. (1986). Dependence on tetrahydrocannabinol in rhesus monkeys. *Journal of Pharmacology and Experimental Therapeutics, 239,* 311–319.

Block, R. I., Farinpour, R., & Schlechte, J. A. (1991). Effects of chronic marijuana use on testosterone, luteinizing hormone, follicle stimulating hormone, prolactin and cortisol in men and women. *Drug and Alcohol Dependence, 28,* 121–128.

Bowersox, J. (1992). PHS cancels availability of medicinal marijuana. *Journal of the National Cancer Institute, 84,* 475–476.

Brecher, E. M. (Ed.). (1972). *Licit and illicit drugs.* Boston: Little, Brown.

Browne, R. G., & Welch, W. M. (1982). Stereoselective antagonism of phencyclidine's discriminative properties by adenosine receptor agonists. *Science, 217,* 1157–1159.

Cami, J., Guerra, D., Ugena, B., Segura, J., & De La Torre, R. (1991). Effect of subject expectancy on the THC intoxication and disposition from smoked hashish cigarettes. *Pharmacology, Biochemistry, and Behavior, 40,* 115–119.

Campbell, K. A., Foster, T. C., Hampson, R. E., & Deadwyler, S. A. (1986). Effects of delta-9-tetrahydrocannabinol on sensory-evoked discharges of granule cells in the dentate gyrus of behaving rats. *Journal of Pharmacology and Experimental Therapeutics, 239,* 941–945.

Caporael, L. R. (1976). Ergotism: The satan loosed in Salem? *Science, 192,* 21–26.

Cohen, S. (1981). *The substance abuse problems.* New York: Haworth Press.

Cunningham, K. A., & Appel, J. B. (1987). Neuropharmacological reassessment of the discriminative stimulus properties of d-lysergic acid diethylamide (LSD). *Psychopharmacology, 91,* 67–73.

Dewey, W. L. (1986). Cannabinoid pharmacology. *Pharmacological Reviews, 38,* 151–178.

Domino, E. F. (1980). History and pharmacology of PCP and PCP-related analogs. *Journal of Psychedelic Drugs, 12,* 223–227.

Eich, J. E., Weingartner, H., Stillman, R. C., & Gillin, J. C. (1975). State-dependent accessibility of retrieval cues in the retention of a categorized list. *Journal of Verbal Learning and Verbal Behavior, 14,* 408–417.

Erard, R., Luisada, P. V., & Peele, R. (1980). The PCP psychosis: Prolonged intoxication or drug-precipitated functional illness? *Journal of Psychedelic Drugs, 12,* 235–245.

Feeney, D. M. (1976). The marijuana window: A theory of cannabis use. *Biobehavioral Biology, 18,* 455–471.

Ferraro, D. P. (1976). A behavioral model of marihuana tolerance. In M. C. Braude & S. Szara (Eds.), *The pharmacology of marihuana* (pp. 475–486). New York: Raven Press.

Ferraro, D. P. (1980). Acute effects of marijuana on human memory and cognition. *NIDA Research Monograph Series 31* (pp. 98–119). National Institute on Drug Abuse, Department of Health and Human Services, Rockville, Md.

Fischer, J., & Taschner, K. L. (1991). Flashback following use of cannabis—A review. *Fortschritte der Neurologie, Psychiatrie, und Ihrer Grenzgebiete, 59,* 437–446.

Foltin, R. W., Brady, J. V., & Fischman, M. W. (1986). Behavioral analysis of marijuana effects on food intake in humans. *Pharmacology, Biochemistry, and Behavior, 25,* 577–582.

Frazer, A., Maayani, S., & Wolfe, B. B. (1990). Subtypes of receptors for serotonin. *Annual Review of Pharmacology and Toxicology, 30,* 307–348.

Freedman, D. X., & Halaris, A. E. (1978). Monoamines and the biochemical mode of action of LSD at synapses. In M. A. Lipton, A. DiMascio, & K. F. Killam (Eds.), *Psychopharmacology* (pp. 347–360). New York: Raven Press.

Fysh, R. R., Oon, M.C.H., Robinson, K. N., Smith, R. N., White, P. C., & Whitehouse, M. J. (1985). A fatal poisoning with LSD. *Forensic Science International, 28,* 108–114.

Gardner, E. L., & Lowinson, J. H. (1991). Marijuana's interaction with brain reward systems: Update 1991. *Pharmacology, Biochemistry, and Behavior, 40,* 571–580.

Glennon, R. A., & Rosecrans, J. A. (1982). Indolealkylamine and phenalkylamine hallucinogens: A brief overview. *Neuroscience and Biobehavioral Reviews, 6,* 489–498.

Greer, G., & Tolbert, R. (1986). Subjective reports of the effects of MDMA in a clinical setting. *Journal of Psychoactive Drugs, 18,* 319–327.

Grilly, D. M. (1981). People's views on drugs and driving: An update. *Journal of Psychoactive Drugs, 13,* 377–379.

Hansen, G., Jensen, S. B., Chandresh, L., & Hilden, T. (1988). The psychotropic effect of ketamine. *Canadian Journal of Psychology, 36,* 527–531.

Harris, L. S. (1978). Cannabis: A review of progress. In M. A. Lipton, A. DiMascio, & K. F. Killam (Eds.), *Psychopharmacology* (pp. 1565–1574). New York: Raven Press.

Heishman, S. J., Huestis, M. A., Henningfield, J. E., & Cone, E. J. (1990). Acute and residual effects of marijuana: Profiles of plasma THC levels, physiological, subjective, and performance measures. *Pharmacology, Biochemistry, and Behavior, 37,* 561–565.

Holden, C. (1980). Arguments heard for psychedelics probe. *Science, 209,* 256–257.

Hollister, L. E. (1986). Health aspects of cannabis. *Pharmacological Reviews, 38,* 1–20.

Hooker, W. D., & Jones, R. T. (1987). Increased susceptibility to memory intrusions and the Stroop interference effect during acute marijuana intoxication. *Psychopharmacology, 91,* 20–24.

Imade, A.G.T., & Ebie, J. C. (1991). A retrospective study of symptom patterns of cannabis-induced psychosis. *Acta Psychiatrica Scandinavica, 83,* 134–136.

Jacobs, B. L. (1976, March). Serotonin: The crucial substance that turns dreams on and off. *Psychology Today,* pp. 70–73.

Jacobs, B. L. (1987). How hallucinogenic drugs work. *American Scientist, 75,* 386–392.

Jacobsen, E. (1968). The hallucinogens. In C.R.B. Joyce (Ed.), *Psychopharmacology: Dimensions and perspectives* (pp. 175–213). Philadelphia: J. B. Lippincott.

Jaffe, J. H. (1985). Drug addiction and drug abuse. In A. G. Gilman, L. S. Goodman, T. W. Rall, & F. Murad (Eds.), *The pharmacological basis of therapeutics* (pp. 532–581). New York: Macmillan.

Johnson, K. M., & Jones, S. M. (1990). Neuropharmacology of phencyclidine: Basic mechanisms and therapeutic potential. *Annual Review of Pharmacology and Toxicology, 30,* 707–750.

Kamien, J. B., Johanson, C. E., Schuster, C. R., & Woolverton, W. L. (1986). The effects of (±)-methylenedioxymethamphetamine and (±)-methylenedioxyamphetamine in monkeys trained to discriminate (+)-amphetamine from saline. *Drug and Alcohol Dependence, 18,* 139–147.

Karniol, J. G. & Carlini, E. A. (1972). The content of (−)delta-9-trans-tetrahydrocannabinol (delta-9-THC) does not explain all biological activity of some Brazilian marihuana samples. *Journal of Pharmacy and Pharmacology, 24,* 833–835.

Lamb, R. J., & Griffiths, R. R. (1987). Self-injection of *d,1*-3,4-methylenedioxymethamphetamine (MDMA) in the baboon. *Psychopharmacology, 91,* 268–272.

Leccese, A. P., Marquis, K. L., Mattia, A., & Moreton, J. E. (1986). The anticonvulsant and behavioral effects of phencyclidine and ketamine following chronic treatment in rats. *Behavioural Brain Research, 22,* 257–264.

Leirer, V. O., Yesavage, J. A., & Morrow, D. G. (1991). Marijuana carry-over effects on aircraft pilot performance. *Aviation Space Environmental Medicine, 62,* 221–227.

Marshall, B. E., & Wollman, H. (1985). General anesthetics. In A. G. Gilman, L. S. Goodman, T. W. Rall, & F. Murad (Eds.), *The pharmacological basis of therapeutics* (pp. 276–301). New York: Macmillan.

Martin, B. (1986). Cellular effects of cannabinoids. *Pharmacological Reviews, 38,* 45–74.

Matsuda, L. A., Lolait, S. J., Brownstein, M. J., Young, A. C., & Bonner, T. I. (1990). Structure of a cannabinoid receptor and functional expression of the clone cDNA. *Nature, 346,* 561–564.

Meyer, R. E. (1978). Behavioral pharmacology of marijuana. In M. A. Lipton, A. DiMascio, & K. F. Killam (Eds.), *Psychopharmacology* (pp. 1639–1652). New York: Raven Press.

Miller, L. L., & Branconnier, R. J. (1983). Cannabis: Effects on memory and the cholinergic limbic system. *Psychological Bulletin, 93,* 441–456.

Neill, J. R. (1987). "More than medical significance": LSD and American psychiatry. *Journal of Psychoactive Drugs, 19,* 39–45.

Nichols, D. E. (1986). Differences between the mechanism of action of MDMA, MBDB, and the classic hallucinogens. Identification of a new therapeutic class: Entactogens. *Journal of Psychoactive Drugs, 18,* 305–313.

Page, J. B., Fletcher, J., & True, W. R. (1988). Psychosociocultural perspectives on chronic cannabis use: The Costa Rican follow-up. *Journal of Psychoactive Drugs, 20,* 57–65.

Peralta, V., & Cuesta, M. J. (1992). Influence of cannabis abuse on schizophrenic psychopathology. *Acta Psychiatrica Scandinavica, 85,* 127–130.

Perez-Reyes, M., White, W. R., McDonald, S. A., Hicks, R. E., Jeffcoat, A. R., & Cook, C. E. (1991). The pharmacologic effects of daily marijuana smoking in humans. *Pharmacology, Biochemistry, and Behavior, 40,* 691–694.

Pfeiffer, A., Brantl, V., Herz, A., & Emrich, H. M. (1986). Psychotomimesis mediated by k opiate receptors. *Science, 233,* 774–775.

Pierce, P. A., & Peroutka, S. J. (1990). Antagonist properties of d-LSD at 5-hydroxytryptamine$_2$ receptors. *Neuropsychopharmacology, 3,* 503–508.

Rasmussen, K., & Aghajanian, G. K. (1986). Effect of hallucinogens on spontaneous and sensory-evoked locus coeruleus unit activity in the rat: Reversal by selective 5-HT$_2$ antagonists. *Brain Research, 385,* 395–400.

Rech, R. H., & Rosecrans, J. A. (1982). Review of mechanisms of hallucinogenic drug action. *Neuroscience and Biobehavioral Reviews, 6,* 481–482.

Ricuarte, G., Bryan, G., Strauss, L., Seiden, L., & Schuster, C. (1985). Hallucinogenic amphetamine selectively destroys serotonin nerve terminals. *Science, 229,* 986–987.

Sanders-Bush, E., & Breeding, M. (1991). Choroid plexus epithelial cells in primary cultures: A model of 5HT$_{1C}$ receptor activation by hallucinogenic drugs. *Psychopharmacology, 105,* 340–346.

Schaeffer, J., Andrysiak, T., & Ungerleider, J. T. (1981). Cognition and long-term use of ganja (cannabis). *Science, 213,* 465–466.

Schmidt, C. J. (1987). Neurotoxicity of the psychedelic amphetamine, methylenedioxymethamphetamine. *Journal of Pharmacology and Experimental Therapeutics, 240,* 1–7.

Siegel, R. K. (1979). Natural animal addictions: An ethological perspective. In J. D. Keehn (Ed.), *Psychopathology in animals.* New York: Academic Press.

Siegel, R. K. (1986). MDMA: Nonmedical use and intoxication. *Journal of Psychoactive Drugs, 18,* 349–354.

Siegel, R. K., & Jarvik, M. E. (1980). DMT self-administration by monkeys in isolation. *Bulletin of the Psychonomic Society, 16,* 117–120.

Silling, S. M. (1980, January). LSD flashbacks: An overview of the literature for counselors. *American Mental Health Counselors Association Journal,* pp. 39–45.

Solowij, N., Michie, P. T., & Fox, A. M. (1991). Effects of long-term cannabis use on selective attention: An event-related potential study. *Pharmacology, Biochemistry, and Behavior, 40,* 683–688.

Stephens, R. C. (1987). *Mind-altering drugs.* Newbury Park, CA: Sage.

Vardy, M. M., & Kay, S. R. (1983). LSD psychosis or LSD-induced schizophrenia? *Archives of General Psychiatry, 40,* 877–883.

Varma, V. K., Malhotra, A. K., Dang, R., Das, K., & Nehra, R. (1988). Cannabis and cognitive functions: A perspective study. *Drug and Alcohol Dependence, 21*, 147–153.

Wallace, B., & Fisher, L. E. (1991). *Consciousness and Behavior* (3rd ed.). Boston: Allyn & Bacon.

Weiner, N. (1985). Atropine, scopolamine, and related antimuscarinic drugs. In A. G. Gilman, L. S. Goodman, T. W. Rall, & F. Murad (Eds.), *The pharmacological basis of therapeutics* (pp. 130–144). New York: Macmillan.

Zablocki, B., Aidala, A., Hansell, S., & White, H. R. (1991). Marijuana use, introspectiveness, and mental health. *Journal of Health and Social Behavior, 32*, 65–79.

Chapter Twelve

Antipsychotics

One of the most common major mental disorders for which drug treatment is almost inevitable is *schizophrenia*. This form of *psychosis* (a general term used to reflect a severe disorganization in personality, thought, emotion, and behavior) may afflict two out of 100 individuals at some point in their lives, and approximately one out of 200 individuals in American society is currently being treated for this disorder with one or more drugs. It seems almost ironic that this chapter, which deals with drugs that we ask or coerce others to take to eliminate psychotic-like effects, would immediately follow a chapter dealing with drugs that some individuals take to purposely induce these kinds of effects. Perhaps, because the biochemical activities of the drugs discussed in Chapter 11 may have something in common with the endogenous condition, by understanding them we can somehow understand and treat schizophrenia and other psychotic disorders.

Schizophrenia is most commonly evidenced in young adulthood. The symptoms may occur suddenly, generally following severe environmental stress (often termed *reactive* schizophrenia), or they may develop gradually over a period of time (often termed *process* schizophrenia). Symptoms include distorted thinking (evidenced in delusions and in speech patterns wandering and failing to lead to their apparent goals), perceptual distortions and hallucinations (mostly auditory), flattened affect or inappropriate expression of emotion, withdrawal of the individual's interest from other people and the outside world, and altered motor behavior (ranging from complete immobilization to frantic, purposeless, or ritualistic activity), among many others. Recently, there has been a tendency for authors to cluster symptoms of schizophrenia into "positive" and "negative" categories (Andreasen, 1988). *Negative symptoms* represent a loss or diminution of functions that should be present, such as blunted affect, lack of energy, inability to experience pleasure, and poverty of speech and thought. *Positive symptoms* include phenomena that are distortions or exaggerations of normal functions, such as hallucinations, delusions, and thought disorder. Although these symptoms vary considerably from individual to individual, they almost always cause severe difficulties in everyday tasks and interpersonal relationships. Therefore, considerable intervention is generally required in order to reduce these difficulties.

People have been using drugs for thousands of years to counteract abnormal mental and emotional states. Unfortunately, though, until about 40 years ago, there was no drug (or any other treatment for that matter) that specifically reduced the symptoms of schizophrenia without severely stupefying the individual and without inducing a strong physical dependence. This all changed with the discovery of the selective effects of chlorpromazine, a drug capable of both calming the excited schizophrenic and animating the totally withdrawn schizophrenic.

Prior to the 1950s, the major nondrug "therapies" for schizophrenia consisted of isolation, restraint, electroshock treatment, and surgery (prefrontal lobotomy). In 1954 there were approximately 600,000 hospitalized patients diagnosed as schizophrenics. Today, with the use of chlorpromazine and related antipsychotic drugs (also called neuroleptics because of the profound neurological symptoms they induce), there are fewer than one-third that number currently in hospitals. Unfortunately, these statistics do not mean that a cure for schizophrenia has been found, that fewer people are developing the disorder, that there are fewer people being admitted to hospitals for the disorder, or that these drugs are a panacea with few side effects or social consequences. The fact is that although these drugs reduce the core symptoms of schizophrenia in three out of four individuals, there is no known cure for the vast majority of them. Proportionally, there are the same number of individuals developing the disorder now as in the past, and the number of admissions to hospitals with the diagnosis of schizophrenia is far higher now than it was 35 years ago. Furthermore, regardless of the drugs used, the side effects associated with their use range from those that involve relatively minor discomfort to those with socially disabling qualities to those that may be lethal.

The basic rationale for the use of antipsychotic drugs is that they generally work better than nothing at all. In many cases they are used in conjunction with various kinds of behavior therapy and psychotherapy, which most clinicians believe would be totally useless without the drugs. Most experts believe that there are many causes of the symptoms of schizophrenia (perhaps the plural, schizophrenias, would be more appropriate in this context)—many of these having some common biochemical denominator. Although the evidence favors a strong hereditary component for the majority of these disorders, it is likely that the symptoms are the result of a complex interaction between environmental factors and genetic susceptibility (Barnes, 1987). In addition to parental and societal factors, chemicals in the environment and nutritional factors, among other things, may be involved. For example, for many years alcohol abuse has been suggested to be an important etiological factor in some schizophrenia-like psychoses (Hays & Aidroos, 1986). Whatever the cause, by altering the biochemical functioning of the brain with drugs we are able to reduce the symptoms.

Biochemical Hypotheses of Schizophrenia

Before describing some of the basic properties of the drugs used to treat schizophrenia, it may be instructive to discuss briefly some of the major hypotheses surrounding this disorder, to provide a context for its treatment with drugs. Perhaps the most prevalent biochemical hypothesis involves the neurotransmitter dopamine (DA) (Seeman, 1987).

The Dopamine Hypothesis of Schizophrenia

Basically, the *dopamine hypothesis* states that there is an overactive or hypersensitive DA system or systems (see Figure 12–1) in many forms of schizophrenia. For example, there might be excessive DA levels or receptors or a deficiency in one or more transmitters that normally modulate dopaminergic activity, such as GABA, serotonin (5-HT), or norepinephrine (NE). Lately, most of the focus has been on the D_2 receptor as the one particularly relevant to schizophrenic symptoms, although recent studies suggest that both D_1 and D_2 receptors in concert play a complex role in their expression. In some cases, D_1 and D_2 receptors have opposing actions (for example, D_1 receptors activate the secondary messenger system involving adenylate cyclase, whereas D_2 receptors inhibit it), and in others they appear to exhibit synergistic actions (Seeman, 1987). There are several possible reasons for this complexity, one of which is that the D_2 receptor performs a role as both an autoreceptor and a postsynaptic receptor whereas the D_1 receptor plays a role as a postsynaptic receptor only. (If you are really confused at this point, you might review the section in Chapter 4 that deals with the relationship between autoreceptors and postsynaptic receptors in the process of neurotransmission.)

The first clue that dopamine may be involved in schizophrenia came from the observation that drugs used to treat schizophrenia (antipsychotics) also induced motor disturbances, called extrapyramidal symptoms, that were indistinguishable from those of Parkinson's disease, which, by the late 1960s, was known to be associated with DA deficiency and controllable with the dopamine precursor L-dopa. Furthermore, it

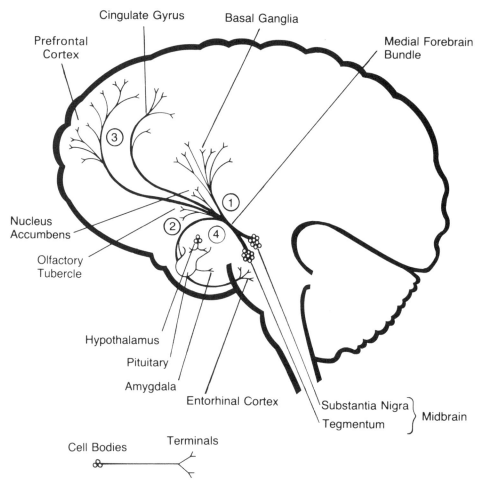

Figure 12–1

Four of the major dopamine pathways of the brain likely to be affected by antipsychotics and believed to be responsible for some of the beneficial effects of these drugs with respect to schizophrenia as well as many of their side effects. (1) The nigrostriatal tract connects the substantia nigra with the caudate-putamen complex of the basal ganglia; (2) the mesolimbic tract connects the midbrain with various limbic structures; (3) the mesocortical tract connects the midbrain with association areas of the frontal cortex; and (4) the tuberoinfundibular tract connects the hypothalamus with the pituitary gland. The presence versus absence of dopamine autoreceptors on the neurons of these different tracts may account for the different time courses for psychosis symptom reduction and motor disturbance onset with antipsychotic drug treatment as well as the differences among antipsychotic drugs in inducing motor disturbances (see text for further discussion).

was observed that when L-dopa was used to control the motor side effects of antipsychotics, it only made the psychosis worse. Within a few years, numerous other observations fell in line with the hypothesis.

First, substances that decrease DA levels tend to decrease the symptoms of schizophrenia (Carlsson, 1978). For example, reserpine prevents the binding of monoamines to the synaptic vesicles, allowing them to be metabolized by the enzyme MAO, and reduces the amount of DA that can be released from the axon. Synthesis of DA from its initial precursor tyrosine can be reduced with the drug alpha-methyl-p-tyrosine (AMPT). Both of these compounds are capable of reducing the symptoms of schizophrenia; however, since neither of these compounds exerts specific enough effects (for example, reserpine reduces the levels of all the monoamines, and AMPT reduces the levels of all catecholamines), they are not used clinically.

Second, substances that inhibit DA release or block its access to DA receptors are all effective in the treatment of schizophrenia. With respect to the traditionally used antipsychotic drugs (phenothiazines, butyrophenones, and thioxanthenes), there is a high correlation between their clinical potency (determined on the basis of the average daily dose of the drug needed to reduce symptoms) and their potency in inhibiting the stimulated release of DA from brain slices (Seeman & Lee, 1975). There is also a high correlation between their clinical potency and their relative ability to bind to D_2 receptors (presumably while occupying the receptors they prevent DA from binding and activating the receptors) (Seeman, 1987).

However, once the DA-blocking properties of antipsychotics became known, the hypothesis required an explanation for the observation that these drugs generally needed to be given several weeks before the full treatment benefits were expressed. The explanation was that, because antipsychotics also block DA autoreceptors, DA neurons initially fired more frequently and released more DA into the synapse; that is, there was an increase in DA turnover. This in turn counteracted the drugs's blockade of postsynaptic DA receptors and prevented the therapeutic benefits. With chronic drug exposure, DA turnover was observed to return slowly to pretreatment levels owing to inactivation of DA neuron firing—a phenomenon referred to as depolarization block (Lane & Blaha, 1987). Thus, as the DA hypothesis predicts, the time course for symptom remission appears to correspond to the time it takes for depolarization block to occur.

Third, substances that are agonists at DA postsynaptic receptors (such as apomorphine), or that increase DA levels (such as L-dopa, MAO inhibitors, and PCP), or that increase DA release (such as amphetamine and methylphenidate), or that block DA reuptake (such as cocaine) have been noted to worsen or produce schizophrenic symptoms (Lieberman et al., 1987; Moskovitz et al., 1978). Interestingly, while high doses of apomorphine may trigger psychotic symptoms, low doses of it may actually reduce schizophrenic symptoms (Tammiga et al., 1978).

This contradictory effect has been attributed to its having a greater affinity for autoreceptors for DA than for postsynaptic DA receptors. Since autoreceptors play an inhibitory role in regulating DA synthesis and release, their activation would decrease the amount of DA normally released from the terminal. However, the reduced DA release is more than compensated for when higher doses of apomorphine are given because the drug directly activates postsynaptic DA receptors. This phenomenon may also occur with L-dopa; that is, low doses may reduce and high doses may exacerbate schizophrenia symptoms (Seeman, 1987).

Fourth, recent studies have noted that the binding of DA agonists and antagonists is greater in the limbic (nucleus accumbens) and caudate (basal ganglia) areas of the brains of deceased schizophrenics than in the brains of normal individuals, suggesting that schizophrenics may have more receptors for DA (Seeman, 1987). In one of these studies, the densities of DA receptors had a bimodal distribution (that is, one group of schizophrenics had DA densities in the normal range and another group had DA densities in the high range), suggesting that there are at least two distinct categories of schizophrenia (Seeman et al., 1984). At first, such findings were suggested to be an artifact caused by patients' previous chronic treatment with antipsychotic drugs, which could have resulted in the up-regulation of DA receptors. However, recent studies using a technique known as *positron emission tomography (PET)* revealed that even schizophrenic patients who had not been exposed to antipsychotics had elevated brain DA receptors, specifically the D_2 type (Wong et al., 1986). PET analysis has also revealed that it is the D_2 receptors to which most antipsychotic drugs specifically bind (Farde et al., 1986).

As indicated earlier, other neurotransmitter systems may be indirectly involved in the DA hypothesis. For example, several NE tracts exist that may serve to dampen DA activity. Thus, if this modulatory role is decreased, DA activity may increase. This process is consistent with some studies suggesting that the brains of deceased schizophrenics may have lower than normal levels of the enzyme DA-beta-hydroxylase, which is necessary for the synthesis of NE from DA[1]. Also, drugs that inhibit DA-beta-hydroxylase, such as disulfiram (Antabuse) and fusaric acid, have been shown to induce schizophrenic-like symptoms in some individuals (Seeman, 1987). Note, however, that DA may be directly involved in these actions because NE is synthesized from DA. Without DA being metabolized into NE, DA levels would increase in neurons that normally release NE. One can only theorize as to what might happen if DA instead of NE were released from these neurons, and, if so, what would happen if DA activated NE receptors.

---

[1]One should remember that DA is found in three types of neurons in the brain: (1) neurons where DA is the primary neurotransmitter; (2) neurons in which DA is the precursor for NE, which is the primary neurotransmitter; and (3) neurons in which DA, and subsequently NE, is the precursor to epinephrine, which is the primary neurotransmitter.

There is evidence that 5-HT released from axons of the reticular formation plays an inhibitory role in dopaminergic activity. The theory that insufficient 5-HT activity may be involved in schizophrenia is consistent with studies showing that depletion of 5-HT can potentiate the stereotypic reaction of rats to amphetamine. This is also consistent with the fact that LSD, which blocks the release of 5-HT in the reticular activating system, can induce some of the characteristics of psychosis. However, as noted in Chapter 11, LSD also stimulates postsynaptic 5-HT$_2$ receptors and exhibits dopamine agonist properties, so the specific mechanism through which LSD provokes psychotic symptoms is still unclear (Seeman, 1987).

Despite several lines of evidence supporting the DA hypothesis of schizophrenia, a number of unresolved questions remained. There was a question of why investigators repeatedly failed to find evidence of increased brain levels of DA or DA metabolites in unmedicated schizophrenics, or why antipsychotics were more effective in reducing the positive symptoms of schizophrenia than the negative symptoms, or why tolerance did not develop to many of the beneficial effects of antipsychotics.

Recently, a model for schizophrenia that attempts to integrate all these observations has been developed (Grace, 1991). Highly simplified, this model proposes that in schizophrenics a prolonged decrease in prefrontal cortical activity (e.g., due to cortical atrophy) reduces the tonic (i.e., sustained) release of DA in subcortical areas. Over time this reduction elicits homeostatic compensations in DA responsivity (e.g., DA receptor up-regulation) in these subcortical areas. These, in turn, increase overall dopamine responsivity in these subcortical areas and cause enhanced phasic (i.e., transient) dopamine release—presumably elicited by behaviorally relevant stimuli—to provoke abnormally large responses. It was further assumed that the tonic decrease in DA activity underlies the negative symptoms of the disorder, whereas the phasic increase in DA activity underlies the positive symptoms.

This model explains why traditional antipsychotics, which are potent D$_2$ receptor blockers, are more effective in reducing positive symptoms than negative symptoms and why the atypical antipsychotic clozapine, which decreases phasic DA release but increases tonic DA levels, reduces both types of symptoms. It also explains why amphetamine induces only positive symptoms, because it enhances both tonic and phasic DA release, whereas PCP induces both types of symptoms because it inhibits reuptake of phasically released DA while inhibiting DA released tonically via its action at NMDA ion channels. Although this model is intriguing and handles a lot of diverse phenomena associated with schizophrenia and its treatment, further verification of its various assumptions is needed. It must also be recognized that some cases or symptoms of schizophrenia may be totally unrelated to disturbances in dopaminergic functions.

Alternatives to the Dopamine Hypothesis

The DA hypothesis has been the most widely researched and accepted hypothesis over the past several years, but several other biochemical hypotheses for schizophrenia have been proposed. One long-standing biochemical hypothesis about schizophrenia is that it is due to improper metabolization of monoamine neurotransmitters. Note that the molecular structures of the psychotomimetic compounds in Figure 11–1 that bear a strong resemblance to the monoamine transmitters all have one or more CH_3 (methyl) groups. Thus the so-called *transmethylation hypothesis* proposes that methylated transmitters, in conjunction with stress, produce the perceptual and thought distortions common to schizophrenia (Gillin et al., 1978).

Evidence for the transmethylation hypothesis of schizophrenia is not nearly as impressive as it is for the DA hypothesis. Although numerous methylated neurotransmitter-like substances have been found in brain tissue, they occur in exceedingly small quantities, and there is no evidence that the brains of schizophrenics contain more of these than normal brains do. Some investigators have reported that substances that can act as methyl donors (such as the amino acid methionine) or cause methylation of DA (like the enzyme COMT) can exacerbate the symptoms of schizophrenia. Others have suggested that adding large amounts of substances that theoretically can act as methyl group acceptors (for example, the B_3 group consisting of niacin, niacinamide, nicotinamide, or nicotinic acid) can reduce the symptoms of schizophrenia, particularly those with an acute onset.

Unfortunately, large-scale studies done in the 1970s in Canada, specifically investigating the transmethylation hypothesis and the efficacy of *megavitamin therapy* (the use of large doses of the vitamins niacin, ascorbic acid, or pyridoxine in the treatment of mental disorders) in schizophrenia, have not been supportive at all (Ban, 1975). These studies found that nicotinic acid, in doses of 3 grams per day, (1) was no more effective than a placebo in newly admitted schizophrenic patients; (2) was less effective than a placebo in newly admitted as well as chronic schizophrenic patients treated with phenothiazines; (3) was less effective when combined with pyridoxine (75 mg/day) in phenothiazine-treated patients; (4) combined with ascorbic acid (vitamin C) was no more effective in phenothiazine-treated patients; and (5) could neither prevent nor counteract the psychopathology induced by the combined administration of a MAO inhibitor and methionine.

These findings also tend to negate the (rather old) hypothesis that schizophrenia is an incipient form of cerebral pellagra (a disease with symptoms of mental illness most commonly found in persons whose diet is low in tryptophan and niacin) based on idiosyncratic needs for exceptional amounts of vitamin B_3.

Another hypothesis is that the symptoms are caused by a reaction to a pathogen (a substance causing disease) in genetically susceptible individuals. Although there is little evidence for this position, some investigators have noted the similarity between symptoms of celiac disease (predominantly an intestinal disturbance) and those of schizophrenia. Since wheat gluten (an insoluble protein) found in cereals exacerbates the symptoms of celiac disease, these investigators attempted to see whether cereal grain proteins were likewise pathogenic in schizophrenics (Singh & Kay, 1976). They found that schizophrenics maintained on a diet free of cereal grain and milk, and receiving optimal treatment with antipsychotics, showed an interruption or reversal of their therapeutic progress when given wheat gluten. Unfortunately, we do not know whether unmedicated schizophrenics will also respond favorably to similar dietary restrictions.

Shortly after the discovery of endorphins, hypotheses related to a defect in endorphin activity were proposed as biochemical explanations for schizophrenia. One hypothesis was that there was too much endorphin activity, while another was that there was too little endorphin activity. However, numerous studies with schizophrenics administered opioid antagonists (e.g., naloxone, naltrexone) or opioid agonists (e.g., beta-endorphin, methadone) produced largely negative findings (Davis et al., 1977; Schmauss & Emrich, 1986), which have pretty much dissipated the enthusiasm for both the overactive and underactive endorphin hypotheses regarding schizophrenia. However, endorphins have not been completely ruled out as a factor in this disorder. Recently, it has been suggested that there exists an opioid-DA interaction that is altered in schizophrenia (Schmauss & Emrich, 1986). This possibility is consistent with several observations: (1) opioid receptors have been located on DA neurons; (2) lesions in nigrostriatal DA pathways (see Figure 12–1) have been associated with enhanced enkephalin levels; and (3) opiates generally reduce DA cell activity and alter behaviors mediated by DA. However, further research is needed before we can determine whether or not there is a direct connection between opioid-DA interactions and schizophrenia symptoms.

Numerous other abnormalities, which have more to do with structural defects than biochemical defects, have been speculated to be involved with schizophrenia, but evidence for them is equivocal or unverified (Barnes, 1987). New techniques for studying living brain structure and functions directly are being employed and will likely improve our understanding of this mental disorder (Andreasen, 1988). These include imaging techniques (such as computerized axial tomography and magnetic resonance imaging) and methods for measuring blood flow, metabolism, and receptor mapping (such as positron emission tomography). For example, these techniques have revealed that many schizophrenics have slightly enlarged cerebral ventricles and subtle anatomical abnormalities in the region of the hippocampus (Suddath et al., 1990). Other studies have found reduced blood flow in the frontal and prefrontal cortex of schizophrenics as well as decreases in metabolism in the basal ganglia that are reversed with antipsychotics (Buchsbaum et al., 1987).

Interpreting these findings is difficult. Some investigators question the methodology of these studies or their clinical significance. Others question whether these effects precede—that is, cause—the disorder or are consequences of the different life-style or treatment often applied to the individuals (Van Kammen et al., 1983). Still others question whether these observations are, in fact, indicative of abnormalties or are even specific to schizophrenia (Barnes, 1987).

There are many other problems with this area of research. Some of these are due to the nature of the illness itself. The diagnosis of schizophrenia is hardly cut-and-dried. Symptoms vary among and within individuals over time. Occasionally, the syndrome appears suddenly; more commonly the symptoms have a gradual onset. Often studies fail to employ the same diagnostic criteria to all patients included in them and fail to differentiate between long-hospitalized patients and recently admitted patients. For example, if one is trying to determine the efficacy of a particular therapeutic intervention and includes chronic, "burned-out" schizophrenics, failures may be due to the fact that some schizophrenics cannot improve because their illness is so chronic.

Related to this issue is the likelihood that schizophrenia is not a single disorder, but is actually a set of symptoms with varying etiology. Therefore, with a heterogeneous sample of individuals, particularly a small sample, it is highly unlikely that any therapeutic intervention, which may only benefit a few individuals in the sample, will result in significant differences between treated and untreated groups. It may be, for example, that there are individuals displaying the symptoms of schizophrenia who respond to megavitamin therapy, but in a large group of schizophrenics they may not be detected.

Other problems in this line of research stem from not using a double-blind procedure (where neither the patient nor the treatment provider knows what treatment condition the patient is in) or from beginning the treatment assessment before a reasonable *washout period*, where the patients stop taking all medication, has occurred. The fact is, the overall psychological functioning of many patients (such as nonresponsive chronic schizophrenics and patients whose symptoms remit regardless of whether antipsychotics are administered or not) actually improves when antipsychotic medications stop (May & Goldberg, 1978). Without a washout period, these patients' improvement would be attributed erroneously to the treatment.

Present-day Antipsychotics

Antipsychotics (also termed neuroleptics and major tranquilizers) in clinical use today are unrelated chemically and pharmacologically to previously known sedative-hypnotics (such as barbiturates) as well as more recently developed anxiolytics. Although they act as sedative-like drugs at times, as the group name implies they are strikingly effective at reducing the symptoms of psychosis, particularly schizophrenia (Baldessarini, 1990). Also, although they may sometimes be used in small doses as a treatment for anxiety, their side effects limit their usefulness in treating this condition. In addition, antipsychotics tend to increase muscle tone and tension, lower the convulsive threshold (which means the potential for seizure activity increases), and have a negligible potential for inducing psychological dependence. Sedative-hypnotics generally decrease muscle tension, increase the convulsive threshold, and have a considerable abuse potential. Antipsychotics have a wide assortment of potential side effects that are not found with sedative-hypnotics—most notably motor disturbances, anticholinergic effects, and allergic reactions. Unlike many sedative-hypnotics (specifically those that are not benzodiazepine derivatives), antipsychotics do not produce anesthesia, although they are often used as preanesthetics to reduce patients' apprehension over pending surgery and to reduce the dose of anesthetic required. By themselves, their lethal potential is very low, but a lethal synergism may occur when they are combined with other sedative-type drugs. Although not particularly effective as antidepressants, these drugs may be beneficial in some cases of depression.

More than a dozen antipsychotics are currently marketed in the United States, comprising six basic molecular groups. Representative drugs in these groups are shown in Table 12–1 (based on Baldessarini, 1990, and Newton et al., 1978), along with their range of clinically effective doses (for schizophrenia) and some of the more common side effects (to be discussed shortly). Despite their very different molecular structures and potencies (in terms of the amount needed to exert therapeutic effects), at the dosages noted these drugs are remarkably similar in their relative effectiveness in reducing the symptoms of schizophrenia. Also, although they generally share the same spectrum of side effects, their relative potential in inducing these at equivalent antipsychotic doses varies considerably. Thus the particular type of antipsychotic used is most likely to be dependent on the physician's familiarity with the drug and on specific characteristics of the patients with regard to their tendency to develop (or ability to tolerate) certain side effects of the drug at therapeutic doses.

Clozapine (Clozaril) is one of the few exceptions to what was just stated. It is the first truly unique and clinically effective antipsychotic drug developed since chlorpromazine (Baldessarini & Frankenburg,

Table 12–1

Relative Incidence of Side Effects to Some Common Antipsychotics

Antipsychotic	Dose Range	EPS	Sedative Activity	Anti-ACH Effects	Hypo-tension	Pigmentary Changes
Phenothiazines						
Acetophenazine (Tindal)	60–120	Mod–High	Low–Mod	Low	Low	Low
Chlorpromazine (Thorazine)	300–800	Mod	High	High	High	High
Fluphenazine (Prolixin)	2.5–20	High	Low	Low–Mod	Low	Low
Mesoridazine (Serentil)	75–300	Low–Mod	Mod–High	Mod	Mod	High
Perphenazine (Trilafon)	8–32	Mod–High	Mod	Low–Mod	Low	Low
Thioridazine (Mellaril)	200–600	Low	Mod–High	High	Mod–High	Mod–High
Trifluoperazine (Stelazine)	6–20	High	Low	Low–Mod	Low	Low
Triflupromazine (Vesprin)	100–150	Mod–High	Mod–High	Mod–High	Mod–High	Mod–High

	Dose range	Sedation	Anti-ACH	EPS	Orthostatic hypotension	Pigmentary changes
Thioxanthenes						
Chlorprothixene (Taractan)	50–400	Mod	High	High	Mod–High	Low
Thiothixene (Navane)	6–30	Mod–High	Low	Low–Mod	Low–Mod	Low
Butyrophenones						
Haloperidol (Haldol)	6–20	High	Low	Very Low	Low	None
Indoles						
Molindone (Moban)	50–225	Low–Mod	Low–Mod	Low	Very Low	Low
Dibenzoxazepines						
Loxapine (Loxitane)	60–100	Mod	Low–Mod	Low	Low	Low
Dibenzodiazepines						
Clozapine (Clozaril)	250–450	Very Low	Mod	Mod–High	Mod	None

Source. Based on Baldessarini (1990), Baldessarini and Frankenburg, (1991), and Newton et al., (1978).
Notes. Dose range refers to the normal daily clinical oral dosage; EPS refers to extrapyramidal symptoms; anti-ACH effects refers to anticholinergic effects. Excluding clozapine, there is a strong positive correlation between the midrange dose for each drug and the drug's tendency to induce sedation ($r = 0.79$), anticholinergic effects, orthostatic hypotension, and pigmentary changes. On the other hand, there is a strong negative correlation between the midrange dose for each drug and the drug's tendency to induce EPS ($r = -0.66$).

1991). It is unique for several reasons. First, in addition to being an effective treatment in many schizophrenics that respond to typical antipsychotics, it can successfully reduce the symptoms of approximately one-third of schizophrenics who do not respond to typical antipsychotics. Second, it may also be more effective in reducing the negative symptoms of schizophrenia than typical antipsychotics. Third, it has minimal extrapyramidal effects. It induces minimal pseudoparkinson effects, and there is no evidence that clozapine induces tardive dyskinesia (Safferman et al., 1991). (In fact, it was this feature of clozapine that led the manufacturer of the drug to question its marketability in the 1960s, because the prevailing view at the time was that a drug's ability to reduce schizophrenic symptoms was closely tied to its ability to induce extrapyramidal motor disturbances.) Fourth, clozapine is much more likely to induce severe agranulocytosis—that is, to suppress white blood cell formation (1–2% incidence per year)—than typical antipsychotics. Because there is a considerable risk of mortality when agranulocytosis occurs, clinicians in most countries, particularly the United States, were reluctant to use the drug in their patients, and the drug's manufacturer was not encouraged to market it. However, now that research has indicated that this problem can be surmounted with appropriate patient monitoring, the FDA has approved its use in the United States. Unfortunately, this monitoring system (termed the Clozaril Patient Management System) costs several thousand dollars a year to implement. This expense, of course, is a major drawback for many patients, whose economic status makes the cost prohibitive. Until alternative systems are developed or allowed by the FDA, cost will continue to be a problem.

As stated earlier in this chapter, inhibitors of the enzyme MAO have been observed to exacerbate both delusions and hallucinations of schizophrenics. This observation had led to the long-standing view that such drugs should never be prescribed for schizophrenics. Recently, however, this view has been challenged by the findings that the MAO inhibitor tranylcypromine (Parnate), when added to the usual dose of chlorpromazine, can significantly reduce the negative symptoms of the disorder, such as emotional withdrawal, depressed mood, motor retardation, and blunted affect (Bucci, 1987). These findings suggest that such treatment is safe and effective and may be useful in preventing the occurrence of motor disturbances.

Pharmacodynamics of Antipsychotics

As indicated earlier, most of the available evidence indicates that the primary biochemical effect of just about all antipsychotics is to competitively block DA's access to its receptors. As DA autoreceptors at the dopaminergic cell bodies and axon terminals are also blocked, the immediate consequences are an increase in dopaminergic cell activity (that is, firing) and an increase in DA synthesis and release. With chronic antipsychotic exposure, many of these effects are reversed; that is, dopaminergic cell activity decreases, and DA synthesis and release are reduced. While the decreased release of DA with chronic antipsychotic exposure has generally been attributed to enhanced DA autoreceptor sensitivity at DA nerve terminals, it has also been suggested that depolarization block of dopaminergic cells (thus leading to a decrease in cell firing) may be the mechanism underlying this effect (Lane & Blaha, 1987). However, evidence from several recent studies has raised considerable doubts as to the importance of depolarization inactivation for the mechanisms of action of antipsychotic drugs in general (Meltzer, 1991).

There is growing evidence that the classical antipsychotics (such as chlorpromazine and haloperidol) and the atypical antipsychotics (such as clozapine and thioridizine) exert differential effects depending on the type of receptors blocked. For example, clozapine's relatively higher D_1 and $5-HT_2$ antagonistic actions and relatively low D_2 receptor blockade appear to be major reasons for its differences from typical antipsychotics in terms of its psychopharmacological profile (Meltzer, 1991). Unfortunately, clozapine and other antipsychotics exhibit actions on numerous neurotransmitter systems, so it is not clear what mixture of actions is most relevant for antipsychotic efficacy.

Dopamine is believed to serve as the neurotransmitter in at least five specific pathways in the brain (Baldessarini, 1985). Four of these are shown in a cross section of the brain in Figure 12–1. The nigrostriatal pathway, often referred to as the extrapyramidal tract, can be thought of as regulating the responsiveness of the basal ganglia to the motor commands of the cortex (Paul, 1977). Thus, if there is insufficient DA input, motor commands are difficult to initiate and carry out. Parkinson's disease is a result of a degeneration of the substantia nigra neurons comprising this pathway. Essentially the same extrapyramidal symptoms, sometimes referred to as *pseudoparkinsonism,* can occur as a result of dopaminergic blockade by antipsychotics.

Mesolimbic and mesocortical fibers terminate in many of the limbic areas known to affect emotions and emotional expressions. Electrical or chemical stimulation of these target areas has been reported to produce hallucinations and thought disturbances. Several behavioral and perceptual changes (for example, paranoid ideation, depersonalization, perceptual distortions, catatonia, and mood and emotional disturbances) accompany stimulation or ablation of various areas of the limbic system in humans (Paul, 1977). Therefore, it is the blockade of DA by antipsychotics in these areas that is most commonly believed to be relevant to their antipsychotic properties.

It appears that the classical antipsychotics exert essentially the same effects on the nigrostriatal, mesocortical, and mesolimbic tracts (namely, an increase in dopaminergic activity with initial drug exposure and subsequent decrease following chronic exposure), whereas the atypical antipsychotics like clozapine exert these effects on the mesolimbic and mesocortical tracts while exerting minimal effects on the nigrostriatal DA cells (Baldessarini & Frankenburg, 1991). These findings suggest that the inability of the atypical antipsychotic drugs to decrease the latter's activity may be related to their lower incidence of motor disturbances (namely, pseudoparkinsonism and tardive dyskinesia). They also indicate that the gradual inactivation of mesolimbic and mesocortical neurons may be involved in the delayed onset of therapeutic effects during antipsychotic treatment.

Differences in the effects of antipsychotics may also be attributable to their differential actions at D_1 and D_2 dopamine receptors. Recent evidence has led to the suggestion that there is an optimal ratio of relative drug activity at these two receptors that contributes to the symptomatic relief in schizophrenia (Walters et al., 1987). Antipsychotics also differ considerably in terms of their binding affinities for dopamine autoreceptors, which in turn differ markedly in their distribution of dopaminergic neurons (Meltzer, 1991). Dopamine neurons comprising some dopaminergic tracts possess somatodendritic autoreceptors, whereas others possess few if any of these. Conversely, some dopamine neurons have autoreceptors that modulate the synthesis and release of dopamine, whereas others do not. Thus the differences in autoreceptor type and number among the prefrontal, mesocingulate, nigrostriatal, and mesolimbic dopamine neurons may be the basis for differences in their basal dopamine activity as well as differences in their response to dopamine agonists and antagonists.

To summarize, while dopaminergic dysfunction remains as a chief culprit in many symptoms of schizophrenia, it is no longer tenable to attribute all the efficacy of antipsychotic drugs to their ability to block D_2 receptors and subsequently induce development of depolarization inactivation of mesolimbic or mesocortical DA neurons. The primary evidence for this position comes from research with clozapine, which does not differ from typical antipsychotics in these regards but does differ on several dimensions in terms of efficacy in treating schizophrenic symptoms (Meltzer, 1991).

Other dopaminergic pathways exist within the hypothalamus (the incertohypothalamic tract) and between the hypothalamus and the pituitary gland (the tuberoinfundibular tract) that are responsible for regulating neuroendocrine function and synthesis and secretion of several pituitary hormones—for example, prolactin. Antipsychotic blockade in these areas is believed to be responsible for numerous endocrine changes and side effects, including abnormal lactation and menstruation, impotence, edema, and weight gain.

Efficacy of Antipsychotics

Numerous clinical trials with antipsychotic drugs have established their effectiveness in all subtypes of schizophrenia, at all stages of the illness, and at all ages (Baldessarini, 1990). Rarely does a patient treated with adequate doses of antipsychotics fail to show some degree of improvement, varying from complete remission of the psychosis to minimal symptomatic change. On the contrary, placebos and other sedatives like phenobarbital produce little mean improvement in large groups of schizophrenics; some individuals improve with these treatments, but an equal number get worse.

Approximately 70% of the patients diagnosed with schizophrenia show great improvement in their symptomatology with antipsychotic treatment, and approximately 20% show minimal improvement (Baldessarini, 1985). (These figures may change significantly once clozapine and related substances come into wider use.) As mentioned earlier, a few patients get worse with antipsychotic medications, perhaps because of toxic reactions at high doses. Neurochemical differences within the schizophrenic population are a likely factor in differential responsiveness to antipsychotics, but pharmacokinetic factors also may be involved (Verghese et al., 1991). This hypothesis is consistent with recent studies on institutionalized patients that have demonstrated that nonresponders may exhibit antipsychotic blood levels far lower (often two to seven times lower) than responders when given the same doses of antipsychotics. Another factor in nonresponse may relate to the difficulties in diagnosing schizophrenia; that is, some patients diagnosed with this disorder may actually be misdiagnosed unipolar or bipolar patients (discussed in Chapter 13) and may be more appropriately treated with lithium or antidepressants (Glazer et al., 1987).

As yet, there are no consistent pretreatment symptomatic predictors of antipsychotic response. Several studies have suggested that, in comparison with poor responders, good responders are more likely to have better social adjustment and less schizoid developmental history, are older at first hospitalization or onset of symptoms, and have higher plasma levels of catecholamine (DA and NE) metabolites (Bowers et al., 1987).

Factors such as antipsychotic dose, major symptom characteristics, and chronicity are important in determining the efficacy of antipsychotics. In spite of the fact that antipsychotics have been used for nearly 40 years, there is no general consensus as to the correct doses to be employed, but many clinicians feel that the doses of these drugs now in use are far in excess of what is required (Verghese et al., 1991). In addition there may be a therapeutic window such that levels below or above the window are associated with poorer outcomes. There is widespread agreement that patients with positive symptoms are more likely to respond to typical antipsychotics, whereas those with negative symptoms respond poorly. It is also clear that a history of chronic hospitalization predicts poor response (Volavka & Cooper, 1987).

Analysis of the psychotic symptoms most affected by antipsychotics indicate a specificity in their activity. Agitated, belligerent, impulsive behavior in patients is markedly reduced, whereas withdrawn or autistic patients sometimes become more responsive and communicative. Generally over a period of days, psychotic symptoms of hallucinations, delusions, and disorganized or incoherent thinking tend to disappear (Baldessarini, 1990). Improvements in sleep, self-care, appetite, and sometimes seclusiveness occur. Improvement in insight, judgment, memory, and orientation are also likely in cases of acute psychosis, whereas in chronic schizophrenics, changes in these are variable and often unsatisfactory (Baldessarini, 1985). On the other hand, nonspecific schizophrenic symptoms such as anxiety, tension, and guilt may remain relatively unaffected by antipsychotics. Indeed, in mild cases of schizophrenia these symptoms may be aggravated. In chronic schizophrenic patients stabilized on an antipsychotic medication who experience moderate to severe symptoms of anxiety, use of a benzodiazepine anxiolytic, such as alprazolam (Xanax), has been shown to be useful as an adjunctive treatment (Morphy, 1986).

General improvement with antipsychotic treatment approximates a learning curve, in that there is a rapid change in the first few weeks of treatment, a slowing of improvement in the sixth to 12th weeks, and a very slow change thereafter. The rate of change for specific symptoms may vary; for example, hyperactive and manic symptoms may disappear after only a few doses of an antipsychotic, whereas delusions or hallucinations may persist with lessened affect after weeks of daily drug exposure. The abnormal thought and poor interpersonal relations of catatonic patients may improve weeks before the pathologic motor pattern is altered (Hollister, 1973).

There are some indications that the high-potency antipsychotics like haloperidol most rapidly control the manic patient. There were some early suggestions that these high-potency drugs given in large doses (for example, 100 mg or more of haloperidol) may be more effective when given at the beginning of treatment, with the dosage reduced considerably when schizophrenic symptoms subside. However, more recent studies have not found large-dose treatment to be any more effective than smaller doses of these drugs (Baldessarini, 1985).

There is uneven development of tolerance to the effects of antipsychotics (Baldessarini, 1985). Their ability to suppress psychotic symptoms is fairly stable, although symptoms can worsen or improve over time. In fact, once the symptoms subside, most authorities suggest that lower antipsychotic doses should be given unless the patient has a clear history of symptom worsening when the medication dose is decreased.

Tolerance does tend to occur to a certain degree with respect to many of the side effects of these drugs, including sedative effects, hypotension, and anticholinergic effects.

Antipsychotic drugs do not generally possess any potential for inducing psychological dependence, primarily because of the numerous side effects associated with this class of drugs. However, they may induce mild abstinence symptoms after abrupt cessation of high doses; in some cases, there may be signs of malaise, gastrointestinal dysfunction, nausea and vomiting, and tremulousness. A transient worsening of psychotic symptoms may occur. Also, motor disturbances similar to those associated with tardive dyskinesia may occur, but then rapidly dissipate. Since most of these drugs have relatively long plasma half-lives or have active metabolites, plasma levels of active drug decline slowly, so that these symptoms are generally not very severe or noticeable.

After a patient has been stabilized with antipsychotic medication, the question of what to do next remains, particularly in light of the potential side effects (some of which may be irreversible) associated with chronic drug exposure. One possibility is to simply stop the medication. However, a recent review of a number of well-controlled studies indicated that although only 30% of the patients maintained on medication showed symptom relapse, approximately 65% of the patients given placebos relapsed within a year (Baldessarini, 1985). Thus there was both good news and bad news. That is, some patients will relapse even if maintained on antipsychotics, whereas other patients will not relapse if taken off these drugs and do not require continued drug exposure. Some patients who relapse when taken off antipsychotics completely may benefit from a significant reduction in their medication dose (for instance, a 50% decrease in dose). In some cases, these patients' overall psychological functioning may actually improve from the dose reduction (Faraone et al., 1986).

Unfortunately, predicting which patients will relapse and which will not is very difficult. Recent studies assessing psychosocial factors in the relapse of patients whose antipsychotic medications have been significantly reduced have suggested that interpersonal variables relating to stress and coping may mediate relapse. Patients may be at a greater risk of relapse if they live with highly critical and overinvolved relatives. Those with reduced risk of relapse either have been involved in behavioral treatments that improve social competence and family problem solving or have social network members with whom they can discuss problems in a helpful manner (Faraone et al., 1986). Patients with good social adjustment who develop symptoms abruptly in response to stress and who usually respond rapidly to antipsychotics probably should not be maintained on them, since they may never develop the symptoms again. Furthermore, chronic hospitalized schizophrenics who respond only minimally to antipsychotics should also not be maintained on antipsychotics, since the risk of tardive dyskinesia outweighs the benefits of these drugs.

Antipsychotic Side Effects

As noted earlier, the primary differences among the drugs in this class are differential tendencies to induce the numerous side effects (see Table 12–1) associated with their use (Baldessarini, 1990). Perhaps the most noticeable and common of these side effects are the movement abnormalities referred to as *extrapyramidal symptoms* (so-called because they result from disturbances in the brain structures affecting bodily movement, excluding motor neurons, the motor cortex, and the pyramidal tract). Because many of these symptoms resemble those associated with Parkinson's disease, antipsychotics are said to induce pseudoparkinsonism. The symptoms consist primarily of tremor, *dystonia* (muscle rigidity), and *bradykinesia* (extreme slowness of movement). Other symptoms include *akathisia* (motor restlessness), *akinesia* (immobility), expressionless face, and subtle motor speech abnormalities.

Signs of motor disturbances usually begin within a few days of initiating antipsychotic medication and are almost always noticed within three months of treatment. As noted earlier, clozapine is an exception; it does not appear to induce extrapyramidal side effects (Baldessarini & Frankenburg, 1991). Extrapyramidal symptoms wax and wane. Acute dystonic reactions tend to dissipate quickly, pseudoparkinsonism symptoms may persist or decrease over several weeks, and tardive dyskinesia symptoms may begin to appear after several months (Baldessarini, 1985).

Extrapyramidal symptoms can usually be controlled by lowering the dosage of antipsychotic or adding antiparkinsonism agents. These are generally drugs with antihistamine and anticholinergic properties (for example, Artane, Benadryl, and Cogentin). The fact that drugs with anticholinergic properties are effective in reducing both pseudoparkinsonism and parkinsonism has suggested to some researchers that these symptoms are due to a dopaminergic-cholinergic imbalance—that is, too little DA activity relative to acetylcholine activity.

Neuroendocrine side effects (weight gain, breast enlargement and tenderness, decreased sex drive, and lack of menstruation) may also occur. Recently, the DA agonist amantadine (Symmetrel) has been used in several clinical trials to successfully reduce both the neuroendocrine side effects and the extrapyramidal symptoms induced by antipsychotics (Correa et al., 1987). Curiously, adding amantadine to antipsychotics was also found to significantly reduce psychotic symptoms. Although this phenomenon appears contrary to the DA hypothesis of schizophrenia, some investigators have argued that this result may be related to amantadine's action as a selective nigrostriatal dopamine agonist—that is, reversing DA blockade at nigrostriatal but not mesolimbic sites. Others argue that amantadine is a mixed agonist-antagonist—that is, an agonist at nigrostriatal and tuberoinfundibular sites and an antagonist at mesolimbic sites (Correa et al., 1987).

Although less disturbing than the extrapyramidal symptoms, the side effects associated with acetylcholine blockade (such as blurred vision, dry mouth, nasal congestion, constipation, and difficulty in urinating) can be unpleasant. The lower-potency compounds also have a higher incidence of orthostatic hypotension and allergic reactions than the high-potency compounds. Examples of such reactions are photosensitivity, dermatitis (skin rash), pigmentary changes (yellow skin and eyes), and agranulocytosis (decrease in white blood cells). The lower-potency compounds may also be more prone to induce epileptic seizure activity (Baldessarini, 1985).

It would appear that one strategy for dealing with side effects would be to change the antipsychotic drug. One might note from Table 12-1 that the antipsychotics requiring higher therapeutic doses (namely, the lower-potency compounds) generally have a lower incidence of extrapyramidal symptoms associated with them. On the other hand, these antipsychotics are more likely to be associated with a higher incidence and a higher degree of anticholinergic side effects. In fact, it is likely that these drugs' potent antimuscarinic properties are the reason for the lower incidence of extrapyramidal symptoms associated with them.

One rare, but potentially fatal, side effect of antipsychotics that has only recently become widely recognized is the so-called *neuroleptic malignant syndrome* (Guze & Baxter, 1985). Core features of this syndrome are severe catatonia, instability of the autonomic nervous system, hyperthermia, and stupor. Early reports indicated that the syndrome was lethal in approximately 20–30% of patients developing this side effect, but recent reports suggest that lethality has decreased to almost zero, perhaps because of earlier diagnosis, rapid drug discontinuation and institution of intensive care, or use of dopamine-augmenting drugs (for example, amantadine, L-dopa, and bromocriptine) (Caroff & Mann, 1988). Although all antipsychotics have been shown to induce this syndrome, it is believed that it is more likely to occur with the use of higher doses of the more potent DA-blocking agents.

The determination of the appropriate antipsychotic and dose depends upon the clinician's experience and his or her familiarity with the various antipsychotics, the ability to regularly monitor the patient's response, the patient's compliance with the drug regimen, and luck. Because the extrapyramidal side effects are generally less tolerated than the others, most patients are more comfortable with those antipsychotics with high antimuscarinic activity, such as thioridazine (Mellaril). Because so many psychiatrists are familiar with the original prototype chlorpromazine (Thorazine), it is still one of the most commonly prescribed antipsychotics. Patients who respond well to chlorpromazine or thiorida-zine, but who find the side effects associated with a low-potency com-pound too disturbing, may respond well to one of the higher-potency phenothiazines like trifluoperazine (Stelazine) or to the high-potency butyrophenone haloperidol (Haldol). For patients who do not take their medications reliably, antipsychotics like fluphenazine decanoate (Prolixin Decanoate), a high-potency phenothiazine with a very long duration of action (perhaps as long as six weeks with a single injection in some pa-tients on maintenance therapy), can be injected intramuscularly or subcu-taneously. The thioxanthenes chlorprothixene (Taractan) and thiothixene (Navane), the indole molindone (Moban), and the dibenzoxazepine loxa-pine (Loxitane) all seem to have a good antipsychotic action with moder-ately well tolerated side effects.

　　Finally, in patients who do not respond to the typical antipsy-chotics, or who tend toward developing extrapyramidal side effects, clozapine (Clozaril) can be used alone or in conjunction with other antipsychotic drugs, provided precautionary measures are taken. White blood cell counts should be performed regularly, particularly in cases of infection, to prevent the risk of agranulocytosis. Although clozapine does not induce extrapyramidal symptoms, it does carry a relatively high risk of inducing grand mal seizures at higher dosages (Baldessarini & Frankenburg, 1991). It may induce autonomic side effects, such as orthostatic hypotension, hypersalivation, constipation, and weight gain. Orthostatic hypotension may be particularly troublesome because it may make patients fall down and severely hurt themselves.

Tardive Dyskinesia

Just about all of the side effects noted in the preceding section go away if antipsychotic medications are reduced in dosage or are eliminated. How-ever, one potential and considerably troublesome side effect that in some cases may not disappear is *tardive dyskinesia* (Tarsy & Baldessarini, 1984). It is common to all the antipsychotics (except the atypical anti-psychotics like clozapine). It is a movement disorder consisting of fre-quent, repetitive, involuntary movements of the lips, tongue, jaw, face, and sometimes trunk or limbs. It usually occurs after prolonged anti-psychotic treatment, and once established, the symptoms may persist for months or years following antipsychotic treatment. The symptoms decrease or disappear altogether with sedation or sleep and increase under emotional stress or during activities requiring repetition of motor activities or attention to fine motor tasks. Attempts to consciously con-trol the symptoms may increase the movements.

　　Age is a factor in recovery from tardive dyskinesia symptoms. With young patients, discontinuation of antipsychotic medication generally increases the symptoms, but there may be steady improvement over a period of months or years, provided the antipsychotics are withheld. Most research shows that mild cases in the young are most easily reversible, with current remission rates of 50–90% being reported. With older patients, there is poor prognosis for recovery.

Estimates of the incidence of tardive dyskinesia vary greatly, with a mean of around 10–15%. Patients with late-onset psychoses, females, and individuals over the age of 50 are more prone to developing the symptoms (Yassa et al., 1986). The onset of the symptoms is typically subtle but may be abrupt when the antipsychotics are suddenly withdrawn. Although clinicians have advocated that drug-free periods be used routinely to reduce the possibility of tardive dyskinesia and to determine whether the symptoms are developing, several recent studies have provided evidence that drug-free periods are actually accompanied by an increased risk of subsequent tardive dyskinesia, for reasons as yet unclear (Nordic Dyskinesia Study Group, 1986; Yassa et al., 1986).

A variety of biochemical pathologies are likely involved in tardive dyskinesia. This side effect is believed to be due predominantly to prolonged DA receptor blockade, leading to supersensitive DA receptors and causing a relative dominance of DA over acetylcholine activity (just the opposite of pseudoparkinsonism) (Baldessarini, 1985). Decreased activity in certain GABAergic striatonigral neurons and noradrenergic hyperactivity have also been suggested to be factors in the pathophysiology of tardive dyskinesia (Nordic Dyskinesia Study Group, 1986).

Early drug treatments for the disorder consisted of either trying to reduce DA activity or enhancing cholinergic activity. Unfortunately, the former tactic (for example, increasing the dose of antipsychotic) leads only to temporary relief and potential worsening of the condition later on. The latter tactic (for example, administering physostigmine, which reduces acetylcholine metabolism, or lecithin, deanol, or choline, which increase brain acetylcholine synthesis) has been shown to exert temporary or negligible benefits or to induce other side effects.

Recent attempts to amplify DA activity (such as with L-dopa or apomorphine) to desensitize DA receptors have led to encouraging findings, but there is the possibility that these treatments may precipitate or aggravate schizophrenic symptoms. A number of other miscellaneous drugs, including lithium, pyridoxine, niacinamide, manganese, estrogen, baclofen, fusaric acid, tryptophan, barbiturates, morphine, naloxone, enkephalins, hydergine, amantadine, and methylphenidate (in other words, just about everything), have been tried and found to be of limited, negligible, or questionable clinical value in the treatment of tardive dyskinesia (Volavka et al., 1986).

It is clear that until a satisfactory treatment for tardive dyskinesia is found, the prevention and early diagnosis of these potentially socially disruptive symptoms must be emphasized. Effective prevention lies in cautious use of antipsychotics. The smallest doses that sustain improvement should be used, and patients who can maintain gains without drugs should be afforded such an opportunity. It is indeed unfortunate that a person exhibiting, and being treated for, one set of socially disruptive behaviors may someday exhibit another set of socially disturbing behaviors for which there is no treatment.

Bibliography

Andreasen, N. C. (1988). Brain imaging: Applications in psychiatry. *Science, 239,* 1381–1388.

Baldessarini, R. J. (1985). *Chemotherapy and psychiatry.* Cambridge, MA: Harvard University Press.

Baldessarini, R. J. (1990). Drugs and the treatment of psychiatric disorders. In A. G. Gilman, T. W. Rall, A. S. Nies, & P. Taylor (Eds.), *The pharmacological basis of therapeutics* (pp. 383–435). New York: Pergamon Press.

Baldessarini, R. J., & Frankenburg, F. R. (1991). Clozapine: A novel antipsychotic agent. *New England Journal of Medicine, 324,* 746–754.

Ban, T. A. (1975). Nicotinic acid in the treatment of schizophrenias. *Neuropsychobiology, 1,* 133–145.

Barnes, D. M. (1987). Biological issues in schizophrenia. *Science, 235,* 430–434.

Bowers, M. B., Swigar, M. E., Jatlow, P. I., Hofman, F. J., & Goicoechea, N. (1987). Early neuroleptic response: Clinical profiles and plasma catecholamine metabolites. *Journal of Clinical Psychopharmacology, 7,* 83–86.

Bucci, L. (1987). The negative symptoms of schizophrenia and the monoamine oxidase inhibitors. *Psychopharmacology, 91,* 104–108.

Buchsbaum, M. S., Wu, J. C., DeLisi, L. E., Holcomb, H. H., Hazlett, E., Cooper-Langston, K., & Kessler, R. (1987). Positron emission tomography studies of basal ganglia and somatosensory cortex neuroleptic drug effects: Differences between normal controls and schizophrenic patients. *Biological Psychiatry, 22,* 479–494.

Carlsson, A. (1978). Mechanism of action of neuroleptic drugs. In M. A. Lipton, A. DiMascio, & K. F. Killam (Eds.), *Psychopharmacology* (pp. 1057–1070). New York: Raven Press.

Caroff, S. N., & Mann, S. C. (1988). Neuroleptic malignant syndrome. *Psychopharmacology Bulletin, 24,* 25–29.

Correa, N., Opler, L. A., Kay, S. R., & Birmaher, B. (1987). Amantadine in the treatment of neuroendocrine side effects of neuroleptics. *Journal of Clinical Psychopharmacology, 7,* 91–95.

Davis, G. C., Bunney, W. E., DeFraites, E. G., Kleinman, J. E., van Kamen, D. P., Post, R. M., & Wyatt, R. J. (1977). Intravenous naloxone administration in schizophrenia and affective illness. *Science, 197,* 74–76.

Faraone, S. V., Curran, J. P., Laughren, T., Faltus, F., Johnston, R., & Brown, W. A. (1986). Neuroleptic bioavailability, psychosocial factors, and clinical status: A 1-year study of schizophrenic outpatients after dose reduction. *Psychiatry Research, 19,* 311–322.

Farde, L., Hall, H., Ehrin, E., & Sedvall, G. (1986). Quantitative analysis of D_2

dopamine receptor binding in the living human brain by PET. *Science, 231,* 258–261.

Gillin, J. C., Stoff, D. M., & Wyatt, R. J. (1978). Transmethylation hypothesis: A review of progress. In M. A. Lipton, A. DiMascio, & K. F. Killam (Eds.), *Psychopharmacology* (pp. 1097–1112). New York: Raven Press.

Glazer, W. M., Pino, C. D., & Quinlan, D. (1987). The reassessment of chronic patients previously diagnosed as schizophrenic. *Journal of Clinical Psychiatry, 48,* 430–433.

Grace, A. A. (1991). Phasic versus tonic dopamine release and the modulation of dopamine system responsivity: A hypothesis for the etiology of schizophrenia. *Neuroscience, 41,* 1–24.

Guze, B. H., & Baxter, L. R. (1985). Current concepts: Neuroleptic malignant syndrome. *New England Journal of Medicine, 313,* 163–166.

Hays, P., & Aidroos, N. (1986). Alcoholism followed by schizophrenia. *Acta Psychiatrica Scandinavica, 74,* 187–189.

Hollister, L. E. (1973). *Clinical use of psychotherapeutic drugs.* Springfield, IL: Charles C. Thomas.

Lane, R., & Blaha, C. D. (1987). Chronic haloperidol decreases dopamine release in striatum and nucleus accumbens in vivo: Depolarization block as a possible mechanism of action. *Brain Research Bulletin, 18,* 135–138.

Lieberman, J. A., Kane, J. M., & Alvir, J. (1987). Provocative tests with psychostimulant drugs in schizophrenia. *Psychopharmacology, 91,* 415–433.

May, P.R.A., & Goldberg, S. C. (1978). Prediction of schizophrenic patients' response to pharmacotherapy. In M. A. Lipton, A. DiMascio, & K. F. Killam (Eds.), *Psychopharmacology: A generation of progress* (pp. 1139–1154). New York: Raven Press.

Meltzer, H. Y. (1991). The mechanism of action of novel antipsychotic drugs. *Schizophrenia Bulletin, 17,* 263–277.

Morphy, M. A. (1986). A double-blind comparison of alprazolam and placebo in the treatment of anxious schizophrenic outpatients. *Current Therapeutic Research, 40,* 551–560.

Moskovitz, C., Moses, H., & Klawans, H. L. (1978). Levodopa-induced psychosis: A kindling phenomenon. *American Journal of Psychiatry, 135,* 669–675.

Newton, M., Godbey, K. L., Newton, D. W., & Godbey, A. L. (1978, July). How you can improve the effectiveness of psychotropic drug therapy. *Nursing78,* pp. 45–55.

Nordic Dyskinesia Study Group (1986). Effect of different neuroleptics in tardive dyskinesia and parkinsonism. *Psychopharmacology, 90,* 423–429.

Paul, S. M. (1977). Movement and madness: Towards a biological model of schizophrenia. In J. D. Maser & M.E.P. Seligman (Eds.), *Psychopathology: Experimental models* (pp. 358–386). San Francisco: W. H. Freeman.

Safferman, A., Leiberman, J. A., Kane, J. M., Szymanski, S., & Kinon, B. (1991). Update on the clinical efficacy and side effects of clozapine. *Schizophrenia Bulletin, 17,* 247–257.

Schmauss, C., & Emrich, H. M. (1986). Dopamine and the action of opiates: A reevaluation of the dopamine hypothesis of schizophrenia with special considerations of the endogenous opioids in the pathogenesis of schizophrenia. *Biological Psychiatry, 20,* 1211–1231.

Seeman, P. (1987). Dopamine receptors and the dopamine hypothesis of schizophrenia. *Synapse, 1,* 133–152.

Seeman, P., & Lee, T. (1975). Antipsychotic drugs: Direct correlation between clinical potency and presynaptic action on dopamine neurons. *Science, 188,* 1217–1219.

Seeman, P., Ulpian, C., Bergeron, C., Riederer, P., Jellinger, K., Gabriel, E., Reynolds, G. P., & Tourtellotte, W. W. (1984). Bimodal distribution of dopamine receptor densities in brains of schizophrenics. *Science, 225,* 728–731.

Singh, M. M., & Kay, S. R. (1976). Wheat gluten as a pathogenic factor in schizophrenia. *Science, 191,* 401–402.

Suddath, R. L., Christison, G. W., Torrey, E. F., Casanova, M. F., & Weinberger, D. R. (1990). Anatomical abnormalities in the brains of monozygotic twins discordant for schizophrenia. *New England Journal of Medicine, 322,* 789–794.

Tammiga, C. A., Schaffer, M. H., & Davis, J. M. (1978). Schizophrenic symptoms improve with apomorphine. *Science, 200,* 567–568.

Tarsy, D., & Baldessarini, R. J. (1984). Tardive dyskinesia. *Annual Review of Medicine, 35,* 605–623.

Van Kammen, D. P., Mann, L. S., Sternberg, D. E., Scheinin, M., Ninan, P. T., Marder, S. R., van Kammen, W. B., Rieder, R. O., & Linnoila, M. (1983). Dopamine-beta-hydroxylase activity and homovanillic acid in spinal fluid of schizophrenics with brain atrophy. *Science, 220,* 974–977.

Verghese, C., Kessel, J. B., & Simpson, G. M. (1991). Clinical pharmacokinetics of neuroleptics. *Psychopharmacology Bulletin, 27,* 541–564.

Volavka, J., & Cooper, T. B. (1987). Review of haloperidol blood level and clinical response: Looking through the window. *Journal of Clinical Psychopharmacology, 7,* 25–30.

Volavka, J., O'Donnell, J., Muragali, R., Anderson, B. G., Gaztanaga, P., Boggiano, W., Whittaker, R., & Sta. Maria, T. (1986). Lithium and lecithin in tardive dyskinesia: An update. *Psychiatry Research, 19,* 101–104.

Walters, J. R., Bergstrom, D. A., Carlson, J. H., Chase, T. N., & Braun, A. R. (1987). D_1 receptor activation required for postsynaptic expression of D_2 agonist effects. *Science, 236,* 719–722.

Wong, D. F., Wagner, H. N., Tune, L. E., Dannals, R. F., Pearlson, G. D., Links, J. M., Tamminga, C. A., Broussoile, E. P., Ravert, H. T., Wilson, A. A., Toung, J.K.T., Malat, J., Williams, J. A., O'Tauma, L. A., Snyder, S. H., Kuhar, M. J., & Gjedde, A. (1986). Positron emission tomography reveals elevated D_2 dopamine receptors in drug-naive schizophrenics. *Science, 234,* 1558–1561.

Yassa, R., Nair, V., & Schwartz, G. (1986). Early versus late onset psychosis and tardive dyskinesia. *Society of Biological Psychiatry, 21,* 1291–1297.

Chapter Thirteen

Antidepressants and Antimanics

The primary symptoms of schizophrenia are most notable in the cognitive and perceptual spheres; distortions in mood and emotions are secondary and variable. However, with the affective disorders—depression, mania, and manic-depression—mood and emotional disturbances are the primary symptoms, and these may be accompanied by distortions in thought patterns. (Unfortunately, these distinctions may not be particularly clear and can lead to variability in clinical diagnoses.) Since depression is a primary factor in tens of thousands of suicides every year, it is a major public health concern requiring intervention. Studies indicate that as many as 15% of the population experience at least one severe depressive episode at some point in their lives. Although mania is much less common, the destructive behaviors accompanying it also require intervention. In many of these cases, drugs are a primary form of intervention, either alone or in combination with other forms of psychotherapy.

The treatment of depression is made difficult by the fact that it is both a normal mood state, which a person encounters during periods of loss and which is generally transitory, and an emotional disorder. Depression can also result from a pattern of drug abuse that the person may be reluctant to change. Symptoms of depression as a disorder may remit spontaneously or may come and go over time. Therefore, it is hard to determine whether intervention is necessary or would even be beneficial. However, depression is viewed as an emotional disorder requiring intervention when the person is profoundly sad for a period of time, loses the ability to experience normal pleasure (anhedonia), denies past accomplishments, feels unworthy of current achievements, or expresses suicidal ideas. Physical complaints of loss of appetite and weight, insomnia, early morning awakenings, aches and pains, and so forth may also be present. Under extreme conditions, a depressed person may severely distort reality and exhibit unusual beliefs or behaviors. Because fear and anxiety may accompany depression, the person may be physically active but may not be able to concentrate on any one task for very long.

In about one-fifth of depressed persons there may be an extreme shift in mood toward mania—sometimes called *manic-depression* or *bipolar disorder* (the current designation in the *Diagnostic and Statistical Manual of Mental Disorders, Third Edition–Revised,* published in 1987 by the American Psychiatric Association). In the large majority of these cases, there is a clear genetic basis (Kolata, 1986). Although manic episodes are not always accompanied by depressive episodes, such cases are extremely rare. During these episodes, the person may exhibit extreme elation, display unusually high activity levels, and be irrationally optimistic and overconfident. However, this mood is brittle—that is, easily and dramatically changed by the specific circumstances—and the person can become irritable if frustrated. The thought patterns during mania are often disturbed, with one thought rapidly following another (referred to as "flight of ideas"). While mild forms of mania, termed hypomania, may be beneficial to the person in social and vocational contexts, extreme forms of mania can be very destructive to the person's career and interpersonal relationships. Some persons with the bipolar disorder may shift back and forth between the two extremes of depression and mania, while others may exhibit long periods of relatively normal functioning between episodes. Because depressive episodes are generally more common in these individuals, it is often difficult to determine whether a unipolar disorder (that is, one in which only depression symptoms are evidenced) or bipolar disorder is present. However, the distinction is important because the types of drugs that are most effective in the two disorders are quite different. Giving a bipolar patient medication appropriate for the unipolar depressive disorder may precipitate a manic episode, whereas giving a unipolar depressed patient medication appropriate for the bipolar patient may not be beneficial and may prolong unnecessary discomfort (Holden, 1986).

Biochemical Hypotheses of Affective Disorders

As is the case with schizophrenia, there are many theories about the causes of affective disorders. However, because this text deals with chemicals that alter cognitions, emotions, and behavior, presumably through altering the biochemistry of the brain, we will deal only with biochemically oriented theories.

As you read this section, it should become clear that we really have little understanding of what causes dysfunctional mood states or how present-day antidepressants or antimanics produce their benefits at a biochemical level. We know a lot about these drugs with respect to their actions on various neurotransmitter systems, but how these actions relate to their beneficial effects is still a puzzle. Clearly, some actions contribute primarily to side effects; others contribute to side effects and possibly to their beneficial effects; and others are probably linked to their beneficial effects. But in reality we just aren't sure. I wish I could give the readers some simple answers to their questions about these issues, but at present simple answers just aren't available.

The hypothesis that has dominated neuroscientists' thought for many years is known as the *catecholamine hypothesis of affective disorders* (McNeal & Cimbolic, 1986). This hypothesis suggests that depression may be related to a deficiency of norepinephrine and/or dopamine (primarily norepinephrine) at functionally important CNS receptors and that mania may be related to the opposite set of conditions. However, as will soon become evident, studies indicated that deficits in serotonergic functioning may also be involved in mood disturbances, so the hypothesis has been broadened and is often referred to as the *monoamine* (or simply *amine*) *hypothesis of affective disorders.*

The role of catecholamines in affect is consistent with a great deal of research indicating that the catecholamines are highly involved in primary motivation and reward. These neurotransmitters are found in high concentrations in the limbic system and are heavily involved in areas of the brain in which electrical stimulation has reinforcing properties (Fibiger & Phillips, 1981). As noted earlier, one of the primary features of depressed individuals is their lack of drive and their inability to experience normal life activities as rewarding.

One of the first pieces of evidence for the hypothesis came from the observation that the drug reserpine not only reduced mania in humans but also precipitated a severe depression in some individuals treated with this drug. These phenomena correlate with the finding that reserpine depletes the brain of catecholamines by preventing their binding to the synaptic vesicles. Outside of the protection of the vesicles, the catecholamines are accessible to the enzyme monoamine oxidase (MAO), which is present intraneuronally; MAO then metabolizes the catecholamines into inactive molecules. Conversely, it was discovered that some drugs that had mood-elevating properties also were capable of inhibiting the action of MAO (thus they are called MAO inhibitors). Theoretically, this inhibiting action should allow catecholamines to accumulate in neuronal tissues and make more neurotransmitters available for release in the process of neurotransmission. Furthermore, MAO inhibitors were found to block the effects of reserpine; that is, even though reserpine prevents the monoamines from binding to vesicles, without MAO activity there would still be a pool of monoamines in the terminal available for release during an action potential.

As noted in Chapter 9, it has long been recognized that the potent psychostimulants like amphetamine and cocaine elevate mood and can induce mania and that these effects correlate with their ability to temporarily increase the levels of catecholamines in the synapse (by increasing the amounts released or blocking their reuptake after release). However, prolonged use of these drugs depletes catecholamines (probably because they are used faster than they are synthesized). This depletion correlates with the depression and lethargy that often occur when the person stops taking these drugs.

Further evidence for the catecholamine hypothesis came with the discovery of the tricyclic antidepressants (so called because of their three-ringed molecular structure). Many studies noted that the primary biochemical action of these drugs was inhibition of the reuptake of catecholamines back into the axon terminal, thus allowing them to stay in the synaptic cleft longer and to have greater access to their receptors. Similar actions occur with more recently developed nontricyclic antidepressants. However, it was with these observations that the catecholamine hypothesis began to fall apart because the biochemical actions of the reuptake-blocking drugs were observed to occur within minutes of exposure, but their mood-elevating effects generally take several days or weeks of chronic exposure.

To resolve this discrepancy, researchers began looking at changes in the receptors of norepinephrine after chronic tricyclic exposure. For example, it is possible that chronic exposure to tricyclics somehow enhances the sensitivity of postsynaptic catecholamine receptors. Their search led to a confusing array of findings. Both presynaptic alpha-2-adrenoceptors (autoreceptors) and postsynaptic beta-adrenergic receptors tend to decline in sensitivity with chronic tricyclic exposure, whereas postsynaptic alpha-1-adrenoceptors tend to increase in sensitivity (McNeal & Cimbolic, 1986). The findings regarding the postsynaptic beta-receptors seem contrary to the catecholamine hypothesis. However, the decreased binding in the population of noradrenergic autoreceptors would be consistent with the hypothesis because it would reduce the inhibitory function of these receptors and allow more norepinephrine to be released or synthesized. This phenomenon may explain why acute treatment with tricyclics has no beneficial effects, whereas chronic treatment does (Garcia-Sevilla & Zubieta, 1986). When reuptake is initially inhibited, norepinephrine would be expected to build up outside the neuron. However, because of excessive activity at the noradrenergic autoreceptors, release of norepinephrine would be decreased, thus counterbalancing the effect of reduced reuptake. With chronic exposure and desensitization in norepinephrine autoreceptors, there would be an enhancement of norepinephrine release. Unfortunately, most of the more recent studies exploring this issue have led to the conclusion that adrenergic autoreceptor subsensitivity is an unproven and unlikely mechanism for producing the antidepressant effects of NE reuptake inhibitors (Meltzer, 1990).

There are other problems with respect to fitting the tricyclic antidepressants into the catecholamine hypothesis. One is that animals administered these drugs show predominantly signs of sedation. Another is that nondepressed humans evidence no signs of mood elevation when these drugs are administered. These effects may be due to the fact that most drugs of this nature also have significant anticholinergic properties that can cause sedation and may be viewed as unpleasant by normal individuals.

Lithium is another drug with actions that on the surface appear to be consistent with the catecholamine hypothesis but that upon close examination are paradoxical. Lithium is a very effective treatment for manic symptoms, and it may also antagonize some effects of amphetamine and cocaine. Furthermore, several studies on the biochemical effects of lithium suggest that it either reduces the amount of catecholamine released from nervous tissue or enhances catecholamine reuptake (Baldessarini, 1990). However, as is the case with the tricyclics, these physiological effects occur rapidly, whereas remission (the clinical term for lessening or abating) of manic symptoms takes several days or weeks to occur. These biochemical actions are also hard to reconcile with the fact that lithium can significantly reduce the likelihood of depressive cycles in the manic-depressive patient.

Other drugs that may be viewed as having properties consistent with the catecholamine hypothesis are the antipsychotics and the antihypertensive drug clonidine. The antipsychotics are very effective in reducing manic symptoms and are known to reduce access of catecholamines, primarily dopamine, to their receptors. Their action in both cases is relatively rapid (Baldessarini, 1990). Clonidine is a noradrenergic autoreceptor agonist. Its primary action is the inhibition of norepinephrine synthesis or release, and in very rare cases, it may result in depression. It has also been shown to reduce mania in some manic patients (Hardy et al., 1986).

Other evidence supporting the catecholamines' involvement in mood comes from studies suggesting that some depressed patients seem to excrete lower amounts of MHPG (McNeal & Cimbolic, 1986), one of the major breakdown metabolites of norepinephrine. In manic patients, MHPG levels have been found in several studies to be elevated in the cerebrospinal fluid (CSF), in comparison with normal subjects or depressed patients (Swann et al., 1987). On the other hand, the CSF levels of the major metabolites of DA and serotonin have not been shown to bear any consistent relationship with manic symptoms. Following lithium treatment (the most common drug treatment for mania), there is a reduction in CSF MHPG levels. Curiously, in one recent study verifying these observations, it was determined that lithium responders (that is, patients whose symptoms decreased on lithium) and nonresponders did not differ in terms of pretreatment mania ratings or neurotransmitter metabolite measures. Nor did they differ in the degree to which CSF MHPG levels decreased during lithium treatment. Thus these findings, although they support a relationship between mania and increased noradrenergic function, suggest that reduced noradrenergic activity may be necessary but not sufficient for successful alleviation of manic symptoms (Swann et al., 1987).

It is unlikely that a single neurotransmitter is responsible for mood and mood disorders. Several drugs in the tricyclic class also effectively reduce serotonin (5-HT) reuptake and, in fact, have a greater affinity for the serotonin reuptake pump than for the norepinephrine pump. Recent studies indicate that chronic exposure to MAO inhibitors down-regulates serotonin autoreceptors, thereby enhancing serotonin neurotransmission (Offord & Warwick, 1987). Recently, some researchers have gone so far as to suggest that "low 5-HT" depressed individuals are those most prone to suicide, because several studies have found that people who commit suicide are likely to have low levels of a serotonin metabolite, 5-HIAA, in their cerebrospinal fluid as well as more $5-HT_2$ receptors in their prefrontal cortex—both of which are consistent with diminished serotonergic transmission (Arango et al., 1990). Thus the monoamine serotonin is also viewed as being important in certain cases of depression. That the symptoms of depression may be the result of either insufficient noradrenergic or serotonergic activity would not be surprising considering the fact that in the CNS both systems greatly overlap in terms of distribution and physiological activity (see, for example, Figure 5–4).

Other versions of the monoamine hypothesis have been proposed. One is that low levels of serotonin "permit" the level of norepinephrine to determine the affective state; that is, a low level of norepinephrine causes depression, and a high level causes mania (Richelson, 1991). This hypothesis would be consistent with the observation that drugs that selectively amplify the activity of either serotonin (e g., fluoxetine) or norepinephrine (e.g., desipramine) are effective antidepressants. It would also tie in with lithium's ability to stabilize mood in manic-depressives, because one of lithium's actions, upon chronic administration, is to stabilize serotonin synthesis (Cooper et al., 1991).

While it is generally accepted that, acutely administered, most antidepressant drugs enhance monoaminergic neurotransmission, it is not clear how their actions are related to depression symptom remission. The inhibition of 5-HT or NE uptake is rapid, but the lifting of symptoms is slow. On the other hand, the time course for symptom remission is highly correlated with the desensitization or down-regulation of NE or 5-HT receptors that results from the increased activity of these neurotransmitters at their receptors (Nelson, 1991). This correlation would suggest that depression is the result of overly sensitive 5-HT or NE receptors—rather than the originally hypothesized deficiency of activity at NE or 5-HT receptors. But if this is the case, why does repeated electroconvulsive shock (the most effective antidepressant treatment available) increase the density of some 5-HT postsynaptic receptors, with a time course that correlates well with the lag time of the appearance of the therapeutic effect (Barbaccia et al., 1988)? It appears that we will have to wait for further research addressing these issues before we can begin to understand the biochemical underpinnings of depression and the mechanism through which antidepressants work.

Acetylcholine has also been implicated in affective disorders. It has been suggested that an overactive acetylcholine system or an imbalance between acetylcholine and norepinephrine is a causative factor in depression (Sitaram et al., 1980). This hypothesis is supported by the clinical finding that physostigmine, an inhibitor of the enzyme that normally inactivates acetylcholine, may aggravate depression and reduce mania (Risch et al., 1980). This is consistent with the fact that many antidepressants, some of which have minimal effects on either norepinephrine or serotonin reuptake, have anticholinergic properties. In the past these properties were only believed to be responsible for some of the side effects of these drugs. However, drugs with comparable potency as antidepressants (for example, amitriptyline and desipramine) may differ in a greater than 35-fold range in anticholinergic potency (Baldessarini, 1990). Thus it is unlikely that these drugs' anticholinergic properties play much of a role in their ability to relieve depression.

Decreased GABAergic function may play a role in various forms of endogenous depressions, because GABA-mimetic drugs have been found to be effective antidepressants. Consistent with this hypothesis are studies noting that the cerebrospinal fluid of severely depressed patients contains significantly higher concentrations of endogenous inhibitors of benzodiazepine agonists than found in age- and sex-matched normal volunteers (Barbaccia et al., 1988).

Finally, endorphins have also been implicated in some cases of depression. They are found in relatively high concentrations in the limbic system and appear to modulate many of its activities. Also, narcotics have long been recognized for their euphoric and antidepressant properties. There has been recent speculation that many narcotic addicts comprise a subclass of depressed individuals who take narcotics to feel "normal" (Khantzian, 1985). Unfortunately, should this hypothesis prove to be valid, it would make drug treatment difficult because all known substitutes for endorphins—both exogenous and endogenous—have the strong potential for inducing tolerance and physical dependence with chronic use.

Pharmacotherapy for Depression

The two major classes of drugs currently used in the United States for the treatment of depression are the **tricyclics** and the **MAO inhibitors**, with members of both classes being introduced in the late 1950s (Baldessarini, 1990). However, the tricyclics are used much more frequently than the

MAO inhibitors because their effectiveness rate is somewhat higher and their toxicity is lower, particularly with respect to interactions with other drugs and certain food substances. A number of compounds that do not belong to either class have recently come into use, most notably the selective serotonin reuptake inhibitors (Goodnick, 1991a). Although many of these appear to be as effective as the tricyclics with less toxicity and fewer side effects, the tricyclics remain the prototype antidepressant drugs against which all newcomers must be compared.

No single antidepressant drug has been shown to be effective in relieving the symptoms of unipolar depression in more than two out of three patients (Davis et al., 1992). However, because there is tremendous variation in the pharmacodynamics of different antidepressants and because depression may be caused by a variety of mechanisms, with sufficient patience and trials with different types of antidepressants, the overall treatment efficacy rate may approach 90%. The best predictor for a positive response to a particular antidepressant is a previous positive response to it by the patient or a close relative who shows similar symptoms (Janowsky et al., 1987). Unfortunately, about one out of four patients will relapse even when maintained on an antidepressant medication; again, shifting to another type of antidepressant will produce symptom remission in many of these patients.

In comparison, about one out of three patients treated with placebos will show significant symptom remission, and about half of these responders will relapse with placebo maintenance. Placebo efficacy rates vary considerably depending on a variety of factors—for example, approximately 40% efficacy in married or mildly depressed patients versus approximately 20% in single or more severely depressed patients (Wilcox et al., 1992). There is some evidence that the difference in efficacy between active medications and placebo may increase after six weeks of treatment, but because of ethical and economic reasons, most studies of this nature do not go much beyond a three- or four-week evaluation period (Prien, 1988). In any case, one must consider the possibility that some patients who improve with these medications do so because of a true drug effect while others do so because of nonspecific (placebo) factors. Recent evidence suggests that a true drug response is more likely to be delayed and more persistent than a nonspecific response and that those patients who relapse with continued antidepressant therapy are more likely to display placebo-response patterns (early onset and/or fluctuating course) (Harrison et al., 1988).

Tricyclic Antidepressants

Tricyclics are so named because they consist of three-ringed molecules. The most common clinically used tricyclic compounds in the United States are imipramine (Tofranil) and a primary metabolite desipramine

(Norpramin), amitriptyline (Elavil) and a primary metabolite nortriptyline (Pamelor), doxepin (Sinequan), amoxapine (Asendin), trimipramine (Surmontil), and protriptyline (Vivactil). These drugs all block reuptake of norepinephrine (NE) and serotonin (5-HT), but they differ considerably in terms of their potency and selectivity in these actions (Richelson, 1991). For example, desipramine exhibits the most potent and selective action on NE uptake, whereas imipramine exhibits considerably lower potency regarding NE uptake and considerably higher potency regarding 5-HT uptake than desipramine. Trimipramine exhibits relatively low potency regarding uptake of NE and 5-HT but exhibits a more select action on 5-HT than NE. These drugs also exhibit wide differences with respect to blocking histamine (H_1), muscarinic, serotonin (5-HT_2), and dopamine (D_2) receptors.

Regardless of these differences, they all are equally effective in relieving depression, and they all take several days or weeks to alter the symptoms of depression. In most cases the core symptoms of depression are relieved with tricyclics. Patients feel more confident, their mood is improved, their physical symptoms are reduced, and their suicidal thoughts are eliminated (Feighner et al., 1985).

Tricyclics appear to be most effective in severe cases of unipolar unremitting depression. Although it has generally been believed that they are more effective in treating endogenous depression (where there is no evidence of obvious precipitating events) characterized by regression and inactivity than exogenous depression (where there are clearly precipitating events, such as loss of a loved one), recent research has not supported the endogenous versus exogenous dichotomy (Holden, 1986). The reason that studies have not found tricyclics to be of much benefit in exogenous depression and mild depression may be that there is a high placebo-response rate or a high spontaneous remission rate in these cases coupled with the slow onset of action by the drugs (Brown, 1988). Tricyclics are not recommended for use in bipolar depression because they may trigger a transition from depression to manic excitement and because this disorder is quite responsive to lithium, which generally induces fewer side effects.

According to a recent multimillion-dollar research treatment program sponsored by the National Institute on Mental Health, the short-term efficacy of tricyclics in the treatment of unipolar depression appears to be comparable to at least two forms of brief psychotherapy—cognitive behavior therapy and interpersonal psychotherapy (Elkin et al., 1989). Some tricyclics have also been shown to facilitate the effects of behavioral treatment in depressed patients whose primary symptoms are those associated with phobias (Telch et al., 1985).

Psychological disturbances that may or may not have a clear link to depression may also show favorable response to some tricyclics. Studies have indicated that tricyclics may be beneficial in cases of *bulimia* (an eating disorder characterized by binge-purge eating and depressive symptoms). However, these drugs tend to induce weight gain and carbo-hydrate craving, both of which are poorly tolerated by bulimics. Clomi-pramine (Anafranil), a tricyclic with potent serotonin-reuptake-inhibiting properties, has been shown to significantly reduce the obsessive and compulsive symptoms of obsessive-compulsive disorder in both adults and children (Ananth, 1986). In many cases, these effects appear to be independent of the drug's antidepressant properties. Tricyclics, particu-larly those that inhibit the reuptake of serotonin, have also been used successfully in the treatment of chronic pain (Sacerdote et al., 1987).

There is no evidence that tolerance develops to the antidepressant properties of tricyclics, but there is some indication that tolerance may develop to the anticholinergic side effects and orthostatic hypotension. There is minimal potential for tricyclics to induce psychological depen-dence, as they are void of primary reinforcing properties and have numerous side effects. As you might expect, nonhumans also will not self-administer these drugs. Unlike the psychostimulants, there is no evidence that abrupt cessation of tricyclics induces depression. How-ever, reduction of tricyclic medication should be gradual because an abstinence syndrome (sleep disturbance, nightmares, nausea, head-ache, and hypercholinergic-type effects) may occur if medication is stopped abruptly (Janowsky et al., 1987).

Tricyclic Side Effects

Tricyclic antidepressants can be extremely toxic, and they have relatively low therapeutic indexes, unfortunate characteristics for drugs used in the treatment of a disorder that can lead to suicide. In fact, tricyclics account for a quarter of all fatal overdoses in the United States, with 70% of tricyclic deaths never reaching the hospital (Jarvis, 1991). Therefore, a prudent approach to the treatment of depressed patients would be to give them no more than a two-week supply of these medications (Janowsky et al., 1987).

As is the case with all current antidepressants, tricyclics have the potential to induce epilepsy-like seizures (Tollefson, 1991). Because of their potent anticholinergic (specifically antimuscarinic) action, tachycar-dia, blurred vision, dry mouth, constipation, and urinary retention are common. Therapeutic doses of these drugs have significant effects on the cardiovascular system, such as orthostatic hypotension (a drop in blood pressure upon standing up). In addition, an increased tendency for arrhythmia (irregularity in the heartbeat) to develop with these drugs has resulted in a number of unexpected deaths. Therefore, great caution must be observed in their use in patients with cardiac problems. Weak-ness and fatigue may also occur infrequently. Although significant mo-tor disturbances are rare, a fine tremor may occur, particularly in elderly patients. The relatively infrequent side effects of jaundice, agranulocytosis, rashes, weight gain, and orgasmic impotence have also been reported to occur with tricyclics.

Since high doses of these drugs can induce CNS-toxic reactions, there is a biphasic relationship between drug plasma levels and efficacy. That is, there is a therapeutic window; below or above a particular plasma level, the drug is not effective in elevating mood (Tollefson, 1991). Unfortunately, when idealized dosages are administered to different individuals, resulting steady-state plasma concentrations may vary tenfold or more (DeVane et al., 1991). These characteristics contribute to difficulties in establishing optimal dosage regimens for individual patients.

Monoamine Oxidase Inhibitors

Monoamine oxidase (MAO) is an enzyme found in cells throughout the body. It is localized predominantly on the outer membrane of subcellular particles called mitochondria. It comes in two forms, designated Type A and Type B, depending on the substances that they act on. MAO is responsible for the intraneuronal metabolic inactivation (through deamination) of serotonin, dopamine, and norepinephrine. The **monoamine oxidase inhibitor (MAOI)** antidepressants comprise a group of heterogeneous drugs that share the ability to block this action of MAO. As one might expect, the efficacy of MAOIs in treating catecholamine-related depressions appears to be related to the normal level of MAO activity in the patient; that is, depressed patients with low MAO activity to begin with are less responsive to MAOIs than patients with higher MAO activity (Georgotas et al., 1987).

Although MAO inhibition is presumed to be the primary one involved in their antidepressant properties, MAOIs have numerous other biochemical effects that may be involved. Furthermore, as was the case with the tricyclics, the MAO-inhibiting actions occur rapidly and precede symptom remission by as much as two or more weeks. One of the first MAOIs, iproniazid, was originally used in the treatment of tuberculosis and was soon found to have mood-elevating properties. However, its toxicity eventually led to its withdrawal from the market, a fate common to many of these types of drugs. The three MAOIs presently used clinically as antidepressants in the United States are tranylcypromine (Parnate), phenelzine (Nardil), and isocarboxazid (Marplan).

Although the antidepressant properties of the first MAOI were noted at about the same time as those of the first tricyclic, until recently the therapeutic use of MAOIs was very limited. Generally they were used only in patients who remained depressed after an adequate trial of one or two different types of tricyclics (Nierenberg & White, 1990). The tricyclics are generally favored over the MAOIs because most early controlled comparisons between MAOIs and tricyclics indicated that MAOIs were significantly less effective in most cases of depression.

In addition MAOIs are less commonly used than tricyclics because MAOIs may induce more toxic reactions when combined with certain drugs or foods. For reasons as yet unclear, hypotension is commonly observed with MAOIs. On the other hand, MAOIs can interact unpredictably with many adrenergic-related chemicals to induce a so-called *hypertensive crisis*—a very serious toxic effect that can lead to headaches, fever, intracranial bleeding, and in some cases death. This can occur when MAOIs are combined with tricyclics, psychostimulants, and L-dopa. For these reasons, the combination of MAOIs and tricyclic antidepressants is generally contraindicated.

MAOIs also interact in a similar fashion with foods containing the amino acid tyramine and other monoamines. Examples of such foods are cheese, yeast products, chocolate, some wines, milk, beer, pickled herring, chicken liver, and large amounts of coffee, among many others. This problem comes about because the MAO inhibition allows these biologically active amines, which hepatic MAO would normally deaminate into inactive molecules, to release catecholamines from axon terminals and produce sympathomimetic effects, which include a marked rise in blood pressure and other cardiovascular changes. MAOIs also interfere with various enzymes to prolong and intensify the effects of nonadrenergic-related drugs (such as sedative-hypnotics, general anesthetics, narcotics, and anticholinergics), and they interfere with the metabolization of various naturally occurring substances.

Because of these interactions, individuals being treated with MAOIs (and their families) are normally given a list of drugs and foods to avoid. (Unfortunately, such information has been used in the past by patients to derive a list of agents through which they can commit suicide.) Typically, these drugs are cleared from the body rapidly, so plasma levels are not correlated with MAO inhibition (Mallinger & Smith, 1991). However, since phenelzine and isocarboxazid bind irreversibly to MAO, it may take up to two weeks after discontinuing their use for the body to resynthesize new enzyme molecules and restore monoamine metabolism to normal. The effects of tranylcypromine are reversed more rapidly because it is not bound irreversibly to MAO. In either case, a period of several days to two weeks is recommended before switching a patient from one MAO inhibitor to another or to a tricyclic (Baldessarini, 1990).

In spite of the long delay in therapeutic response, a number of toxic reactions to overdoses of MAOIs can occur within hours (Baldessarini, 1990). These may consist of agitation, hallucinations, high fever, convulsions, and hypotension or hypertension. Treatment of these symptoms is difficult because of the numerous interactions between MAOIs and other drugs that normally might be useful in dealing with these symptoms. The long duration of MAO inhibition requires that the patient be monitored for several days after a toxic reaction. Several side effects have been noted with doses of MAOIs lower than those inducing acute toxicity—for example, cellular damage to liver cells, tremors, insomnia, agitation, hypomania, hallucinations, dizziness, and anticholinergic-like effects. It is obvious from the list of potential toxic effects of the MAOIs that they are greater and more serious than those of most other psychotherapeutic drugs. Thus it is not surprising that their use is reserved for patients who are not responsive to other drugs, or who perhaps refuse electroconvulsive shock therapy.

For reasons just discussed, the MAOIs have generally been considered to be a second- or third-line defense against most cases of depression, generally being used only after unsuccessful treatment with an adequate dosage of one or two different monoamine reuptake inhibitors (e.g., tricyclics). However, recent research on MAOIs has indicated that they have much more versatility than previously assumed (Rudorfer, 1992). For example, with adequate dosage in nonpsychotic depressed patients, MAOIs may be as effective in the treatment of typical major depressions as tricyclics. They have also been shown to be effective in the treatment of bipolar patients, if combined with lithium to prevent treatment-emergent mania or hypomania. Recent clinical reports have documented the safety of switching patients who have not responded to tricyclics to an MAOI without a washout period, thus potentially shortening the misery a depressed patient must undergo before a successful treatment is found. In fact, if done carefully, MAOIs can be combined with tricyclics or lithium to enhance treatment efficacy. Although the dangerous interactions between MAOIs and other substances remain a limiting factor in MAOI use, new understanding into the mechanisms, prevention, and treatment of these toxicities has led to streamlining of instruction to patients, which enhances compliance and acceptability of MAOI treatment.

MAOIs have also been found to be potentially efficacious in a wider spectrum of atypical depressions than previously recognized—for example, agoraphobia, bulimia, borderline personality disorder, and posttraumatic stress disorder. Finally, more selective or reversible MAOIs have been developed and may enhance the treatment of specific types of depression. Standard MAOI antidepressants reduce both subtypes of the MAO enzymes (MAO-A and MAO-B) and do so irreversibly; that is, the enzymes must be resynthesized by the body before some other antidepressants can be given safely (e.g., fluoxetine) or dietary restrictions can be removed. Clinical tests are now being conducted with MAOIs that are specific to MAO-B (e.g., *l*-deprenyl) or MAO-A (e.g., clorgyline) to determine whether they may be useful as second-line MAOIs in patients unable to tolerate the standard MAOI side effects. Reversible MAOIs, such as moclobernide and toloxatone, which do not require synthesis of the enzyme after drug discontinuation, are also under clinical investigation. Preliminary reports suggest that these drugs are less likely to interact with other substances, like tyramine, that may cause hypertensive effects and may induce more rapid symptom remission than older antidepressants.

Depressions of the type most responsive to MAOIs are sometimes referred to as *nonresponding atypical depressions* in the clinical literature. Atypical depressed patients may also exhibit a reversal of the usual diurnal variation; that is, rather than feeling worse in the morning and improving somewhat as the day goes on, they may feel worse toward the end of the day. Atypical symptoms of oversleeping, overeating, and gaining weight may be present. Such patients may also be phobic, obsessional, and more agitated than the more typical depressed patient (Janowsky et al., 1987).

A recent comparison between imipramine and the MAOI phenelzine in patients with these characteristics suggested that phenelzine was superior to imipramine in patients who also experienced panic attacks, and was comparable to imipramine in those patients without panic attacks (Davidson et al., 1987). Another form of atypical depression that appears to respond well to phenelzine is termed *hysteroid dysphoria* (Kayser et al., 1985). Patients with this disorder (usually women) are characterized by immaturity, self-centeredness, attention-getting behavior, manipulativeness, and quite often vague seductiveness. They experience depressions that are often precipitated by rejection, especially the loss of a romantic attachment. Their depressed episodes are characterized by a tendency to oversleep or spend more than normal amounts of time in bed, to overeat or crave sweets, and a labile mood that temporarily improves when attention or praise is given.

MAOIs have also been shown in many recent studies to be as effective as tricyclics in elderly depressed patients (Janowsky et al., 1987) and may be used as an alternative treatment in elderly patients who cannot tolerate some of the side effects of tricyclics. Like the tricyclics, the MAOIs may exert considerable improvement in the moods and eating behavior of bulimics, although their use in a condition whose primary symptoms involve uncontrollable eating behavior may not be advisable (because of the dietary constraints already mentioned) (Walsh et al., 1984).

MAOIs may also exert a favorable response in people with certain neurotic illnesses with depressive features and in people who suffer from acute anxiety, phobias, and panic attacks (in which the person may experience light-headedness, dizziness, "rubbery" legs, choking, difficulty in breathing, a racing or palpitating heart, tingling sensations, and extreme fright) (Buigues & Vallejo, 1987). Disabling obsessive thoughts that are characteristic of the obsessive-compulsive disorder may also respond to MAOIs, whether major symptoms of depression are present or not. The effectiveness of these types of antidepressants in disorders whose primary symptoms are more appropriate to an anxiety or fear condition is most curious.

As is the case with the tricyclic antidepressants, there is little potential for tolerance development or psychological dependence with the MAOIs. Abstinence symptoms associated with MAOI cessation have not been identified.

New Generation Antidepressants

Following one or more trials with adequate dosages of the tricyclics and MAOIs described in the preceding section (that is, after several different types of drugs have been tried), 85–90% of the patients with major depression will show significant symptom reduction. However, these drugs have a slow onset of action, numerous side effects, and a significant lethal potential. Over the past 15 years or so, a number of compounds with antidepressant properties have been developed that have more specific actions, potentially greater efficacy, and significantly fewer side effects and toxicity. Because these drugs are presently coming into use, or will likely be used in the near future, let us briefly review some of the key properties of these compounds.

The most promising new type of nontricyclic antidepressant consists of highly selective serotonin reuptake blockers that are void of anticholinergic and antihistaminic side effects associated with traditional antidepressants. These drugs may produce other undesirable side effects, including anxiety, headaches, nausea, and insomnia, but these are generally better tolerated than are the side effects induced by older antidepressants (Meltzer, 1991). The serotonin reuptake blockers also have considerably higher therapeutic indexes than previous antidepressants.

Of this group, fluoxetine (Prozac), approved for clinical use by the FDA in 1987, has become one of the most frequently prescribed antidepressants on the market. Although comparable to older antidepressants in relieving the symptoms of depression, fluoxetine's side-effect profile makes it more effective in the treatment of some patients, for example, the elderly (because it exerts minimal cardiovascular side effects). It also has a higher therapeutic index (greater than 50) and is better tolerated in combination with most medicines (notable exceptions are lithium and MAOIs) or alcohol (Goodnick, 1991a). Research also indicates that fluoxetine may be helpful in promoting weight loss in obese patients, in cutting down alcohol consumption in heavy drinkers, and in reducing the symptoms of severe premenstrual syndrome (a constellation of emotional and behavioral symptoms experienced during a specific phase of the menstrual cycle) (Stone et al., 1990).

Recently, a number of anecdotal reports have suggested that fluoxetine may induce suicidal thoughts or actions in a small portion of patients. However, because these patients typically exhibit characteristics, such as depression, for which suicidal ideation is not uncommon, it is difficult to assess the degree to which fluoxetine is responsible for it. Whether causal or not, the incidence of violent suicidal preoccupation with fluoxetine treatment is rare (e.g., less than 5% of patients treated) and does not appear to be significantly different from that which occurs with other antidepressants (Fava & Rosenbaum, 1991; Beasley et al., 1991). In fact as one might expect from an antidepressant, reduction in suicidal ideation is much more likely to occur.

With fluoxetine becoming the most popular first-line treatment for depression, a number of other recently developed, potentially promising antidepressants have been relegated to the sidelines. However, because they may be useful as alternatives to fluoxetine, traditional tricyclics, and MAOIs, several of these will be discussed (summarized from Feighner, 1983; Fuller, 1986; and Hollister, 1986).

Other antidepressants without the typical tricyclic structure or MAO-inhibitory properties that have been developed include maprotiline (Ludiomil) and its analogue oxaprotiline. They are potent norepinephrine reuptake blockers with no serotonergic effects. Their efficacy appears comparable to that of earlier compounds. They have less sedative and anticholinergic side effects than amitriptyline, but they may cause seizures, even at therapeutic doses.

Trazodone (Desyrel) has a pharmacological profile atypical of earlier antidepressants in that it has little effect on catecholamine activity, no anticholinergic effects, and no MAO inhibition. It selectively inhibits serotonin reuptake but may also enhance serotonin release apparently via a mechanism that is unrelated to reuptake inhibition (Gross et al., 1987). It lacks anticholinergic side effects and possesses low cardiovascular toxicity. Claims that trazodone appears to have a more rapid onset of symptom remission than the older antidepressants with equivalent efficacy have been difficult to prove. It has some sedative-hypnotic activity, which may be useful in patients with agitation, anxiety, and insomnia. It may also be useful in schizophrenics with secondary depression and bipolar depressives, as it does not appear to exacerbate psychotic or manic symptoms. Its primary side effects are lethargy, headaches, nausea, and mild gastrointestinal disturbances.

Some benzodiazepines such as alprazolam (Xanax), may be used as antidepressants. Alprazolam has a potent GABA-enhancing effect similar to other benzodiazepines, but unlike others in this class, it has antidepressant efficacy comparable to older tricyclics with a faster onset of action. However, tolerance may develop to its antidepressant properties after a few weeks. Like the benzodiazepines, it has a low incidence of anticholinergic side effects, low cardiotoxicity, and minimal potential for lethality with overdose. However, drowsiness and lethargy are common, but generally well-tolerated, side effects. Because of alprazolam's relatively short plasma half-life and its tendency to induce physical dependence with chronic use, dosages should be gradually tapered over several weeks when treatment with alprazolam is discontinued (Rickels et al., 1990).

Bupropion (Wellbutrin) has antidepressant efficacy comparable to the tricyclics, but it differs from previous antidepressants because it appears to exert no noradrenergic or serotonergic activity but weakly facilitates dopaminergic transmission, and this ability may account for its exerting mild amphetamine-like effects (Goodnick, 1991b). (Its structure resembles that of amphetamine.) In addition, double-blind, placebo controlled studies have demonstrated that a majority of patients who were intolerant to or resistant to tricyclics responded favorably when treated with bupropion (Preskorn, 1991). It possesses no MAO-inhibition effects and minimal anticholinergic or antihistaminic actions, which result in its producing a low incidence of side effects, sedation, orthostatic hypotension, and adverse cardiac effects. Also, its tendency to induce hypomanic or manic episodes in unipolar depressives appears low, although it may trigger manic episodes in bipolar patients. The major problem with bupropion is its tendency to induce seizures and other forms of CNS toxicity— for example, delirium, psychosis, and extrapyramidal side effects—with high levels of bupropion (Preskorn, 1991). It may also induce mild dryness of the mouth, headache, nausea, constipation, and tremor.

Finally, the nonbenzodiazepine anxiolytic buspirone (BuSpar) has been shown to be effective in relieving symptoms of depression (Charney et al., 1990). Although its efficacy is more moderate than other drugs discussed in this section, its low toxicity and side effects, lack of dependence liability, and minimal interactions with other drugs (e.g., alcohol) make it an attractive alternative to these other drugs.

It should be clear from the preceding summary that there is a whole spectrum of new drugs that may be useful in the treatment of depression. Most of these have a lower incidence of side effects and less toxicity than earlier compounds. In addition, some of these may have a faster onset of action or may be effective in patients who do not respond favorably to these compounds. These drugs appear to be particularly valuable in the treatment of geriatric depressives, patients with cardiovascular disease, and patients who do not tolerate anticholinergic side effects well. However, because many of these drugs have only been tried in limited clinical trials, it may be some time before their actual impact on pharmacotherapy is realized.

Psychostimulants

Drugs like amphetamine and cocaine have several properties, particularly their fast onset of action, that would appear to make them ideal antidepressants. Although some clinically depressed patients do experience feelings of calmness, well-being, or euphoria when given these drugs, the majority of such patients experience mixed mood effects, or experience dysphoric feelings of tension and increased sadness (Post et al., 1974). Thus their effects cannot be described as simply antidepressant. Furthermore, as was noted in Chapter 9, their euphoric effects in normal individuals show tolerance, and their chronic use can worsen or induce depression when drug exposure ceases. In fact, the rebound following cocaine use involves such a severe depression that it can be life-threatening by causing, or at least precipitating, suicidal behavior. Thus these types of drugs are an outmoded and contraindicated treatment for severe depression (however, see next paragraph).

Drug Combinations in the Treatment of Depression

There is a very good chance that a major depression can be effectively treated with one of the drugs that are currently available. However, there are still a small number of patients who are treatment-resistant. There may be a complete lack of response to medication, a tendency to relapse after an initial response, or an inability to tolerate the drugs' side effects. If a number of tricyclics, MAOIs, and new-generation antidepressants (e.g., fluoxetine) have been tried in adequate doses for at least six weeks each and the patient still has not responded, or if the side effects cannot be tolerated, it may be fruitful to try some combinations of drugs and/or psychotherapy (Nierenberg & White, 1990). For example, lithium has been shown to augment the effectiveness of tricyclic antidepressants in some patients refractory to tricyclics alone. Some studies have reported that combining L-tryptophan, thyroid hormone (T_3), or a psychostimulant (amphetamine) with a tricyclic antidepressant can be beneficial in patients who have shown an inadequate response to a tricyclic alone. Although the combination of tricyclics and MAOIs has generally been avoided in the United States because of potential drug interactions that may induce hypertensive crises, several clinicians have suggested that with close monitoring these drugs can be combined with relative safety (Feighner et al., 1985). Considering the high risk of suicide in severely depressed individuals, such approaches should not be routinely dismissed.

Conclusions

Present-day antidepressants differ considerably in terms of their molecular structure, their metabolic activities, and their specificity of actions, both within and between neurotransmitter systems. When selecting a particular antidepressant for treatment, at least four factors should be considered: symptom-profile efficacy, onset of action or latency of response to treatment, potential side-effect profile, and toxicity. There is general agreement that most antidepressants differ little with regard to efficacy and the period of time for onset of action; significant differences do occur with regard to side-effect profiles and potential toxicity (Tollefson, 1991). Side effects are of considerable clinical importance, not only because they may represent a health risk to the patient but also because they may deter patient compliance, which in turn may lead to suboptimal outcome and can limit the clinician's ability to adjust the dosages into an adequate therapeutic range.

Pharmacotherapy in Mania and Bipolar Illnesses

The effectiveness of a particular treatment for mania may depend on whether the patient experiences only manic symptoms, which occur intermittently between episodes of normal mood, or experiences cycles of mania and depression. Treatment efficacy may also depend on whether episodes of mania and depression occur infrequently and separately (typical bipolar disorder), or involve rapid cycling (e.g., patients experience four or more episodes per year), or involve dysphoric (mixed) mania in which manic and depressive symptoms occur together. Lithium is generally the initial drug used in all these cases, but its effectiveness is most apparent in cases of typical bipolar disorder. Tricyclic or other antidepressants are commonly used in combination with lithium if the patient does not respond to lithium after several weeks or is experiencing a severe depressive episode. Carbamazepine (Tegretol), either alone or in combination with lithium, appears to be somewhat more effective than lithium in the treatment of rapid-cycling or mixed bipolar patients. A number of other drug treatments (e.g., calcium blockers, cholinergic agents, adrenergic blockers) and nondrug treatments (e.g., electroconvulsive shock, phototherapy, psychosurgery) have been explored as alternatives to these, but research supporting their efficacy is very limited, and none have gained widespread acceptance (Prien & Potter, 1990).

Lithium

The properties of lithium are so unique that it stands alone among all the psychotherapeutic drugs (Baldessarini, 1990). Although the first report of its antimanic effects by Australian psychiatrist John Cade in 1949 would seem to put it at the forefront of the psychopharmacological revolution begun in the 1950s, it had little impact in the United States until 20 years later. One reason was its high toxicity, particularly when combined with low sodium intake. Several months prior to Cade's report, a number of deaths were reported in patients with kidney and heart problems who were given lithium salt as a substitute for ordinary table salt (sodium chloride). Thus, despite its remarkable antimanic properties, physicians were reluctant to use such a toxic drug. Furthermore, a few years later, chlorpromazine was noted to possess antimanic effects as well as considerably lower toxicity. A rapid succession of similar compounds, as well as antidepressants, new stimulants, sedatives, and hypnotics, came into being, each requiring considerable study with respect to their safety and efficacy. Another factor in the lack of enthusiasm for lithium was its minimal marketability because, as an element of nature, it was unpatentable. Eventually, however, lithium's remarkable properties became well recognized, and its use has become commonplace.

Lithium is unique for several reasons (Baldessarini, 1990). First, it is a light metal ion (positively charged) that exists in nature as a salt (lithium carbonate, lithium chloride). Although the ion is found in trace amounts in animal tissues, it plays no known physiological role. Second, therapeutic levels of lithium have almost negligible psychotropic effects in normal individuals—that is, there are no sedative, depressant, stimulant, or euphoriant effects. Third, and most important, it is highly specific in relieving manic symptoms without oversedating the person (a common problem with antipsychotics) or inducing depression (as was the case with reserpine). Furthermore, continued treatment with lithium salt can prevent or decrease the severity of future episodes of mania and depression in most bipolar patients (this is what experts mean when they say lithium has prophylactic properties).

Pharmacokinetics of Lithium

Since lithium's therapeutic index can be as low as 2 or 3, it is important to monitor its concentrations in the body on a regular basis, at least until stable levels can be assured (Baldessarini, 1990). Lithium is usually administered orally in a salt form, most commonly lithium carbonate (the particular salt used is not important in the therapeutic action since the anionic partner serves only as an inert vehicle for transport). It is readily absorbed from the G.I. tract, with almost complete absorption occurring within 8 hours. Passage through the blood-brain barrier is slow, but once plasma levels have stabilized, cerebrospinal fluid levels stabilize at approximately half that of plasma concentrations. Plasma concentration of lithium ion is generally determined in milliequivalent units per liter of blood (mEq/L) (milliequivalent refers to the number of grams of solute dissolved in 1 milliliter of a normal solution). Therapeutic doses are achieved when plasma levels of lithium reach 0.6 to 1.5 mEq/L (generally achievable with two to three 300-mg tablets of lithium carbonate per day).

Above these levels toxic signs of diarrhea, vomiting, drowsiness, confusion, and muscular weakness may occur (Annitto, 1979). At levels above 2.0 mEq/L, ataxia, tinnitus, and interference with kidney function can occur, and levels above 3.0 mEq/L may result in coma, respiratory depression, and death. Even at therapeutic levels, side effects of fine hand tremors, nausea, thirst, and excessive sweating may occur. In comparison to most other drugs requiring chronic exposure, the side effects of therapeutic levels of lithium are rather mild or uncommon. Nevertheless, idiosyncratic reactions can occur; for instance, its use has been associated with diabetes, seizure activity, and neurological disturbances, particularly when combined with other drugs.

The pharmacokinetics of lithium may vary considerably among individuals, but they are relatively stable over time within individuals. Although lithium has a relatively long plasma half-life (about 20–24 hours), it is generally given in divided doses because of its low therapeutic index. Slow-release preparations have recently been developed that produce smoother lithium plasma level curves, allow administration once a day or every other day, and may have fewer side effects (Goodnick & Schorr-Cain, 1991). Concentration levels of lithium are heavily dependent on sodium intake. Lithium is generally excreted more readily with high sodium intake, but critically high concentrations of lithium may occur with low sodium intake or drug-induced sodium depletion (as might occur with diuretics) as a result of enhanced retention. Also, lithium's urinary retention and elimination half-life may double during mania (Goodnick & Schorr-Cain, 1991).

Pharmacodynamics of Lithium

Our understanding of lithium's neuropharmacological properties with respect to its ability to stabilize mood is particularly weak. As an ion, lithium has the potential for altering the distribution and exchange of ions involved in the process of conduction (see Chapter 4). Therefore, there has been some speculation that such interactions may account for lithium's mood-stabilizing properties, although it is uncertain whether important interactions with these ions occur at therapeutic concentrations of lithium (Tosteson, 1981). In brain tissue at therapeutic concentrations, lithium reduces the stimulation-produced and calcium-dependent release of catecholamines (but not serotonin) from nerve endings (Baldessarini, 1990). It may also enhance the reuptake of catecholamines. These actions are consistent with the catecholamine hypothesis of mania but do not really fit the opposite side of the hypothesis regarding catecholamines and depression. Lithium appears to have no direct influence on postsynaptic catecholamine receptors because it does not affect enzyme activity normally triggered by receptor activation nor does it affect the binding of ligands to catecholamine receptors.

In studies attempting to determine whether lithium is able to reduce the effects of amphetamine (which you should recall initially amplifies catecholamine release and reduces their reuptake), there have been a variety of outcomes. Although studies have found that lithium attenuates several of amphetamine's behavioral effects, in other tests it has either produced no change or has intensified amphetamine's effects (Cox et al., 1971; Flemenbaum, 1974; Furukawa et al., 1975; Matussek & Linsmayer, 1968).

The problem with these studies, in terms of trying to understand the relationship between lithium's actions and its ability to lessen manic symptoms, is that they are all acute studies. It is well established that a minimum of 7–10 days of chronic lithium administration is usually required before therapeutic benefits are observed. This time period corresponds to the time it takes for lithium to "stabilize" the relationship between tryptophan uptake in the brain and its synthesis into 5-HT (mentioned earlier in the discussion of the biochemical basis of affective disorders). Once this new equilibrium state has been achieved, the actions and effects of drugs like amphetamine and cocaine are greatly reduced (Cooper et al., 1991). So it may be this action of lithium that is most critical for its therapeutic effects.

Recent studies have also indicated that therapeutic concentrations of lithium interfere with the formation of a precursor of a secondary messenger (phosphoinositide) through which a variety of neurotransmitters act (Worley et al., 1988). These findings led to the hypothesis that the dampening action on phosphoinositide-associated neurotransmission could prevent excessive shifts of individual neurotransmitter systems from their basal activity. If different phosphoinositide-linked transmitters were separately involved in manic and depressive episodes, it could explain the normalizing effect of lithium. Which of the specific transmitter systems are most important, and whether or not the symptoms of the disorder are in fact mediated by separate systems, remain to be determined.

Efficacy of Lithium in Mood Disturbances

The efficacy of lithium in treating acute mania and preventing subsequent episodes of both mania and depression in bipolar disorder is unquestioned, with approximately 60 to 80% of such cases displaying partial to complete symptom remission (Prien & Potter, 1990). The action of lithium in these cases is more specific than that found with phenothiazines and related antipsychotics. However, since manic symptom remission does not generally occur for several days with lithium alone, combining lithium with a traditional antipsychotic drug during severe manic episodes is common practice. Recent studies have suggested that persons with a strong genetic link to manic-depression—for example, patients in whose families the disorder has occurred—may show the most favorable response to lithium (Campbell et al., 1984).

In some individuals maintained on lithium, there is an unusual mood stability, which might be viewed unfavorably by these patients (Johnson, 1979). Most bipolar patients probably do not want to experience the uncontrolled onset of depressive or manic moods, but would like to experience normal emotions. However, lithium patients often report being emotionless in situations where mood shifts are expected, or at least appropriate.

Although lithium appears to have little antidepressant activity in persons experiencing a depressive episode, it can prevent depressive episodes in some patients with recurrent unipolar depression. Several studies have reported impressive results indicating that patients who are refractory to traditional antidepressants (including lithium) may respond favorably to lithium in combination with traditional antidepressants (Goodnick & Schorr-Cain, 1991).

Side effects are not generally a factor in lithium's efficacy. Although the majority of patients experience some adverse consequences—such as tremor, thirst, fluid retention, weight gain, and frequent need to urinate—these are relatively minor problems. Lithium's potential interactions with other drugs that patients may also likely be taking (e.g., antipsychotics, diuretics, and nonsteroidal antiinflammatory drugs) may limit its efficacy (Tollefson, 1991).

Lithium salts have also been used with varying degrees of success in other disorders with an affective component that have a cyclical nature to them, such as recurrent hyperactivity in children (however, not in the attention deficit disorder described in Chapter 14) (Campbell et al., 1984), the premenstrual syndrome, and episodic anger or aggression. The benefits of lithium in these cases have been attributed to lithium's ability to reduce impulsiveness or explosiveness—as if a delay mechanism or filter device were inserted between stimulus analysis and decision mechanisms in patients who previously went automatically from stimulus to response (Johnson, 1979).

Alternatives to Lithium in the Treatment of Mania

Antipsychotic drugs have been used successfully in the acute treatment of mania for almost 35 years. Both low-dose (for example, haloperidol) and high-dose (for example, chlorpromazine) antipsychotics have been shown to be effective in treating mania, although haloperidol is more likely to be used. They are often used concomitantly with the institution of lithium therapy. In many cases it is not practical to attempt to manage a manic patient with lithium alone during the first week of the illness, so antipsychotics, which suppress manic symptoms faster than lithium, are often combined with lithium (Prien & Potter, 1990). Once the patient has stabilized, the antipsychotic is withdrawn. Although chronic treatment with antipsychotics may be just as effective as lithium in preventing subsequent manic episodes, their vast spectrum of potentially debilitating side effects makes them less desirable than lithium for this purpose.

If a bipolar patient suffering from moderate depression has not responded to lithium treatment alone for several weeks, many, but not all, authorities recommend that a tricyclic or other antidepressant be combined with lithium (Prien & Potter, 1990). The rationale for giving lithium alone before adding an antidepressant is based on the presumption that standard antidepressants may precipitate mania, hypomania, or rapid cycling. This is also the reason that typical antidepressants by themselves are not recommended for use in bipolar patients.

In manic-depressive patients for whom lithium, alone or in combination with an antidepressant, has not been effective, the antiepileptic drug carbamazepine (Tegretol) has been found to both reduce mania and prevent depression. A recent double-blind study comparing lithium and carbamazepine in manic patients found no significant difference between their antimanic effects, but it was suggested that lithium may be more consistently effective in a heterogeneous population of manic patients while carbamazepine may be specifically effective in lithium-nonresponsive rapid-cycling bipolar patients or patients with dysphoric mania (Prien & Potter, 1990). Whether carbamazepine works better when combined with lithium is not clear. Carbamazepine is related chemically to the tricyclic antidepressants, but it is not clear that this relationship has anything to do with its mechanism of action in manic-depressives. Its anticonvulsant properties may be involved, because some studies have indicated that anticonvulsant drugs, such as sodium valproate, may also have antimanic as well as antidepressant prophylactic properties.

Nondrug Treatments for Depression

Clearly, not all grief, misery, and general disappointments associated with life in human society call for drug intervention. Most episodes of these types, even severe cases, evidence a very high rate of spontaneous remission with sufficient time passage. Psychological intervention that changes the person's interpersonal relationships or belief structures may be beneficial in these cases. One extensive study conducted by the National Institute of Mental Health concluded that some forms of brief psychotherapy may be as effective in the treatment of depression as pharmacotherapy (Elkin et al., 1989). The researchers in this study are now attempting to determine which types of patients respond best to which types of therapies. Some severe depressions may not respond to drug therapy, or a patient may be so suicidal that waiting for a drug to take effect would be inadvisable (Feighner et al., 1985). In such cases, electroshock therapy may be considered, because it remains the most rapid and effective treatment for severe acute depression and is potentially lifesaving for the suicidal patient.

Although physicians play the most direct role in pharmacotherapy for depression, those of you who will work or are now working in the mental health field outside of medicine may also serve important functions. Because you are the one most likely to deal initially with a depressed client, or to have the most contact with such an individual during his or her treatment, you may serve as an information gatherer to determine whether drug therapy may be a useful adjunct to traditional psychotherapies. You may also oversee the progress of a client who is under drug treatment. Your interaction with the patient during the evaluation and your reassurances may in themselves prove therapeutic. You can determine whether there are precipitating events underlying the client's symptoms, assess how chronic the problem is and whether there is a cyclical nature to it, determine whether the client is suicidal, gather family history, and so on. This is valuable information in establishing whether or not a person may be a good candidate for drug intervention. Mere inquiry into the nature of your clients' dysphoria can challenge them to confront their lives and their inability to respond appropriately to these events. If your clients are taking medication for their disorders, you can look for side effects of the drugs and signs of drug toxicity. Your optimism over the likely benefits of a prescribed medication may have tremendous value in alleviating distress, guilt, and hopelessness in the patient and may be the difference between a patient's compliance or noncompliance in sticking with a drug regimen that may take two to four weeks before any benefits are realized. Those of you who practice psychotherapy may find that antidepressants make your clients more amenable to your particular therapeutic techniques.

Bibliography

Ananth, J. (1986). Clomipramine: An antiobsessive drug. *Canadian Journal of Psychiatry, 31*, 253–258.

Annitto, W. J. (1979, March). Recognizing lithium-associated neurotoxicity. *Drug Therapy*, pp. 45–51.

Arango, V., Ernsberger, P., Marzuk, P. M., et al. (1990). Autoradiographic demonstration of increased serotonin 5-HT$_2$ and beta-adrenergic receptor binding sites in the brain of suicide victims. *Archives of General Psychiatry, 47*, 1038–1047.

Baldessarini, R. J. (1990). Drugs and the treatment of psychiatric disorders. In A. G. Gilman, T. W. Rall, A. S. Nies, & P. Taylor (Eds.), *The pharmacological basis of therapeutics* (pp. 383–435). New York: Pergamon Press.

Barbaccia, M. L., Costa, E., & Guidotti, A. (1988). Endogenous ligands for high-affinity recognition sites of psychotropic drugs. *Annual Review of Pharmacology and Toxicology, 28,* 451–476.

Beasley, C. M., Dornseif, B. E., Bosomworth, J. C., et al. (1991). Fluoxetine and suicide: A meta-analysis of controlled trials of treatment for depression. *British Medical Journal, 303,* 685–692.

Brown, W. A. (1988). Predictors of placebo response in depression. *Psychopharmacology Bulletin, 24,* 14–17.

Buigues, J., & Vallejo, J. (1987). Therapeutic response to phenelzine in patients with panic disorder and agoraphobia with panic attacks. *Journal of Clinical Psychiatry, 48,* 55–59.

Campbell, M., Perry, R., & Green, W. H. (1984). Use of lithium in children and adolescents. *Psychosomatics, 25,* 95–106.

Charney, D. S., Krystal, J. H., Delgado, P. L., & Heninger, G. R. (1990). Serotonin-specific drugs for anxiety and depressive disorders. *Annual Review of Medicine, 41,* 437–446.

Cooper, J. R., Bloom, F. E., & Roth, R. H. (1991). *The biochemical basis of neuropharmacology,* 6th ed. New York: Oxford University Press.

Cox, C., Harrison-Read, P. E., Steinberg, H., & Tomkiewicz, M. (1971). Lithium attenuates drug-induced hyperactivity in rats. *Nature, 232,* 336–338.

Davidson, J., Raft, D., & Pelton, S. (1987). An outpatient evaluation of phenelzine and imipramine. *Journal of Clinical Psychiatry, 48,* 143–146.

Davis, J. M., Janicak, P. G., Wang, Z., Gibbons, R. D., & Sharma, R. P. (1992). The efficacy of psychotropic drugs: Implications for power analysis. *Psychopharmacology Bulletin, 28,* 151–156.

DeVane, C. L., Rudorfer, M. V., & Potter, W. Z. (1991). Dosage regimen for cyclic antidepressants: A review of pharmacokinetic methods. *Psychopharmacology Bulletin, 27,* 619–632.

Elkin, I., Shea, T., Watkins, J. T., et al. (1989). National Institute of Mental Health treatment of depression collaborative research program. *Archives of General Psychiatry, 46,* 971–982.

Fava, M., & Rosenbaum, J. F. (1991). Suicidality and fluoxetine: Is there a relationship? *Journal of Clinical Psychiatry, 52,* 108–111.

Feighner, J. P. (1983). The new generation of antidepressants. *Journal of Clinical Psychiatry, 44,* 49–55.

Feighner, J. P., Herbstein, J., & Damlouji, N. (1985). Combined MAOI, TCA, and direct stimulant therapy of treatment-resistant depression. *Journal of Clinical Psychiatry, 46,* 206–209.

Fibiger, H. C., & Phillips, A. G. (1981). Increased intracranial self-stimulation in rats after long-term administration of desipramine. *Science, 214,* 683–685.

Flemenbaum, A. (1974). Does lithium block the effects of amphetamine? *American Journal of Psychiatry, 131,* 820–821.

Fuller, E. (1986, March). When to use the new antidepressants. *Patient Care, 20,* pp. 21–55.

Furukawa, T., Ushizima, I., & Ono, N. (1975). Modifications by lithium of behavioral responses to methamphetamine and tetrabenazine. *Psychopharmacologia, 42,* 243–248.

Garcia-Sevilla, J. A., & Zubieta, J. K. (1986). Activation and desensitization of presynaptic alpha-2-adrenoceptors after inhibition of neuronal uptake by antidepressant drugs in the rat vas deferens. *British Journal of Pharmacy, 89,* 673–683.

Georgotas, A., McCue, R. E., Friedman, E., & Cooper, T. (1987). Prediction of response to nortriptyline and phenelzine by platelet MAO activity. *American Journal of Psychiatry, 144,* 338–340.

Goodnick, P. J. (1991a). Pharmacokinetics of second generation antidepressants: Fluoxetine. *Psychopharmacology Bulletin, 27,* 503–512.

Goodnick, P. J. (1991b). Pharmacokinetics of second generation antidepressants: Bupropion. *Psychopharmacology Bulletin, 27,* 513–520.

Goodnick, P. J., & Schorr-Cain, C. B. (1991). Lithium pharmacokinetics. *Psychopharmacology Bulletin, 27,* 475–492.

Gross, G., Hante, K., & Gothert, M. (1987). Effect of antidepressant and neuroleptic drugs on the electrically evoked release of serotonin from rat cerebral cortex. *Psychopharmacology, 91,* 175–181.

Hardy, M., Lecrubier, Y., & Widlocher, D. (1986). Efficacy of clonidine in 24 patients with acute mania. *American Journal of Psychiatry, 143,* 1450–1453.

Harrison, W., Stewart, J. W., McGrath, P. J., Tricamo, E., & Quitkin, F. M. (1988). Is loss of antidepressant effect during continuation therapy related to a placebo effect? *Psychopharmacology Bulletin, 24,* 9–17.

Holden, C. (1986). Depression research advances, treatment lags. *Science, 233,* 723–726.

Hollister, L. E. (1986). Current antidepressants. *Annual Review of Pharmacology and Toxicology, 26,* 23–37.

Janowsky, D. S., Addario, D., & Risch, S. C. (1987). *Psychopharmacology case studies* (2nd ed.). New York: Guilford Press.

Jarvis, M. R. (1991). Clinical pharmacokinetics of tricyclic antidepressant overdose. *Psychopharmacology Bulletin, 27,* 541–550.

Johnson, F. N. (1979). The psychopharmacology of lithium. *Neuroscience and Biobehavioral Reviews, 3,* 15–30.

Kayser, A., Robinson, D. S., Nies, A., & Howard, D. (1985). Response to phenelzine among depressed patients with features of hysteroid dysphoria. *American Journal of Psychiatry, 142,* 486–488.

Khantzian, E. J. (1985). The self-medication hypothesis of addictive disorders: Focus on heroin and cocaine dependence. *American Journal of Psychiatry, 142,* 1259–1263.

Kolata, G. (1986). Manic depression: Is it inherited? *Science, 232,* 575–576.

Mallinger, A. G., & Smith, E. (1991). Pharmacokinetics of monoamine oxidase inhibitors. *Psychopharmacology Bulletin, 27,* 493–502.

Matussek, N., & Linsmayer, M. (1968). The effect of lithium and amphetamine or desmethylimipramine-RO 4-1284 induced motor hyperactivity. *Life Sciences, 7,* 371–375.

McNeal, E. T., & Cimbolic, P. (1986). Antidepressants and biochemical theories of depression. *Psychological Bulletin, 99,* 361–374.

Meltzer, H. Y. (1990). Presynaptic receptors: Relevance to psychotropic drug action in man. *Annals of the New York Academy of Sciences, 604,* 353–371.

Meltzer, H. Y. (1991). Beyond serotonin. *Journal of Clinical Psychiatry, 52* (suppl.), 58–62.

Nelson, J. C. (1991). Current status of tricyclic antidepressants in psychiatry: Their pharmacology and clinical applications. *Journal of Clinical Psychiatry, 52,* 193–200.

Nierenberg, A. A., & White, K. (1990). What next? A review of pharmacologic strategies for treatment resistant depression. *Psychopharmacology Bulletin, 26,* 429–460.

Offord, S. J., & Warwick, R. O. (1987). Differential effects o2 nialamide and clomipramine on serotonin efflux and autoreceptors. *Pharmacology, Biochemistry, and Behavior, 26,* 593–600.

Post, R. M., Kotin, J., & Goodwin, F. K. (1974). The effects of cocaine on depressed patients. *American Journal of Psychiatry, 131,* 511–517.

Preskorn, S. H. (1991). Should bupropion dosage be adjusted based upon therapeutic drug monitoring? *Psychopharmacology Bulletin, 27,* 637–643.

Prien, R. F. (1988). Methods and models for placebo use in pharmacotherapeutic trials. *Psychopharmacology Bulletin, 24,* 4–8.

Prien, R. F., & Potter, W. Z. (1990). NIMH workshop report on treatment of bipolar disorder. *Psychopharmacology Bulletin, 26,* 409–428.

Richelson, E. (1991). Biological basis of depression and therapeutic relevance. *Journal of Clinical Psychiatry, 52* (suppl.), 4–10.

Rickels, K., Amsterdam, J., Clary, C., et al. (1990). Buspirone in depressed outpatients: A controlled study. *Psychopharmacology Bulletin, 26,* 163–168.

Risch, S. C., Cohen, R. M., Janowsky, D. S., Kalin, N. H., & Murphy, D. L. (1980). Mood and behavioral effects of physostigmine on humans are accompanied by elevations in plasma beta-endorphin and cortisol. *Science, 209,* 1545–1546.

Rudorfer, M. V. (1992). Monoamine oxidase inhibitors: Reversible and irreversible. *Psychopharmacology Bulletin, 28,* 45–57.

Sacerdote, P., Brini, A., Mantegazza, P., & Panerai, A. E. (1987). A role for serotonin and beta-endorphin in the analgesia induced by some tricyclic antidepressant drugs. *Pharmacology, Biochemistry, and Behavior, 26,* 153–158.

Sitaram, N., Nurnberger, J. I., & Gershon, E. S. (1980). Faster cholinergic REM sleep induction in euthymic patients with primary affective illness. *Science, 28,* 200–202.

Stone, A. B., Pearlstein, T. B., & Brown, W. A. (1990). Fluoxetine in the treatment of premenstrual syndrome. *Psychopharmacology Bulletin, 26,* 331–336.

Swann, A. C., Koslow, S. H., Katz, M. M., Maas, J. W., Javaid, J., Secunda, S. K., & Robins, E. (1987). Lithium carbonate treatment of mania. *Archives of General Psychiatry, 44,* 345–354.

Telch, M. J., Agras, S., Taylor, C. B., Roth, W. T., & Gallen, C. C. (1985). Combined pharmacological and behavioral treatment for agoraphobia. *Behavioral Research and Therapy, 23,* 325–335.

Tollefson, G. D. (1991). Antidepressant treatment and side effect consideration. *Journal of Clinical Psychiatry, 52* (suppl.), 4–13.

Tosteson, D. C. (1981). Lithium and mania. *Scientific American, 244,* 164–174.

Walsh, B. T., Stewart, J. W., Roose, S. P., Gladis, M., & Glassman, A. H. (1984). Treatment of bulimia with phenelzine. *Archives of General Psychiatry, 41,* 1105–1109.

Wilcox, C. S., Cohn, J. B., Linden, R. D., et al. (1992). Predictors of placebo response: A retrospective analysis. *Psychopharmacology Bulletin, 28,* 157–162.

Worley, P. F., Heller, W. A., Snyder, S., & Baraban, J. M. (1988). Lithium blocks a phosphoinositide-mediated cholinergic response in hippocampal slices. *Science, 239,* 1428–1429.

Chapter Fourteen

Pharmacotherapy for Miscellaneous Mental Disorders

Schizophrenia, affective disorders, and problems associated with anxiety are the conditions in which chemical intervention is most likely, but there are a number of other mental or emotional conditions in which the use of psychotropic drugs may also be involved. This chapter will deal briefly with some of the more common ones, paying particular attention to those that occur predominantly in children and the aged.

Because this book is chiefly concerned with psychotropic drugs, the interventions discussed will necessarily deal with drugs. However, as a psychologist, I would strongly suggest that any interventions in these disorders also include a variety of psychotherapies, such as cognitive or behavior therapy, family therapy, or group therapy. In many cases, these should be tried before pharmacotherapy. When drugs and psychotherapy are combined, the two may complement each other. They may be synergistic; for example, a drug may be used to achieve a mood or mental state in patients that makes them more amenable to a particular form of psychotherapy (Telch et al., 1985). The combination of pharmacotherapy and psychotherapy may work better than either one alone simply because one is more effective in one subset of patients while the other is more effective in another subset of patients—despite the fact that both sets appear to share the same overt symptoms. Such is the vagary of diagnostics and etiology of most psychopathology.

Disorders in Children

There are a number of childhood mental or behavioral problems for which drugs are used, and until behavior modification techniques came into general use, the only "therapy" available for them involved the use of psychotropic substances. The major categories of childhood disorders for which drugs have been used are (1) the attention deficit disorder; (2) organic brain damage and retardation; (3) childhood schizophrenia; (4) infantile autism; and (5) affective disorders (generally in postpubertal children). (See Gadow, 1992, for a more complete review of these areas.)

Unfortunately, there are a number of major problems in evaluating the effectiveness of drugs in these disorders. First, accurate diagnoses are difficult to make. Verbal behavior, which is often crucial in determining the type of problems evidenced in adults, may be absent or poorly developed in a child, so that communication with the child is difficult or impossible. Also, the behavior of even normal children is pretty "psychotic"— they talk to nonexistent people, think inanimate objects have feelings and emotions, exhibit perceptual inconsistencies, have very weird senses of humor, tend to be self-centered, and have little regard for personal appearance or hygiene. Second, with children, one does not usually have any past stable history to look back on, as one has with adults. Children generally change, typically at a relatively rapid rate, and go through a number of different qualitative cognitive and physical changes during the developmental process. Therefore, it is often unclear whether behavioral changes that accompany drug treatment are due to the drug or to natural maturational processes. Finally, information about a treatment's effectiveness comes less from the patient being treated and more from the observers of the patient—that is, parents, teachers and clinicians—who often disagree on the outcome of the drug trial.

Although the psychotropics used in children are the same ones used in adults, special considerations for the pharmacokinetics of children and adolescents must be made (Geller, 1991). Children, for their size, have a greater hepatic capacity than adults and, therefore, more rapidly eliminate drugs that utilize hepatic pathways—for example, antipsychotics, tricyclic antidepressants, pemoline, and methylphenidate. Compared to adults, children have relatively less adipose tissue and, therefore, may have less ability for long-term storage of parent drugs and their metabolites. Finally, because of relatively greater total body water and more efficient renal mechanisms, children may more rapidly eliminate drugs that use primarily renal pathways, such as lithium. The functional significance of all this is that the mean plasma half-lives of most psychotropic drugs will be considerably shorter in children and adolescents and that young people will be able to tolerate higher dosages—per unit of body weight—than adults.

Attention Deficit Disorder

The most common childhood disorder for which medication is most likely to be used is the *attention deficit disorder* (*ADD*). It is also known as *hyperactivity,* the *hyperkinetic syndrome,* and *minimal brain dysfunction,* among other terms. ADD may be evidenced in 0.1 to 6% of the school-age population (the wide range is indicative of the difficulties in diagnosis and the differences in criteria used in diagnosis of the disorder), with a male to female ratio of approximately 5:1 (Weiss & Hechtman, 1979). The primary symptoms are lack of investment, organization, and maintenance of attention and effort in completing tasks; inability to delay gratification; and impulsive responding without attention to relevant stimuli in the environment (Dulcan, 1986). Hyperactivity is common but not always present in ADD.

Since these symptoms present a number of difficulties in learning situations, the disorder is of considerable concern in classroom settings. Other characteristics that may be evidenced are extreme aggressiveness and rapid mood swings. These are most often seen in times of stress or in groups, but they may be absent in some calm situations. The children generally show little evidence of fear, and their behavior is refractory to punishment involving aversive stimulation (that is, pain). Many symptoms of ADD tend to induce dominating and negative controlling responses on the part of teachers, parents, and peers (that is, they yell and scold a lot). These in turn may compound the ADD child's difficulties (Cunningham et al., 1985).

Neurological signs are sometimes evidenced along with these behavioral symptoms. These may include abnormal EEG patterns; mild visual or auditory impairments; crossed eyes; fine, jerky, lateral eye movements; poor visual-motor coordination; or handedness confusion. The etiology of the disorder (if indeed it is one disorder) is unclear, although there is sometimes evidence of notable birth trauma or abnormalities during pregnancy. There is often a family history of the disorder. Some evidence has been presented that there is insufficient catecholamine activity in the CNS of hyperactive children. Despite the common popular belief that sugar worsens hyperactive behavior in children, the majority of well-controlled experimental studies have failed to provide any support for this belief (Spring et al., 1987). A largely carbohydrate meal does tend to disrupt children's concentration, but that effect is common with just about everybody.

Before drug intervention is resorted to, a complete physical and neurological examination of the child should be conducted to establish that he or she is not suffering from hypoxia (insufficient blood supply to the brain), low calcium levels, low blood sugar levels, or hyperthyroidism, all of which can result in hyperactive symptoms. It is also important to determine whether or not the child is actually hyperactive. Surprisingly, this is not always easy because the term is broadly defined and no norms for child activity levels exist. For example, in a 1958 report based on questionnaires submitted to parents, approximately half of the children were noted to be overactive. A similar rate of distractibility and hyperactive symptoms in children was noted in a 1971 report based on questionnaires submitted to teachers. These reports suggest that parents and teachers may have unrealistic views as to what normal behavior in children is (Weiss & Hechtman, 1979).

Psychostimulants are the most common drug treatment for ADD, with methylphenidate (Ritalin) being the drug of choice, followed by *d*-amphetamine (Dexedrine) (Dulcan, 1986). There is no empirical evidence that one is better than the other with respect to the target symptoms of the disorder, but methylphenidate may induce less growth suppression. Pemoline (Cylert) has been shown to be slightly less effective than methylphenidate but may exert fewer side effects. Caffeine, often preferred by laypersons who do not believe in giving a "drug" to children, has virtually no efficacy but does have side effects. Some studies have indicated that perhaps as many as 20% of ADD children who do not respond to one type of psychostimulant may respond to another. There is no way as yet of predicting which child will respond to which drug.

MAO inhibitors have been shown to possess efficacy comparable to methylphenidate and amphetamine, but because of the precautions required of MAO inhibitors regarding diet and use of other drugs, they would only be clinically useful in children with idiosyncratic negative responses to these other stimulants or in cases where stimulant abuse might be of concern (Zametkin et al., 1985). Tricyclic antidepressants have been shown to have some efficacy in ADD, but the overall percentage of responders appears less than with psychostimulants. There is some evidence that many adolescents who do not respond to psychostimulants may respond to the tricyclic desipramine (Norpramin) (Gastfriend et al., 1985). Tricyclics may induce a very rapid symptom remission, but in some cases the effects may disappear with time. Their long-term safety in children, especially with respect to growth and development, is not well established. Sedative-hypnotics, such as barbiturates, induce no beneficial effects with respect to any of the target symptoms of the disorder and oftentimes prove to be worse than placebos.

A recent study demonstrating that clonidine was effective in reducing the core symptoms of ADD in 7 out of 10 children (Hunt et al., 1986) adds considerable confusion to the pursuit of understanding the pathophysiology of this disorder. Whereas psychostimulants have been determined to amplify noradrenergic activity (by enhancing norepinephrine release and blocking its reuptake), clonidine (Catapres) is an alpha-2-adrenergic receptor agonist (that is, it activates noradrenergic autoreceptors). Theoretically, this action should reduce the release of norepinephrine. Thus we have a most curious paradox: Drugs that amplify and drugs that reduce noradrenergic functioning have both been shown to be beneficial in reducing ADD symptoms.

Approximately 70–80% of the children diagnosed with ADD respond favorably to psychostimulants—in some cases dramatically—

with significant increases in attention span and significant decreases in motor activity and restlessness. However, if one tries both methylphenidate and dextroamphetamine and uses a wide range of doses, some degree of behavioral improvement almost always occurs in ADD children (Elia et al., 1991). This is reflected in better learning of rote material and improved performance of fine motor tasks like handwriting. Also, aggression and impulsivity are decreased. The amount and quality of the child's interpersonal relationships with both peers and teachers are generally improved, thus increasing the child's self-esteem and normalizing student/teacher interactions (Cunningham et al., 1985).

Psychostimulant intervention should be accompanied by elimination of disturbing influences in the family or classroom through counseling and psychotherapy, implementation of behavior modification and cognitive training programs, and enrollment of the child in learning disabilities classrooms (to help restore the confidence of the child, whose experiences are typically failures). In some cases these interventions alone may be sufficient to ameliorate the condition. However, in general, the benefits of nondrug interventions have been less substantial than those of drug treatment (Brown et al., 1985). There is also evidence that the positive reinforcers used in behavior modification programs may actually take the ADD child's attention away from the task at hand and direct it toward the reinforcing agent. Finally, there are economic factors that must be considered. Unfortunately, most psychological treatments are rather arduous and costly to implement, particularly in comparison to the few cents a day it costs for d-amphetamine.

If improvement with psychostimulants is going to occur, it will be apparent immediately. If these drugs produce only doubtful benefits in a few days (or at most a couple of weeks), their use should be terminated. Unfortunately, determining whether benefits occur may sometimes be difficult, because not all ADD children respond to the same dose and not all of the different target symptoms may respond equally to the same doses of these drugs. In fact, the effects of methylphenidate (the most commonly studied psychostimulant) on cognitive function in ADD children interact with and are interdependent on a host of variables—for example, dose, time course following administration, child characteristics, type of information processing required, task factors, and prevailing social-environmental conditions (Rapport & Kelly, 1991). In general, children's performance on tasks requiring primarily vigilance appears most benefited with low (0.1–0.4 mg/kg) doses (or shortly after the drug is administered). For highly effortful tasks that require greater behavioral inhibition, optimal benefits are most likely with high (0.6–0.9 mg/kg) doses (or 3–4 hours after the drug is administered). For tasks requiring nearly equal degrees of vigilance and inhibition, such as learning tasks, optimal performance is most likely with intermediate (0.3–0.7 mg/kg) doses (or 2–4 hours after drug administration). Thus whether one observes benefits or not may depend on what the observer is looking for, what dose has been given, and the time after the drug is given.

Unfortunately, routine monitoring of the plasma concentrations of any of the drugs used to treat ADD does not appear to be clinically useful, because of wide variations in optimum plasma concentration as well as a poor correlation between behavioral improvement and plasma levels (Elia, 1991), although several studies have found reliable correlations between psychostimulant plasma levels and clinical improvement during the first 1–4 hours of the absorption phase (Geller, 1991). Fortunately, there is a lack of effect of food on psychostimulant absorption in ADD children, which eliminates the need for a fasting state for drug efficacy.

It has long been believed that the response to psychostimulants of ADD children with hyperactivity is different from that of "normal" children and adults, or that it is paradoxical because hyperactive children appear to be calmer, rather than more excited, under their influence. However, studies have found that normal children and hyperactive children respond in a qualitatively similar way to psychostimulants; the effect may just be more apparent in hyperactive children (Rapoport et al., 1980). In a variety of measures, both types of children respond to psychostimulants as adults do, with the exception of mood. Adults tend to report mood elevation or euphoria with psychostimulants, whereas children tend to say that these drugs make them feel "funny" or "strange." Finally, ADD children without hyperactivity benefit as much with psychostimulant treatment as those children with hyperactivity, although the latter children may require somewhat higher doses because they have greater difficulty in the area of behavioral inhibition (Barkley et al., 1991).

The paradoxical reduction in motor activity with psychostimulants may be resolved by noting that sustained attention and high motor activity are incompatible; when attention increases, activity is most likely going to decrease. (Have you ever noticed how "zombielike" children look when they are watching their favorite Saturday morning cartoon?) Another possibility is that hyperactive children may actually be physiologically underaroused, and that psychostimulants bring arousal up to normal while sedative-hypnotics decrease arousal even further and worsen the symptoms. (You may notice that many of the characteristics of the hyperactive child are analogous to those of a moderately drunken adult—that is, inattentiveness, belligerence, and unresponsiveness to normal social controls).

Despite the consistent improvement in the symptoms of the disorder, which should theoretically allow the children to learn more efficiently, there seems to be no evidence that long-term learning and academic achievement are affected by psychostimulants (Dulcan, 1986). Although this paradox has not been resolved, it may be due in part to the practice of using doses that most facilitate classroom behavior but have the least effectiveness with respect to learning. It is also possible, because of the long duration of exposure to these drugs, that much of the learning accomplished under the drug was state-dependent (Swanson & Kinsbourne, 1976). If such is the case, then it is not surprising that individuals who were treated with drugs do not show any long-term gains from the treatment when they are later tested as adolescents or adults without the drugs. Although there has been no definitive study of this possibility, there is evidence that adults who were hyperactive as children (and treated with psychostimulants) do respond favorably in some psychomotor tasks with psychostimulants (Wender, 1978).

One recent study compared young adults who had been treated for hyperactivity with psychostimulants during childhood with a similar group of unmedicated individuals and a control group (Hechtman et al., 1984). They found that the adults who had been hyperactive as youths differed greatly from the control group, regardless of their therapy as children. However, the adults who had been treated with psychostimulants as youths differed from the untreated adults on only a few variables. It seemed that the treated young adults had fewer car accidents, viewed their childhood more positively, stole less in elementary school, and generally had better social skills and self-esteem. The authors suggested that the medicated individuals may have suffered less from early social ostracism and subsequently developed better feelings toward themselves and others.

It is generally believed that ADD is eventually outgrown in puberty and that the effectiveness of psychostimulant medication ceases at this time. Therefore, some experts suggest that these medications should be withdrawn at puberty. However, neither belief is supported by empirical evidence. Although the symptoms do tend to dissipate at puberty, impulsivity, poor social skills, and lower educational achievement often continue into adulthood (Hechtman, 1985). Furthermore, several studies have indicated that adolescents and adults diagnosed with ADD can benefit markedly from psychostimulant drug therapy (Gadow, 1992). It is possible that the decreased positive response to psychostimulants over time in some individuals is due to tolerance.

The most common side effects of psychostimulants in hyperactive children are insomnia and anorexia, which may result in small, temporary effects on normal weight gain. Less common, but more problematical, are symptoms of social withdrawal (as noted above, interpersonal relationships are generally improved with psychostimulant treatment) or acute psychotic reactions. Also, psychostimulants may exacerbate or cause the onset of severe motor and phonic tics in individuals predisposed to Tourette's syndrome (to be described shortly). Clinicians and people who deal with children should be particularly aware of this possibility because early signs of Tourette's syndrome may be difficult to distinguish from hyperactivity and would only get worse with psychostimulants (Caine et al., 1984).

Psychostimulant treatment in hyperactive children does not appear to increase their risk for drug dependency later on. Clinical experience has not revealed any association between the use of these drugs in preadolescents and their later drug abuse. This finding may be due to the fact that hyperactive children do not experience any pleasurable effects from these drugs and are quite willing to terminate this therapy when the suggestion to do so is made. The fact that ADD children dislike taking these medications can lead to noncompliance, which some authorities have suggested may be partially responsible for the variable and conflicting results from drug studies and the lack of long-term efficacy of psychostimulants in this disorder. Therefore, children should not be given sole responsibility for taking their medication and should not be allowed to take it to school with them (since they may "forget" to take it or succumb to pressure from peers to "share" their medication) (Dulcan, 1986).

Over the past decade there has been considerable discussion about the benefits of nutritional interventions for the treatment of hyperactivity, such as elimination of foods containing artificial colors and flavors, natural and artificial salicylates (aspirin-like substances), preservatives, and sugar. This is sometimes referred to as the Feingold diet, named after Ben Feingold, the allergist who initially proposed the association between these substances and many cases of hyperactivity. Although recent empirical studies have not supported Feingold's contention that as many as 50% of hyperactive children may benefit from such dietary restrictions, they have indicated that some hyperactive children, perhaps between 5 and 10%, show behavioral improvements from them (Kolata, 1982).

Infantile Autism

Infantile autism is currently diagnosed by the presence of severe disturbances that are generally noted during the first 30 months of life. The primary symptoms are failure to develop interpersonal relationships, inability to use communicative speech, the presence of bizarre motor behaviors such as rocking and head banging, and an anxious desire for sameness in the child's surroundings. There is an absence of delusions, hallucinations, and loosening of associations common to schizophrenia. Some autistic children show evidence of a very high level of cognitive functioning in a specific area, such as rote memory, but in general, intellectual functioning is significantly below average. I.Q.s are below 50 in 60% of autistic children, between 50 and 70 in 20%, and above 70 in only 20%. Approximately 5 out of 10,000 children are diagnosed with the disorder, and it is four to five times more prevalent in males than in females (Ritvo & Freeman, 1984).

Divergent lines of evidence indicate that autism is a syndrome of heterogeneous origins with similar behavioral manifestations, although research consistently favors neurological abnormalities with a genetic inheritance pattern (Ritvo & Freeman, 1984). A number of electrophysiological and neurochemical findings have suggested that autistic patients are in a state of chronic hyperarousal. Unfortunately, the procedures used in determining these results may be sufficiently fear-arousing in these patients to create the abnormalities found. There is no evidence that the symptoms and developmental delays of autism are due to psychological trauma, physical abuse, bad parenting, or separation.

The primary goals of intervention with autistic children are to promote development of rudimentary or nonexistent functions such as language and adaptive social and self-care skills, and to decrease behavioral symptoms such as stereotypies, withdrawal, hyperactivity, self-mutilation, and aggressiveness directed toward others. Structured educational programs, designed to systematically teach the child higher and wider skills in developmental problem areas, are the preferred mode of treatment. Most pharmacological interventions are used to control behaviors such as assaultiveness, self-mutilation, and unmanageable hyperactivity. However, more recently, chemicals have been used in attempts to correct presumed neurological deficits underlying the symptoms.

Antipsychotics have been used for many years in treating this disorder and have been shown to effectively reduce the symptoms of hyperactivity, stereotypy, and aggressiveness. However, the low-dosage (that is, higher-potency) antipsychotics, such as haloperidol (Haldol), thiothixene (Navane), and trifluoperazine (Stelazine) are more effective than the higher-dosage drugs like chlorpromazine (Thorazine) since the latter drugs' strong sedative properties can interfere with performance and learning (Campbell, 1978). The use of antipsychotics in this disorder may also lead to what has been called an *akathisia frenzy* (what might appear to be a severe case of "ants in the pants"), which begins a cycle in which behavioral disturbances are exacerbated. This may lead to escalating the dose of the antipsychotic, which can produce an increase in akathisia-induced impulsive behavior.

Recent studies with haloperidol have found it to be significantly superior to a placebo in reducing withdrawal and stereotypies in autistic children and, combined with contingent reinforcement, to be an effective method of facilitating the acquisition of imitative speech (Anderson et al., 1984). In addition, lithium may have some value in the treatment of aggression, explosive affect (emotion/mood), and hyperactivity. However, the potentially severe side effects of these drugs, noted in Chapters 12 and 13, make their long-term use a questionable practice.

A wide variety of drugs have been tried with autistic children, with mixed, mostly negative, results (Campbell, 1978). Back in the days when LSD was being used in psychotherapeutic contexts, LSD was suggested to have some beneficial effects in that it seemed to assist the child in retaining eye contact and to prolong his attention span. LSD's inhibition of serotonin activity may have been a factor in these effects (see the discussion of fenfluramine below). Amphetamines have been shown to slightly increase attention span and verbal production and to decrease hyperactivity in some autistic children, but numerous and common side effects of these drugs (such as worsening of withdrawal and stereotypies and loss of appetite) are such that these drugs should not be used as a treatment in this disorder. On the other hand, antagonists at adrenergic beta receptors (for example, propranolol (Inderal) have recently been shown to significantly reduce impulsive, aggressive, and self-abusive behaviors, as well as the need for sameness, in adult autistics (Ratey et al., 1987). These findings support the notion that some autistics are in a chronic state of hyperarousal.

Sedative-hypnotics have not been found to be any better than placebo in controlling autistic symptoms. Administrations of L-dopa, the precursor to dopamine, and 5-hydroxytryptophan, the precursor to serotonin, have been shown to have no beneficial effects in autistic children. In fact, these treatments may actually be counterproductive in that there is speculation that there is excessive activity of these neurotransmitters in some autistic children. Studies investigating the effects of megavitamin therapy with niacin and pyridoxine have been inconclusive with respect to autism (Sloman, 1991).

Recently, the use of the nonamphetamine appetite suppressant fenfluramine (Pondimin) in the treatment of autism has created a great deal of excitement. This drug, which reduces the levels of serotonin in the brains of animals, has been shown in several studies to have both long-lasting and reversible effects in autistic children. Its use was suggested from research indicating that perhaps a third of autistic children have abnormally high levels of blood serotonin (you might recall that this is a primary neurotransmitter in the reticular activating system, which modulates sensory input, activity level, attention, and arousal) (Hashino et al., 1984). Initial studies conducted with autistic children indicated that fenfluramine treatment for several weeks or months was accompanied by notable improvements in both intellectual and social functioning (Gadow, 1992). Significantly, in one study, one of the patients who responded favorably to fenfluramine had an autistic twin brother, not treated with fenfluramine, who showed no improvement in his condition (Geller et al., 1982). Although there was a considerable regression in the patients' symptoms when they were subsequently administered placebos, sustained improvement was noted for several weeks after they were taken off the active drug.

Other studies indicated that fenfluramine-treated autistic children showed a decrease in hyperactivity, distractibility, and motor disturbances but indicated no effect of fenfluramine treatment on intellectual functioning or communication skills (August et al., 1985; Beisler et al., 1986). However, it was suggested that the improvements in the other behavioral areas could make the child more accessible to other forms of interventions, such as behavior modification or special education (August et al., 1985). Except for some patients exhibiting lethargy when first introduced to fenfluramine, mild to moderate weight loss, and irritability and restlessness for the first few days back on the placebo, there were no notable adverse effects of fenfluramine treatment in these studies (Campbell et al., 1986).

Unfortunately, more recent investigations of fenfluramine on severely and profoundly developmentally disabled autistic children and adults have not supported these earlier observations. In addition to finding no significant clinical improvements in autistic symptoms, several side effects (weight loss, moderate tension and agitation, and insomnia) were observed both during and shortly after fenfluramine treatment (Sloman, 1991). The use of fenfluramine in the treatment of autism has become more controversial with the discovery that fenfluramine may be a neurotoxin. Although people have been taking fenfluramine as an appetite-suppressant for more than 20 years without any observable toxic effects, recent studies point to fenfluramine-induced serotonergic toxicity in rats given five times the human dose (Barnes, 1989). (You might recall that the same type of potential toxicity was noted to occur with "ecstasy" and was one of the factors leading to it being categorized as a Schedule I controlled substance.) Thus more research will have to be conducted to determine whether there is a particular subtype of autistic child that responds favorably to fenfluramine, whether more permanent changes accompany even longer exposures to the drug, and whether chronic exposure to the drug results in adverse effects.

As has been the case with so many other disorders, the endorphins have been implicated in childhood autism. In this case, elevated endogenous opioids have been suggested to be a factor in the etiology of the disorder (Goldberg, 1987; Sahley & Panksepp, 1987). It was theorized that parental warmth or contact may stimulate opioid activity as a way of strengthening the bond between parent and child. However, some autistic children who already have elevated opioid levels may not need the surge of opioids induced by parental contact. Therefore, these children may avoid attachment and parental warmth. This may also be the reason why these children do not appear to experience normal pain, which would stop them from engaging in self-injurious behaviors. This theory was supported by recent studies in which the long-acting opiate antagonist naltrexone was administered to autistic children (Campbell et al., 1988; Gadow, 1992). These studies revealed that naltrexone induced several beneficial effects in most of the children. These included significant reductions in withdrawal, fidgetiness, negative/uncooperative behavior, and stereotypies and significant increases in verbal production, relatedness to others, social interactions, and eye contact. There was also evidence that aggressiveness and self-injurious behavior were reduced by naltrexone. Obviously, these preliminary findings must be viewed with caution until they are replicated with larger samples, but they are certainly intriguing.

Childhood Schizophrenia

Pharmacological interventions for the symptoms of schizophrenia in childhood are essentially the same as those for adults (Gadow, 1992). With the antipsychotics there is maximal improvement in two to four weeks, and the degree of improvement is comparable to that of adult improvement. Children seem to tolerate many of the adverse effects of these drugs better than adults do (Engelhardt & Polizos, 1978). Drowsiness is more likely to occur with the higher-dosage antipsychotics, while extrapyramidal effects are more likely with the lower-dosage drugs. Weight gain is generally above normal. After several months of exposure to antipsychotics, withdrawal effects involving involuntary movements, ataxia, or oral dyskinesia may occasionally be evident upon abrupt drug cessation, but these dissipate within a week or two. Tardive dyskinesia may also occur, but the frequency of occurrence is unknown. Following cessation of drug treatment, most children, unlike adults, relapse into schizophrenic symptoms in one to two weeks. As is the case with adults, children in the early stages of the illness are generally more responsive to these medications.

Some children with schizophrenic symptoms also show signs of hyperactivity. Unfortunately, however, as one might expect, the symptoms of these children get worse when treated with psychostimulants. There is some evidence that aggressive psychotic children, with or without periodicity, may respond favorably to lithium (Campbell et al., 1984).

Mental Retardation

Mentally retarded children, roughly defined as those having I.Q.s of 75 or less, often evidence symptoms of impulsivity, hostility, aggressiveness, hyperactivity, poor manageability, and self-mutilation. A wide variety of chemical interventions have been used in the treatment of these children (including sedative-hypnotics, nutritional supplements, anticonvulsants, anxiolytics, and antidepressants), none of which has proven to be effective (Lipman et al., 1978). Although antipsychotics may be used to treat these symptoms, for the most part their efficacy is minimal. In cases where these drugs do appear to induce socially appropriate behavior, one should be careful that the effects are not simply due to a general reduction of behavior to meet the demands of the institutional environment. Furthermore, antipsychotics are likely to interfere with the already minimal performance and learning skills of these children. Also, considering the numerous side effects of antipsychotics (such as extrapyramidal effects, drowsiness, and tardive dyskinesia), it is unlikely that a severely mentally retarded child will benefit from antipsychotic intervention.

The psychostimulants such as amphetamine have not been found to improve the target symptoms associated with mental retardation. Methylphenidate may improve alertness and reduce hyperactivity, but it does not appear to exert any other benefits in this disorder. Unfortunately, the investigations of these drugs with respect to the disorder have been rather limited, or have lacked sufficient controls. Thus one cannot rule out the potential benefits of psychostimulants in some cases of mental retardation in light of the fact that the description of many mental retardation study samples fits well with the symptom picture of the attention deficit disorder. Individuals in both groups are hyperactive, distractible, impulsive, emotionally labile, and aggressive, and they have short attention spans, low tolerance for frustration, and learning difficulties.

Affective Disorders in Adolescents

It has only recently been appreciated that adolescents may exhibit affective disorders (mainly depression) and that drug therapy may be warranted. Drug treatments for affective disorders in adolescents are essentially the same as those for adults (Biederman, 1988). Unfortunately, the efficacy of these treatments in adolescents is much less apparent than with adults (Gadow, 1992), partially because the rate of placebo response in these individuals is quite high. It has also been suggested that the dramatic changes in sex and growth hormones and differences in neurotransmitter activity that accompany adolescence may account for the less than satisfactory response to antidepressant drugs.

Most studies with depressed adolescents have utilized tricyclic antidepressants. There is some evidence, however, that monoamine oxidase inhibitors (MAOIs) may be effective in adolescents who do not respond to tricyclics. As yet, no large-scale, double-blind studies with MAOIs and newer-generation antidepressants (e.g., fluoxetine, bupropion) have been conducted to determine their efficacy in the treatment of depressed adolescents.

Parkinson's Disease

Parkinson's disease is a degenerative brain disorder that afflicts some half million people in the United States. The main symptoms are difficulty in initiating voluntary movements, slowness of movement, muscular rigidity, tremors, and inability to maintain an upright posture while standing or walking. In addition, approximately a third of the cases have accompanying dementia. In 90% of the cases, the symptoms develop after the age of 55.

Properly controlled family studies have failed to document a family concentration of Parkinson's disease, and the concordance rates for the disease among identical twins are no higher than those among fraternal twins. Thus there is no support for the theory that heredity plays a role in the disease (Duvoisin, 1986).

The recent discovery that a metabolite of the compound MPTP (MPP+, discussed in Chapter 10) is capable of inducing both CNS lesions and symptoms that are almost indistinguishable from Parkinson's disease (Kopin & Markey, 1988) has focused attention on environmental pollutants with similar structures, such as industrial chemicals. For example, pesticides like paraquat (a compound in the news over the last 15 years because of its controversial use in controlling marijuana growth) are being explored as potential causative agents in the disease (Lewin, 1985).

The environmental cause hypothesis has been bolstered recently by studies showing a high correspondence between area use of insecticides and the incidence of Parkinson's disease (Lewin, 1985). Also, studies have indicated that more patients are developing Parkinson's disease at a young age and that in many families in which more than one member develops the disease, the onset occurs at roughly the same time within the family, but at very different ages for parents and offspring. Both of these phenomena are inconsistent with a pure genetic mechanism (Lewin, 1987b). For reasons unknown, epidemiological studies have repeatedly shown that Parkinson's disease occurs less frequently among chronic cigarette smokers than among nonsmokers (Yong & Perry, 1986); these results suggest that there may be a compound in tobacco smoke that somehow protects the individual from the toxic consequences of an environmental agent (however, I wouldn't use these findings as an excuse for smoking cigarettes).

Whatever the cause, it has been well established that the symptoms are due to the destruction of dopaminergic neurons in the basal ganglia. The symptoms generally appear when approximately 80% of these neurons have been lost (Dakof & Mendelsohn, 1986). It is believed that tracts in this region of the brain, important for the smooth control of voluntary movements, normally contain balanced dopaminergic (inhibitory) and cholinergic (excitatory) inputs and that any imbalance in these two systems results in specific movement disorders. Therefore, most of the chemical interventions in the treatment of Parkinson's disease involve attempts to balance these by either decreasing the cholinergic system or enhancing the dopaminergic system (Bianchine, 1985).

As mentioned in Chapter 1, drugs with anticholinergic properties were one of the first to be used in the treatment of Parkinson's disease, and until the 1960s they were the most effective drugs available for the disorder. However, more effective drugs developed recently have relegated them to a supportive role. They may still be very useful in patients with minimal symptoms, patients who do not respond to the newer drugs, or those who cannot tolerate their side effects. Anticholinergic side effects, such as mental confusion, sleepiness, and delirium, have also limited their usefulness. Antihistamines with anticholinergic properties may also be used, since they produce fewer side effects, but they are less effective than anticholinergics.

Almost immediately after the discovery of the association between dopamine deficiency and Parkinson's disease, attention turned to the use of L-dopa as a treatment for the disorder. L-dopa (for levodihydroxyphenylalanine) is the immediate precursor to dopamine and, once it enters the brain, it is enzymatically converted into dopamine (administering dopamine itself is not of value because it cannot pass through the blood-brain barrier). Theoretically, this provides for higher levels of this neurotransmitter for use by the remaining dopaminergic neurons. In approximately 80% of the patients, this treatment induces dramatic reductions in all symptoms of the disorder, except for the symptoms of dementia (Bianchine, 1985). In addition, L-dopa partially relieves the changes in mood characteristic of Parkinson's disease, and feelings of apathy are replaced by increased vigor and a sense of well-being. Lost sexual potency may be regained.

L-dopa was clearly the miracle drug of the 1960s and 1970s. Unfortunately, though, as its use became more and more widespread, more and more problems with its use emerged. Although the majority of patients respond well to L-dopa initially, after about 3 to 5 years on L-dopa therapy the drug begins to lose its effectiveness and patients return to pretreatment levels of functioning. There is no evidence that long-term results are markedly improved when low-dose L-dopa regimens are used (Poewe et al., 1986). Therefore, it seems rational to adjust the L-dopa dosage to the individual patient's needs rather than to adhere to a policy that assumes the lowest dose is the best dose. Sometimes the responses of patients fluctuate abruptly between symptom control and no control; this pattern is often referred to as the on-off phenomenon because the control is switched on and off like a light.

In addition, patients often develop distressing and incapacitating problems with chronic L-dopa therapy, including abnormal involuntary movements, and may exhibit psychiatric symptoms such as hallucinations, paranoia, mania, insomnia, anxiety, nightmares, and emotional depression (Bianchine, 1985). Whether the psychiatric disturbances and intellectual decline are the result of the continued progression of the disease or are the result of long-term L-dopa exposure is not clear

(Lewin, 1987a), although most of the side effects are reversible by a reduction in dosage. In any event, some clinicians are now suggesting that individuals who can function adequately in their occupations and social interactions should not be treated with L-dopa until their condition begins to deteriorate. Until this time, drugs that are less effective than L-dopa can be given, so that the beneficial effects of L-dopa may be saved until they are truly necessary.

L-dopa's optimal effect comes from keeping concentrations of the drug within a therapeutic window that becomes increasingly narrow with time; thus pharmacokinetic factors are critical for its efficacy (LeWitt, 1992). The most commonly used formulation of L-dopa is Sinemet, a combination of L-dopa and carbidopa, which prevents the peripheral conversion of L-dopa to dopamine. This formulation produces more-reliable brain concentrations, but even with multiple daily doses, plasma concentrations may increase too fast, producing motor disturbances and adverse psychic effects, or fall off too quickly, allowing the disease symptoms to appear suddenly. Recently, this problem has been reduced considerably by putting Sinemet in an erodible matrix (called Sinemet CR) that retards gastric tablet dissolution and allows plasma level concentrations to be maintained longer and more smoothly.

L-dopa's efficacy is also influenced by when it is taken and what types of food it is taken with. If taken with meals, this drug's peak plasma levels take longer to be achieved and are reduced. Also, large amounts of amino acids following high-protein meals can interfere with its absorption from the gut as well as into the brain, because the amino acids compete with L-dopa for the transport system that allows it to cross the blood-brain barrier (Montgomery, 1992).

Because of the restricted efficacy of L-dopa therapy, researchers have been searching for ways to decrease the amount of L-dopa needed to control symptoms as well as for more direct means of amplifying dopamine activity. Several drugs have been investigated for this purpose (Campanella et al., 1987). Anticholinergic drugs act synergistically with L-dopa, thereby lowering the dosage needed, but they can decrease the absorption of L-dopa to the point that it is no longer therapeutically beneficial. Amantadine (Symmetrel), which is believed to release dopamine from intact terminals, has been found to be somewhat more effective than anticholinergics but considerably less effective than L-dopa. It is sometimes used for short periods as a supplement to L-dopa therapy. Bromocriptine (Parlodel) is one of several ergot derivatives with demonstrated dopaminergic activity that may be useful in the control of Parkinson's symptoms. It appears to be equivalent to L-dopa in therapeutic efficacy, and it may manage the on-off phenomenon more smoothly than L-dopa and induce less dyskinesia. However, visual and auditory hallucinations, hypotension, and purplish discolorations of the skin are more common with bromocriptine. Other adverse effects of bromocriptine may occur with short- or long-term treatment. Selegiline (also called L-deprenyl and marketed as Eldepryl), a selective inhibitor of the MAO-B enzyme, has been shown to enhance L-dopa's effectiveness in Parkinson's patients without potentiating the hypertensive effects of sympathomimetic drugs (Kopin & Markey, 1988). Some studies have indicated that selegiline by itself may also increase the life expectancy of Parkinson's patients (discussed in the final paragraph of this section).

Unfortunately, none of the drugs currently used in Parkinson's disease is able to reverse the course of the disease. With further degeneration of the dopaminergic tracts responsible, eventually no drugs exert beneficial effects, or they exert side effects that cannot be tolerated. However, these drugs have been beneficial in extending the useful lives of individuals with the disease for up to five years.

A potentially new drug approach to the treatment of Parkinson's disease involves attempting to reduce the destruction of dopamine neurons by using MAOIs (such as selegiline) or general antioxidant drugs, such as vitamin E (Kopin & Markey, 1988). The reasoning behind this approach comes from the previously mentioned hypothesis concerning environmental toxins in the lesioning process, which might well be speeded up by the oxidation enzyme MAO or the presence of harmful oxidative molecules. While recent studies have found selegiline to delay the need for L-dopa therapy in early Parkinson's disease patients, possibly by slowing progression of the disease (Tetrud & Langston, 1989), it will probably take a few more years of research to determine the true efficacy of this approach.

Gilles de la Tourette's Syndrome

The symptoms of *Tourette's syndrome* are, to some extent, opposite to those of Parkinson's disease. Rather than reflecting an inability to voluntarily initiate motor activities, they reflect an inability to suppress unwanted motor activities (Shapiro & Shapiro, 1980). The syndrome is characterized by involuntary motor and verbal tics; the former involve the head, torso, and limbs, and the latter involve grunts, sounds, words, or phrases, often of a vulgar or obscene nature (known as coprolalia). (In earlier times, it was thought that persons with these symptoms were victims of demonic possession, as depicted in the movie "The Exorcist.") Its onset is generally noted in childhood and early adolescence, and the symptoms persist throughout the person's lifetime with spontaneous remissions and exacerbations. The symptoms of obsessive-compulsive disorder (discussed shortly) and attention deficit disorder often accompany Tourette's disorder syndrome (Golden, 1990).

As with Parkinson's disease, the basal ganglia have been implicated in the etiology of Tourette's syndrome, but with dopaminergic overactivity being involved, rather than underactivity. Thus the pharmacological modes of treatment for Tourette's syndrome are essentially the opposite of those for Parkinson's disease. The antipsychotics, such as phenothiazines and haloperidol (Haldol), are the only ones that have been observed to consistently reduce the symptoms of the disorder (Campanella et al., 1987). The most recent of these is pimozide (Orap), which some studies have indicated may induce fewer side effects (Regeur et al., 1986). Anxiolytics do not appear to be any more effective than placebos. Although there are no clear data supporting one antipsychotic over the other in efficacy, the phenothiazines appear to exert less stable long-term effects than haloperidol or pimozide. Either of these is the drug of choice in the vast majority of cases.

Drugs that lower dopamine synthesis (such as alpha-methyl-p-tyrosine) or dopamine depletors (for example, tetrabenazine) have produced beneficial effects in the disorder, but they exert troublesome side effects and are not believed to be as useful as haloperidol or pimozide. However, these may be combined with an antipsychotic because of their synergistic effects. Excessive noradrenergic functioning may also be a factor in Tourette's syndrome, because clonidine (the alpha-2-adrenoceptor agonist mentioned on several earlier occasions) has been shown to reduce the symptoms of the disorder. Clonidine has also been found to be useful in alleviating some of the abstinence symptoms (essentially a worsening of Tourette's symptoms) associated with cessation of antipsychotics after chronic use (Max & Rasmussen, 1986). Clonidine does not appear to be as efficacious as haloperidol or pimozide in the treatment of Tourette's symptoms, but many clinicians prefer it as the initial drug in treatment because of its lower incidence of serious side effects. In addition, clonidine may be beneficial in reducing attention deficit disorder symptoms in Tourette's patients who exhibit them (Golden, 1990). Drug treatments attempting to amplify acetylcholine activity (for example, by administering choline chloride or lecithin) have resulted in some clinical improvement in the disorder, but the magnitude of their effect is clearly less than that obtained with haloperidol or pimozide. Finally, for reasons as yet unclear, there have been several reports indicating the usefulness of *calcium blockers* in the treatment of Tourette's disorder (Walsh et al., 1986).

Epilepsy

Epilepsy is a term used to categorize a number of diverse chronic disorders characterized by sudden attacks of brain dysfunction (seizures) usually associated with some alteration of consciousness. The seizures are almost always correlated with abnormal and excessive discharges in the EEG and are often accompanied by violent muscle spasms (convulsions) (Rall & Schleifer, 1985). (By now you are probably aware that essentially the same symptoms may accompany withdrawal from sedative-hypnotics after chronic exposure.) Several lines of evidence suggest that in most of these disorders the seizure begins with and is sustained by the synchronous firing at high frequency of a relatively localized group of neurons, which then spreads to adjacent neurons. A reduction in inhibitory components of neuronal circuits (such as GABA activity) is a likely mechanism for this action (Dichter & Ayala, 1987). For example, a reduction in GABA levels because of a diet deficient in pyridoxine (vitamin B_6), which is required for GABA synthesis, can result in seizures; the problem can be successfully reversed by adding pyridoxine to the diet (Cooper et al., 1991). Modulatory substances such as norepinephrine and opioid peptides may also play a role.

Since there are a variety of disorders involved, the etiology varies considerably, with suspected causes ranging from hereditary factors to head injuries, infectious diseases, allergies, and nutritional abnormalities, among others. As is the case with numerous brain disorders, neurotoxicity resulting from overactivity of the excitatory amino acid neurotransmitters at NMDA receptors has been proposed as a mechanism for promoting seizure activity (Olney, 1990). However, in many cases, no cause for the seizures can be identified (idiopathic epilepsy). In approximately three-fourths of the cases, the symptoms are evidenced prior to adulthood. Seizures may be partial (focal seizures), with various manifestations depending upon the particular cortical area producing the abnormal discharge, or they may be generalized throughout the CNS (Rall & Schleifer, 1985).

The most common types of epilepsy, which can be further subdivided into more detailed descriptions of the symptoms, are *grand mal*, *petit mal* (both involving generalized seizures), and *psychomotor* (focal seizures). Grand mal seizures (sometimes referred to as tonic-clonic seizures because of the sequence of maximal tonic spasms of all body musculature followed by synchronous clonic jerking movements) are characterized by generalized convulsions of the entire body accompanied by the loss of consciousness. Peripheral manifestations may consist of bluing of the lips, face, and fingernails (resulting from deficient oxygenation of the blood), drooling, discharge of urine and feces, and tongue biting. Before the convulsions begin, many grand mal patients often describe an aura, which may consist of an unexplainable fear, an unpleasant or unusual odor, peculiar sounds, tingling of the skin, or spots before the eyes. After the episode, the person is in a weakened and confused state.

Petit mal seizures (also referred to as *absence* seizures because they may not be accompanied by clear motor disturbances) are associated with periods of blank stares. They are most prevalent in children and are often mistaken for daydreaming. Rapid eye blinking and twitching movements sometimes accompany the seizures. There is no aura associated with the seizures, and the person is able to resume normal activity immediately following them. Although they are of short duration (approximately 5 to 20 seconds), several dozen may occur daily.

Psychomotor (temporal lobe) seizures generally stem from temporal lobe dysfunction, and their manifestations take on various forms. They are characterized by an aura, a duration of one to two minutes, and postseizure confusion and amnesia. During a seizure, the person may make purposeless movements, such as lip smacking, chewing, fumbling with clothing, or rubbing of the hands or legs.

Since seizures appear to involve a hyperexcitability of neuronal tissue, it is not surprising that most sedative-hypnotic drugs are anticonvulsants and that most anticonvulsants have sedative-hypnotic properties. However, since the sedative-hypnotic properties are not necessary for antiseizure efficacy and are viewed as undesirable, drugs that are most effective in the treatment of epilepsy are those that can reduce or eliminate seizure activity without inducing sedation or sleep (Rall & Schleifer, 1985). Furthermore, the efficacy and type of drug treatment is heavily dependent upon the type of seizure experienced; that is, a drug effective with one type of seizure may not be effective with another.

From 1857 to 1912 sodium bromide was used to control epilepsy. However, the bromide salts cause mental sluggishness, and prolonged treatment may cause chronic toxicity, which is manifested by sedation, psychotic disturbances, increased glandular secretion, and gastric distress. In 1912 the barbiturate phenobarbital was discovered to be useful in reducing seizures without inducing as many side effects as sodium bromide. To this day it remains a cheap and effective treatment for many forms of epilepsy.

In 1938 phenytoin (diphenylhydantoin [Dilantin]), which is structurally related to the barbiturates (the initial basis for its use in epilepsy), was found to be effective for both grand mal and psychomotor seizures without inducing sedation (refuting the then-current hypothesis that an effective anticonvulsant had to have sedative properties). It is still one of the most commonly used drugs for these types of seizures.

In 1954 primidone (Mysoline), structurally related to phenobarbital (one of its metabolites in the body is phenobarbital), was found to be an effective treatment for epilepsy. Ethosuximide (Zarontin), which has a relatively low incidence of toxicity, came into use in 1960 as one of the more effective treatments of petit mal epilepsy. Carbamazepine (Tegretol), related chemically to the tricyclic antidepressants, was approved for use in the United States as an antiepileptic agent in 1974. Valproic acid (Depakene), approved for use in the United States in 1978, is the most recent of the more common compounds now in use for the chronic treatment of epilepsy. Interestingly, its effectiveness was discovered accidentally when it was used as a vehicle for other compounds that were being screened for antiepileptic activity.

Many other compounds have been determined to have anticonvulsant activity, but they have shown no greater efficacy than those already noted, or they have been found to exert unacceptable side effects, or they have not been approved for use in the United States. Two of the most promising of the latter are progabide, a GABA receptor agonist presently on the market in France, and vigabatrin, an inhibitor of the enzyme responsible for the metabolic breakdown of GABA in the CNS. Several studies testing a number of therapy-resistant epileptics suffering from a variety of types of seizures have revealed that progabide or vigabatrin added to standard antiepileptic medications can significantly reduce seizure frequency. There was no tolerance to their effects, and side effects were mild and transient (Musch et al., 1987; Tartara et al., 1986).

The mechanisms of action of anticonvulsants have not been clearly delineated. All have been suggested to amplify somehow the activity of GABA, the major inhibitory neurotransmitter in the CNS (Zorumski & Isenberg, 1991). Phenytoin has been found to exert a stabilizing effect on all neuronal membranes. It decreases the flow of sodium ions during both resting and action potentials, delays the activation of outward potassium flow during an action potential (which leads to an increased refractory period), and reduces the calcium-dependent, depolarization-linked release of acetylcholine and norepinephrine (Pincus & Kiss, 1986). Other mechanisms are likely involved in these drugs' antiseizure activity; for example, in contrast to phenytoin, some of carbamazepine's anticonvulsant activity has been suggested to be due to its capacity to increase (rather than decrease) discharge of noradrenergic neurons (Rall & Schleifer, 1985).

Overall, the drugs that we have discussed abolish seizure activity in approximately 50% of the cases, and significantly reduce seizure frequency in another 25% (Rall & Schleifer, 1985). Phenytoin, phenobarbital, carbamazepine, and primidone are most effective in psychomotor and grand mal seizures and are not effective in petit mal seizures. While there is no clear difference among these drugs in their efficacy in these cases, some patients refractory to one compound may respond to another. Also, lower-than-effective dosages of these drugs may be combined to decrease the relative incidence or degree of side effects induced by larger doses of the individual drugs.

Petit mal seizures are most effectively treated with ethosuximide, valproic acid, or the benzodiazepine clonazepam (Klonapin). Valproic acid may also be effective in grand mal seizures as well as in other seizures that have not been described here. Multiple drug therapy may also be required in cases where more than one type of seizure activity occurs in the same patient. In cases of *status epilepticus* (a condition in which one major attack of epilepsy succeeds another with little or no intermission), a rapid-onset benzodiazepine such as diazepam is generally given intravenously (in conjunction with mechanical supports for preventing asphyxiation).

All of the drugs used in the treatment of epilepsy have a number of potential side effects that may limit their usefulness in certain patients. Many of these, such as dizziness, loss of balance, slurred speech, and visual difficulties, may be attributable to their sedative-hypnotic properties. Other reactions may involve gum enlargement, rashes, allergic reactions, liver damage, endocrine alterations, and gastrointestinal complaints. The type and degree of reaction vary considerably among these drugs, and the particular drugs administered often depend on these, rather than the relative efficacy with respect to antiseizure activity.

Although epilepsy is viewed as a chronic disorder requiring continuous drug treatment, it may be desirable at some point to withdraw medication (very gradually over a period of months, since the risk of status epilepticus is great with abrupt cessation). Medication may be withdrawn because of evidence of unacceptable side effects or to prevent potential side effects from occurring or if the patient has been seizure-free for a considerable length of time. Studies have indicated that the majority of patients who have been free of seizures for several years with medication will not show a recurrence of symptoms when the medications are withdrawn. However, since a history of a single recent seizure may be detrimental to one's employment or access to a driver's license, the decision to withdraw medication must be made with some deliberation.

Geriatric Psychopharmacology

Although I would like to emphasize that growing old is not considered a disease in and of itself, the fact remains that as we grow older a number of drugs are often used to treat cognitive, emotional, or behavioral deficits that are alleged to be caused by the normal aging process. Also, drugs may be used to treat a disease or condition that is found solely, or at least more frequently, among the elderly. Although most persons over the age of 65 are in good mental health, close to a quarter of this population suffer from disorders ranging from depression (which is reflected in a high suicide rate within this group) to *dementia*. Aging is often accompanied by CNS changes that lead to memory deficits, confusion, irritability, apathy, or disturbed behavior (Domino et al., 1978; Finch, 1982).

Reduction in blood flow to the brain as a result of cerebral arteriosclerosis may cause progressive mental impairment. Specific neurological lesions in the brain can cause such disorders as Parkinson's disease and

Alzheimer's disease. The latter condition is characterized by loss of intellectual abilities including memory, judgment, abstract thought, and higher cortical functions, as well as changes in personality and behavior. Although senile onset occurs after age 65 and presenile onset usually occurs between the ages of 50 and 65, these two conditions are indistinguishable forms of dementia with respect to cellular pathology. Mental depression is also common among the elderly (Ban, 1984). Some of the symptoms of these disorders respond well to drug therapy, but in many cases drugs do little good and may even make psychogeriatric illnesses worse.

There are special problems in treating the elderly with drugs. The first of these centers on diagnoses (Ban, 1984). For example, the treatment of dementia is likely to include psychotropic medication. However, dementia is defined by changes in behavior, not by laboratory tests, or CAT or PET scans. Since mental capacities tend to decline with age, it is difficult to decide when normal aging ends and dementia begins. Furthermore, virtually every type of disease and medication can induce symptoms of dementia: antihypertensive and antiulcer drugs, depression, altered thyroid function and kidney failure, isolation, vascular disease, AIDS and other viral infections, brain tumors, vitamin deficiencies, alcoholism and other drug abuse—the list is endless (Kolata, 1987). Diagnosing other behaviors or emotional problems amenable to psychotropic drug treatment is equally difficult. To compound this problem, because of numerous health problems, geriatric patients often take many drugs (prescription, over-the-counter, and social), a practice which not only makes diagnosis difficult but also puts the elderly at a much higher risk for complex and harmful drug interactions than younger patients.

Another problem, or set of problems, is related to the alteration of pharmacokinetics that occurs with aging (Friedel, 1978). The increase in percentage of body fat means that psychotropic drugs, which for the most part are lipid-soluble, are more widely distributed throughout the body and may have a larger volume of distribution. There is the possibility that psychotropics may accumulate in adipose tissue in older persons, which could result in a longer duration of action and an increased sensitivity to the drugs. Decreased plasma proteins may lead to less plasma binding and an increased possibility of toxicity. The potential for reaching toxicity is further enhanced by the decreased efficiency of metabolism of drugs in the liver and reduced filtration of drugs by the kidneys. Thus higher levels of a drug may be present in the body for a longer period of time than would be the case in younger subjects. For these reasons, it is generally recommended that pharmacologic treatment should commence with one-third to one-half the recommended adult dosage with most drugs, and the dosage should be increased only very gradually (Ban, 1984)—start low and go slow.

A classic example of these difficulties can be seen in the treatment of depression—the most commonly diagnosed psychological disorder in the elderly (Ban, 1984). The anticholinergic side effects of many antidepressants, which may be merely troublesome to most younger individuals, can be very annoying and possibly life-endangering in the elderly. Examples would be aggravation of prostate hypertrophy, precipitation of glaucoma, or bowel impaction. Antidepressants may cause delirium or confusional states in geriatric patients whose symptoms are misdiagnosed (and dismissed) as symptoms of dementia. Reduced cardiovascular functioning of the elderly person, in combination with antidepressant medication, can lead to bradycardia, orthostatic hypotension, severe arrhythmias, or complete disruption of cardiac conduction. The coexistence of chronic medical illness with depression or mental disturbances in many geriatric persons makes psychotropic treatment particularly complex.

Fortunately, and in spite of the potential hazards and discomforts of using antidepressants in elderly patients, they are effective in some 70 to 90% of the cases (Ban, 1984). If the drug is cautiously selected and the initial dosage is one-third to one-half the amount given to younger patients, and plasma levels are carefully monitored, then antidepressant treatment can be safe and effective. Antidepressants may also reduce symptoms similar to those of early senile dementia, which occur secondary to depression (for example, pseudodementia). Furthermore, the development of some of the newer antidepressants with lower toxicity and fewer anticholinergic side effects should only improve the prospects for more effective treatment of this population.

For those psychiatric or psychological dysfunctions common to both younger and older individuals (such as anxiety, sleep disturbances, psychotic reactions, and manic-depression), as long as the pharmacokinetic considerations that we have noted are taken into account, pharmacological interventions are essentially the same for both groups (Ban, 1984). For example, benzodiazepines are recommended for anxiety-related symptoms, but the shorter-acting benzodiazepines, such as oxazepam, should be used to prevent excessive accumulation of these compounds.

Drug intervention for sleep disturbances in the elderly should take into consideration the fact that the need for sleep normally decreases with age. Hypnotic doses of chloral hydrate are less likely to cause persistent effects in the elderly than other hypnotic agents, and drug "hangover" may be less common with chloral hydrate than with most barbiturates and some benzodiazepines. However, chloral hydrate may exert both peripheral side effects (gastric distress, vomiting, and flatulence) and undesirable CNS effects (malaise, light-headedness, ataxia, and nightmares). It should definitely be avoided in patients with marked liver or kidney impairment and should probably be avoided in patients with severe cardiac disease.

Antipsychotics are legitimately used in cases where there is a recurrence of a psychotic episode or in patients who are extremely agitated to the point of hurting themselves or others (Salzman, 1988). However, unless there is evidence of symptoms specific to psychosis, antipsychotics are likely to overly sedate the patients. Unfortunately, antipsychotics tend to be overused in most nursing homes and institutions, and they are more likely given for the benefit of the staff than of the patients. Lithium treatment for manic-depression symptoms is just as effective in elderly patients as it is in younger patients, although with considerably lower doses (approximately 15–20% of normal).

With respect to the primary sources of the cognitive and memory dysfunctions common to the geriatric population, drug interventions have yet to produce clear successes in clinical trials. Psychostimulants such as amphetamines, methylphenidate, magnesium pemoline, and pipradol have not been found to benefit cognitive functioning in geriatric patients (Galizia, 1984). Furthermore, while psychostimulants may be useful in the treatment of apathetic, withdrawn, disheartened, or demoralized older people (Salzman, 1985), these drugs may produce an increase in agitation and psychotic thinking and behavior when the demented states are severe (Salzman, 1988). At one time it was believed that cerebrovasodilators might be beneficial by increasing blood flow; however, such interventions have not produced reliable results (Ban, 1978). For example, a popular drug of this type, Hydergine (ergoloid mesylates), has been touted as having vasodilating and cerebral metabolic activity with concomitant cognitive improvement, but several studies have found contrary results. There is some evidence that Hydergine may improve a subset of cognitive functions (such as short-term memory) in elderly patients with mild dementia (Thienhaus et al., 1987). The issue of efficacy is clouded by the possibility that Hydergine acts as a mood elevator, such that improvement in cognitive function may be secondary to the antidepressant effects.

Neuropeptides have been investigated but are generally ineffective in reducing mild cognitive impairment resulting from age, dementia, or other trauma (Galizia, 1984). ACTH 4-10 (a fragment of adrenocorticotropic hormone) may increase arousal and improve cognitive functioning in some areas in the elderly (Koob, 1987). Vasopressin (a peptide found in the pituitary gland) has resulted in improvement in tests of concentration, attention, and memory, including storage and retrieval of information in humans (Crook, 1988). However, it is not clear whether these effects are directly linked to memory or are simply due to improvements in mood, attentiveness, or some other aspect of performance. For example, vasopressin causes hypertension via its action at peripheral blood vessel receptors. It has been argued that, because the behavioral effects of vasopressin can be blocked by antagonists of these receptors, the apparent CNS effect of vasopressin is indirectly mediated by an arousal secondary to the inappropriate hypertension (Cooper et al., 1991).

Some GABA derivatives such as piracetam (Nootropil) have been tested in elderly patients with mixed results (Crook, 1988; Krueger et al., 1992). Should piracetam prove to be beneficial in cognitive activities, it would be particularly useful because it is devoid of any sedative, analgesic, neuroleptic, or autonomic effects.

Despite the lack of conclusive beneficial drug effects regarding the intellectual dysfunctions of the elderly, there is a rapidly growing body of evidence concerning the potential causes for these dysfunctions that has considerably heightened the future prospects for the development of effective drug interventions. For example, although the specific relationship between age-related CNS dysfunctions and cognitive loss will prove complex, recent evidence suggests that a deterioration in cholinergic neurotransmitter systems is involved in Alzheimer's disease (Coyle et al., 1983). This evidence has stimulated clinical trials attempting to compensate pharmacologically for the presumed cholinergic disturbance by increasing the availability of acetylcholine precursors (for example, by administering choline or lecithin), reducing acetylcholine metabolic degradation with drugs that inhibit the enzyme acetylcholinesterase, such as tetrahydroaminoacridine (THA or tacrine) and physostigmine, or administering muscarinic agonists, such as arecoline (Branconnier et al., 1992). Although the effects of these treatments on memory performance in aged subjects have been neither robust nor consistent, a few studies have indicated that a narrow range of doses of cholinomimetics may significantly reduce the memory impairments in some individuals (Crook, 1988; Krueger et al., 1992).

Whereas initial attempts to treat Alzheimer's patients involved compounds thought to influence cholinergic systems in the brain, the recognition that structural and functional disturbances in noradrenergic, dopaminergic, serotonergic, and other systems also occur in Alzheimer's patients (Crook, 1988) has led to approaches that attempt to address these deficiencies. Antipsychotics, lithium, beta-adrenergic blockers, antidepressants (monoamine uptake inhibitors and monoamine oxidase inhibitors), anticonvulsants, and anxiolytics have been advocated as being useful in reducing certain symptoms in elderly demented patients (Schneider & Sobin, 1992). Unfortunately, the majority of such patients do not respond to such treatments, and the ones that do appear to respond often experience side effects that severely limit the long-term usefulness of these drugs.

The reason for the failure of drug treatments to reverse Alzheimer's disease symptoms may be that neuronal death is so severe that the affected systems are incapable of responding to pharmacologic manipulation. As a result, it has been suggested that pharmacological strategies designed to slow neuronal death rate may have therapeutic value. Although neuronal cell death may occur because of a wide variety of pathological and toxicological processes (e.g., insufficient oxygen or low blood glucose levels), as well as normal gene-programmed processes, in most of them the final common pathway for the activation involves a sustained elevation of free intracellular Ca^{++} concentration (Branconnier et al., 1992). Thus chronic treatment with calcium-channel blockers or antagonists of NMDA receptors (which mediate Ca^{++} flow into cells), such as PCP-like drugs, may have therapeutic value in preventing or delaying the onset of the disease (Johnson & Jones, 1990).

Obsessive-Compulsive Disorder, Phobias, and Panic Attacks

Obsessive-compulsive disorder (OCD) is a condition characterized by recurrent unpleasant thoughts (obsessions) or behaviors (compulsions) that the person cannot suppress or control. It typically begins in adolescence or early adulthood. Both obsessions and compulsions may occur in the disorder, or they may occur separately. *Phobias* are fairly common in the general population and are characterized by irrational fears concerning specific objects or situations—in spite of the fact that the person often recognizes that the fear is disproportionate to the actual degree of danger involved. *Panic disorder* is related to phobias but is much less common. It is characterized by recurrent panic attacks, which are accompanied by heart palpitations or chest pain, a choking or smothering feeling, dizziness, numbness and tingling in the hands or feet, sweating, and trembling. The symptoms come on quite suddenly and unpredictably. Long-term sufferers may begin to feel anxious in anticipation of an attack.

These three categories of psychopathology all share a common affective state characterized by high psychological arousal ranging from anxiety to extreme fear. Thus it would seem that these disorders would be most amenable to treatment with anxiolytics. Curiously, however, while most research indicates that benzodiazepines, now the most commonly used anxiolytics, can reduce the symptoms of these disorders, other drugs, which are not commonly viewed as anxiolytics, have been shown to be equally or more effective in the treatment of these disorders (Davis & Gelder, 1991).

Another affective state that is often evidenced in these disorders is depression. Thus a variety of antidepressants have been used in their treatment, with some degree of success (Lelliott & Monteiro, 1986). While all of the classes of antidepressants described in Chapter 13 appear to be effective in many patients with these disorders, not all are effective in all patients with what appear to be very similar symptoms. The selective serotonin reuptake blockers—for example, sertraline (Zoloft), clomipramine (Anafranil), and fluoxetine (Prozac)—are currently the drugs of choice for OCD (Insel, 1990). Tricyclics and monoamine oxidase inhibitors may also be effective in some patients. Though all these drugs have antidepressant effects and many patients with OCD exhibit symptoms of depression, the efficacy of these compounds does not appear to be related to whether or not the patient is depressed. Also, the treatment of OCD should be distinguished from the usual pharmacological treatment of depression. OCD patients generally require higher doses and longer treatment, and they exhibit improvement in symptoms that is far short of total symptom relief. Thus drug treatment should be integrated with behavioral techniques as well as psychosocial interventions for more effective relief of this disorder.

The tricyclic antidepressants, such as imipramine (Tofranil), or high-potency benzodiazepines such as alprazolam (Xanax) have been shown to be effective treatments for the panic and phobic disorders (Mattick et al., 1990). However, because of potential psychological and physical dependency associated with benzodiazepines, some clinicians have expressed concerns over their chronic use in disorders that may be effectively treated with psychologically based therapies or with drugs that do not have abuse potential. The MAOIs have also been recommended for treatment of these disorders, but their use may be limited by potential interactions with other drugs or the dietary precautions that are necessary for preventing a hypertensive crisis. If panic attacks or phobic reactions are controlled by an MAOI or tricyclic but residual anxiety over experiencing symptoms is present, a benzodiazepine may be added to the drug regimen and then gradually removed as the patient becomes less fearful of suffering from another attack. As an adjunctive therapy to reduce the peripheral manifestations of these disorders (heart pounding and increased blood pressure), beta-adrenergic–blocking drugs, such as propranolol, may be tried. Unless the symptoms of these disorders are accompanied by clear signs of psychosis, antipsychotics are not appropriate in their treatment.

Because all three sets of disorders present very specific behavioral symptoms, behavior therapy techniques such as biofeedback, systematic desensitization, and progressive relaxation may be useful in their treatment. Considerable research suggests this to be the case. Therefore, behavior therapy programs should definitely be involved in the treatment of these disorders, either in lieu of or in conjunction with drug therapy (Davis & Gelder, 1991; Lelliott & Monteiro, 1986).

Sexual Dysfunction

It has often been said that the major sex organ in humans is the brain (Taberner, 1985). Thus it is not surprising that as many as one half of all human sexual difficulties are psychological in origin (Montague et al., 1979), or that they may respond favorably to everything from ground-up rhinoceros horns to Tabasco sauce or oysters. Belief is a powerful drug. Unfortunately, the vast majority of substances taken to alleviate sexual dysfunctions have no direct effects on sexual potency or the ability to achieve orgasm. Other than testosterone, which enhances sexual motivation in both men and women (Sherwin, 1988), there are very few, if any, true **aphrodisiacs**—that is, substances that generally enhance libido and sexual performance. In fact, more often than not, drugs that humans take tend to inhibit the sex drive and sexual performance.

Alcohol is perhaps the drug most frequently used by people to try to enhance the sex drive. However, as Shakespeare stated long ago, "Lechery, sir, it provokes, and unprovokes; it provokes the desire, but it takes away the performance" (*Macbeth*, Act 2, scene 3). Modern science has verified this hypothesis. Although alcohol's ability to disrupt our cortical control over our inhibitions may lead to increased psychological sexual arousal (at low doses), it tends to decrease physiological measures of sexual arousal (that is, vaginal and penile vasocongestion) in both males and females in a dose-dependent fashion (Leavitt, 1982). With chronic use, a variety of sexual difficulties often occur. These may include impotence, atrophy of the testicles, lower testosterone levels, and impaired sperm production.

Spanish fly, a general term for several species of beetles, has long been renowned for its aphrodisiac qualities. At best, it irritates the urethra (and a variety of other organs) and leads to inflammation of the bladder; at worst, it causes death by shock from bleeding (Taberner, 1985).

Other drugs commonly attributed with sexual-enhancing properties include the P/P/H drugs discussed in Chapter 11, particularly marijuana (Leavitt, 1982). Again, however, most of this enhancement comes from belief and expectation (Taberner, 1985). There may also be some physiological basis for this observation with marijuana. In Chapter 11 a study with mice was mentioned that indicated an acute increase in plasma testosterone levels with THC exposure. However, following this increase, there was a considerably longer period of time during which testosterone levels were decreased. Similarly, the vast majority of studies with humans indicate that marijuana may have an estrogen-like effect and that chronic marijuana users often exhibit lower testosterone levels, more sexual impotency, and lower sperm production than nonusers. Fortunately, these effects are readily reversible if marijuana use ceases.

Cocaine was the aphrodisiac of the 1980s. By itself, if injected or smoked, it can elicit a reaction described as a whole-body orgasm and can induce spontaneous ejaculation without genital stimulation. It also has the reputation of enhancing sexual pleasure and "staying power" (Leavitt, 1982). However, because of its vasoconstrictive properties, it, like amphetamine, may decrease the ability to achieve erection in males and orgasm in females. With chronic use, it often leads to impotence and frigidity (Taberner, 1985).

Nonrecreational drugs are also a common source of sexual difficulties. Many medications used to treat cardiac dysfunctions and high blood pressure can cause loss of sexual desire and/or potency. In the aged, who commonly take such medications, this loss can be construed as one of the "inevitable" consequences of aging (the word "inevitable" is in quotes because the declines in sexual desire and potency in the elderly are greatly exaggerated). Antidepressants and antipsychotics may decrease sexual desire in some individuals, although the mood elevation with antidepressants may allow some individuals to enjoy sexual activities again.

In conclusion, when there is evidence of sexual dysfunction, the person's drug-taking practices should be assessed. If he or she is taking a drug, it may be the culprit, and ceasing taking the drug or shifting to an alternative may very well clear up the problem.

Under some circumstances and in some individuals, there are drugs that can enhance sexual desire and reduce impotence. In patients with Parkinson's disease, the use of L-dopa often restores sexual potency (Taberner, 1985). When this effect was first observed, many individuals concluded that L-dopa was an aphrodisiac. But it does not work with normal individuals, and even if it did, the potential negative side effects would outweigh the benefits.

One drug that may work with normal individuals is yohimbine, a substance derived from the bark of an African tree. A recent study has revealed what West African witch doctors have known for centuries—that yohimbine can be effective in the treatment of certain cases of impotence (Reid et al., 1987). Yohimbine is an alpha-2-adrenergic (noradrenergic autoreceptor) antagonist. Its primary effect is to block the inhibitory feedback system via noradrenergic autoreceptors and allow more norepinephrine synthesis and/or release. Whether the problem was psychological or physiological in origin, almost half the male subjects given yohimbine overcame difficulties in erection and regained the ability to perform sexually. Curiously, the beneficial effects were noted two to three weeks after the start of therapy; this response latency is not compatible with the rapid onset of yohimbine's known pharmacological properties or autonomic effects. Whatever the mechanism, the drug is not a panacea. Among other side effects is a significant elevation in blood pressure, which could be fatal. Sweating, nausea, and vomiting may also occur. Again, the costs versus the benefits of this drug need to be weighed carefully.

Eating Disorders

Obesity is a major problem in many cultures. In some cases it has psychological consequences in terms of one's self-esteem and social interaction. In extreme cases, it can lead to severe physiological consequences, such as inability to regulate glucose plasma levels and high blood pressure. Thus a multitude of treatments for obesity have been developed, and often these treatments include psychotropic drugs.

Appetite-control medications, both prescription and nonprescription, are big business. Unfortunately, most of these are amphetamines or are related structurally to amphetamine, and these are easily abused. Furthermore, most do not do much for weight control (perhaps they enhance the person's mood temporarily), or if they do, tolerance develops fairly rapidly. Most studies that have investigated weight losses with these drugs have found the average weight loss to be rather modest, and in most cases, the losses are not maintained for very long. These drugs also have side effects, such as elevated blood pressure. Thus the consensus is that these drugs are of little value in the area of weight control.

The nonsympathomimetic antidepressant fluoxetine (Prozac), which has recently come on the market, has been shown to suppress food cravings in many individuals. Its abuse potential remains to be established, but no drugs with fluoxetine's biochemical properties (namely, those that inhibit serotonin reuptake) have been shown to be self-administered by animals—a good indication that it will have low abuse potential in humans. In high doses, opiate antagonists have been shown to reduce eating in a variety of animal species, but studies with humans have failed to demonstrate significant weight losses with these drugs (Hatsukami et al., 1986).

On the other side of the coin, there has been focus recently on eating disorders that may result in persons becoming severely underweight. The two disorders receiving the most attention are *anorexia nervosa* and *bulimia*. While individuals with these disorders may share certain characteristics, they are viewed by most experts as separate disorders. In both disorders, the individuals are predominantly females who fear becoming obese and believe that one must be thin in order to be physically attractive. Depression and anxiety are common symptoms, but they may not be clearly evident. In most cases their weights are below what is considered normal for their age group.

Anorexics are generally severely underweight (as much as 50% below normal), whereas the weight of bulimics may be in the normal range. Despite their extreme thinness, anorexics may actually perceive themselves as overweight or gaining weight. Bulimics commonly experience food binges, eating everything in sight, but then purge themselves by self-induced vomiting or by taking laxatives. This is rarely the case with anorexics, who generally are on a self-starvation diet. Because of malnutrition-induced disruption in metabolism and hypothalamic functions, anorexics may actually not feel hungry at all.

In addition to the direct problems associated with malnutrition (such as lowered resistance to disease, death by starvation, and absence of menstruation), there are a number of other consequences of these disorders, such as deterioration of the teeth and esophagus (due to stomach acid upon vomiting), constipation, and drug dependence. (One recent study indicated that a third of the cocaine abusers who called a cocaine hot line met the criteria for anorexia or bulimia [Jonas et al., 1987].) Thus, although these disorders are not very common, some kind of intervention is definitely called for when they occur.

A variety of psychological and physiological etiologies and treatments have been explored (the discussion of which is beyond the scope of this text) with, as yet, no consensus as to how these disorders come about or how they should be treated. Many pharmacological interventions have been tried with very limited success. Most studies in this area have not been methodologically sound; for example, they used small samples, did not use a control group, used inconsistent criteria for symptoms, or mixed a variety of psychological and drug treatments.

As mentioned in Chapter 13, the antidepressants may be useful in the treatment of these disorders, especially if there are clear signs of concomitant depression (Pope et al., 1983; Walsh et al., 1984). Tricyclics may induce carbohydrate craving, which can exacerbate the individuals' fear of losing control over their eating behavior, and drug regimens using MAOIs must be closely monitored because of the dietary restrictions that are involved. Anxiolytics, lithium, and antipsychotics have all been shown to reduce some of the symptoms in some individuals with these disorders, but their well-known side effects considerably limit their usefulness. Opiate antagonists have recently been shown to reduce binge eating in bulimics (Mitchell et al., 1986), but further trials are necessary for determining their overall efficacy in this disorder. Basically, there is, as yet, no drug treatment regimen that carries a promise for a sustained and speedy recovery from these eating disorders.

For anorexia, the consensus in the field is that drug therapy has little to offer and that supportive psychotherapy and behavioral intervention used in inpatient programs are the best methods for producing weight gain (Nelson, 1991). A similar belief is held for the treatment of bulimia. Although antidepressant drugs have been shown to reduce patients' frequency of binging significantly, perhaps only 10% of patients treated with drugs are viewed as cured of the disorder.

Bibliography

Anderson, L. T., Campbell, M., Grega, D. M., Perry, R., Small, A. M., & Green, W. H. (1984). Haloperidol in the treatment of infantile autism: Effects on learning and behavioral symptoms. *American Journal of Psychiatry, 141,* 1195–1202.

August, G. S., Raz, N., & Baird, T. D. (1985). Effects of fenfluramine on behavioral, cognitive, and affective disturbances in autistic children. *Journal of Autism and Developmental Disorders, 15,* 97–107.

Ban, T. A. (1978). Vasodilators, stimulants and anabolic agents in the treatment of geropsychiatric patients. In M. A. Lipton, A. DiMascio, & K. F. Killman (Eds.), *Psychopharmacology* (pp. 1525–1534). New York: Raven Press.

Ban, T. (1984). Chronic disease and depression in the geriatric population. *Journal of Clinical Psychiatry, 45,* 18–23.

Barkley, R. A., DuPaul, G. J., & McMurray, M. B. (1991). Attention deficit disorder with and without hyperactivity: Clinical response to three dose levels of methylphenidate. *Pediatrics, 87,* 519–531.

Barnes, D. M. (1989). Neurotoxicity creates regulatory dilemma. *Science, 243,* 29–30.

Beisler, J. M., Tsai, L. Y., & Stiefel, B. (1986). Brief report: The effects of fenfluramine on communication skills in autistic children. *Journal of Autism and Developmental Disorders, 16,* 227–233.

Bianchine, J. R. (1985). Drugs for Parkinson's disease, spasticity, and acute muscle spasms. In A. G. Gilman, L. S. Goodman, T. W. Rall, & F. Murad (Eds.), *The pharmacological basis of therapeutics* (pp. 473–490). New York: Macmillan.

Biederman, J. (1988). Pharmacological treatment of adolescents with affective disorders and attention deficit disorder. *Psychopharmacology Bulletin, 24,* 81–87.

Branconnier, R. J., Branconnier, M. E., Walshe, T. M., McCarthy, C., & Morse, P. (1992). Blocking the Ca^{2+}-activated cytotoxic mechanisms of cholinergic neuronal death: A novel treatment strategy for Alzheimer's disease. *Psychopharmacology Bulletin, 28,* 175–182.

Brown, R. T., Borden, K. A., & Clingerman, S. R. (1985). Pharmacotherapy in ADD adolescents with special attention to multimodality treatments. *Psychopharmacology Bulletin, 21,* 192–211.

Caine, E. C., Ludlow, C. L., Polinsky, R. J., & Ebert, M. H. (1984). Provocative drug testing in Tourette's syndrome: *d*- and *l*-amphetamine and haloperidol. *Journal of the American Academy of Child Psychiatry, 23,* 147–152.

Campanella, G., Ror, M., & Barbeau, A. (1987). Drugs affecting movement disorders. *Annual Review of Pharmacology and Toxicology, 27,* 113–136.

Campbell, M. (1978). Use of drug treatment in infantile autism and childhood schizophrenia: A review. In M. A. Lipton, A. DiMascio, & K. F. Killman (Eds.), *Psychopharmacology* (pp. 1451–1462). New York: Raven Press.

Campbell, M., Adams, P., Small, A. M., Tesch, L. M., & Curren, E. L. (1988). Naltrexone in infantile autism. *Psychopharmacology Bulletin, 24,* 135–139.

Campbell, M., Deutsch, S. I., Perry, R., Wolsky, B. B., & Palij, M. (1986). Short-term efficacy and safety of fenfluramine in hospitalized preschool-age autistic children: An open study. *Psychopharmacology Bulletin, 22,* 141–146.

Campbell, M., Perry, R., & Green, W. H. (1984). Use of lithium in children and adolescents. *Psychosomatics, 25,* 95–106.

Cooper, J. R., Bloom, F. E., & Roth, R. H. (1991). *The biochemical basis of neuropharmacology*, 6th ed. New York: Oxford University Press.

Coyle, J. T., Price, D. L., & DeLong, M. R. (1983). Alzheimer's disease: A disorder of cortical cholinergic innervation. *Science, 219,* 1184–1190.

Crook, T. (1988). Pharmacotherapy of cognitive deficits in Alzheimer's disease and age-associated memory impairment. *Psychopharmacology Bulletin, 24,* 31–38.

Cunningham, C. E., Siegel, L. S., & Offord, D. R. (1985). A developmental dose-response analysis of the effects of methylphenidate on the peer interactions of attention deficit disordered boys. *Journal of Child Psychology and Psychiatry, 26,* 955–971.

Dakof, G. A., & Mendelsohn, G. A. (1986). Parkinson's disease: The psychological aspects of a chronic illness. *Psychological Bulletin, 99,* 375–387.

Davis, J. D., & Gelder, M. (1991). Long-term management of anxiety states. *International Review of Psychiatry, 3,* 5–17.

Dichter, M. A., & Ayala, G. F. (1987). Cellular mechanisms of epilepsy: A status report. *Science, 237,* 157–164.

Domino, E. F., Dren, A. T., & Giardina, W. J. (1978). Biochemical and neurotransmitter changes in the aging brain. In M. A. Lipton, A. DiMascio, & K. F. Killman (Eds.), *Psychopharmacology* (pp. 1507–1516). New York: Raven Press.

Dulcan, M. K. (1986). Comprehensive treatment of children and adolescents with attention deficit disorders: The state of the art. *Clinical Psychology Review, 6,* 539–569.

Duvoisin, R. C. (1986). Etiology of Parkinson's disease: Current concepts. *Clinical Neuropharmacology, 9,* S3–S11.

Elia, J. (1991). Stimulants and antidepressant pharmacokinetics in hyperactive children. *Psychopharmacology Bulletin, 27,* 411–416.

Elia, J., Borcherding, B. G., Rapoport, J. L., & Keysor, C. S. (1991). Methylphenidate and dextroamphetamine treatments of hyperactivity: Are there true nonresponders? *Psychiatry Research, 36,* 141–155.

Engelhardt, D. M., & Polizos, P. (1978). Adverse effects of pharmacotherapy in childhood psychosis. In M. A. Lipton, A. DiMascio, & K. F. Killman (Eds.), *Psychopharmacology* (pp. 1463–1471). New York: Raven Press.

Finch, C. E. (1982). The neurobiology of aging. *Science, 216,* 49–50.

Friedel, R. O. (1978). Pharmacokinetics in the geropsychiatric patient. In M. A. Lipton, A. DiMascio, & K. F. Killman (Eds.), *Psychopharmacology* (pp. 1499–1506). New York: Raven Press.

Gadow, K. D. (1992). Pediatric psychopharmacotherapy: A review of recent research. *Journal of Child Psychology and Psychiatry, 33,* 153–195.

Galizia, V. J. (1984). Pharmacotherapy of memory loss in the geriatric patient. *Drug Intelligence and Clinical Pharmacy, 18,* 784–791.

Gastfriend, D. R., Biederman, J., & Jellinek, M. S. (1985). Desipramine in the treatment of attention deficit disorder in adolescents. *Psychopharmacology Bulletin, 21,* 144–145.

Geller, B. (1991). Psychopharmacology of children and adolescents: Pharmacokinetics and relationships of plasma/serum levels to response. *Psychopharmacology Bulletin, 27,* 401–410.

Geller, E., Ritvo, E. R., Freeman, B. J., & Yuwiler, A. (1982). Preliminary observations on the effect of fenfluramine on blood serotonin and symptoms in three autistic boys. *New England Journal of Medicine, 307,* 165–168.

Goldberg, J. R. (1987). Healthy addiction. *Health, 19(8),* 18.

Golden, G. S. (1990). Tourette syndrome: Recent advances. *Pediatric Neurology, 8,* 705–714.

Hashino, Y., Yamamoto, T., Kaneko, M., Tachibana, R., Watanabe, M., Ono, Y., & Kumashiro, H. (1984). Blood serotonin and free tryptophan concentration in autistic children. *Neuropsychobiology, 11,* 22–27.

Hatsukami, D. K., Mitchell, J. E., Morley, J. E., Morgan, S. F., & Levine, A. S. (1986). Effect of naltrexone on mood and cognitive functioning among overweight men. *Biological Psychiatry, 21,* 293–300.

Hechtman, L. (1985). Adolescent outcome of hyperactive children treated with stimulants in childhood: A review. *Psychopharmacology Bulletin, 21,* 178–191.

Hechtman, L., Weiss, G., & Perlman, T. (1984). Young adult outcome of hyperactive children who received long-term stimulant treatment. *Journal of the American Academy of Child Psychiatry, 23,* 261–269.

Hunt, R. D., Minderaa, R. B., & Cohen, D. J. (1986). The therapeutic effect of clonidine in attention deficit disorder with hyperactivity: A comparison with placebo and methylphenidate. *Psychopharmacology Bulletin, 22,* 229–236.

Insel, T. R. (1990). New pharmacologic approaches to obsessive compulsive disorder. *Journal of Clinical Psychiatry, 51* (suppl.), 47–51.

Johnson, K. M., & Jones, S. M. (1990). Neuropharmacology of phencyclidine: Basic mechanisms and therapeutic potential. *Annual Review of Pharmacology and Toxicology, 30,* 707–750.

Jonas, J. M., Gold, M. S., Sweeney, D., & Pottash, A.L.C. (1987). Eating disorders and cocaine abuse: A survey of 259 cocaine abusers. *Journal of Clinical Psychiatry, 48,* 47–50.

Kolata, G. (1982). Consensus on diets and hyperactivity. *Science, 215,* 958.

Kolata, G. (1987). Panel urges dementia be diagnosed with care. *Science, 237,* 725.

Koob, G. F. (1987). Neuropeptides and memory. In L. Iverson, S. Iverson, & S. Snyder (Eds.), *New directions in behavioral pharmacology* (pp. 531–573). New York: Plenum Press.

Kopin, I. J., & Markey, S. P. (1988). MPTP toxicity: Implications for research in Parkinson's disease. *Annual Review of Neuroscience, 11,* 81–96.

Krueger, R. B., Sackeim, H. A., & Gamzu, E. R. (1992). Pharmacological treatment of the cognitive side effects of ECT: A review. *Psychopharmacology Bulletin, 28,* 409–424.

Leavitt, F. (1982). *Drugs and behavior* (2nd ed.). New York: John Wiley & Sons.

Lelliott, P. T., & Monteiro, W. O. (1986). Drug treatment of obsessive-compulsive disorder. *Drugs, 31,* 75–80.

Lewin, R. (1985). Parkinson's disease: An environmental cause. *Science, 228,* 257–258.

Lewin, R. (1987a). Dramatic results with brain grafts. *Science, 237,* 245–247.

Lewin, R. (1987b). More clues to the cause of Parkinson's disease. *Science, 237,* 978.

LeWitt, P. A. (1992). Clinical studies with and pharmacokinetic considerations of sustained-release levodopa. *Neurology, 42* (suppl. 1), 29–32.

Lipman, R. S., DiMascio, A., Reatig, N., & Kirson, T. (1978). Psychotropic drugs and mentally retarded children. In M. A. Lipton, A. DiMascio, & K. F.

Killman (Eds.), *Psychopharmacology* (pp. 1437–1450). New York: Raven Press.

Mattick, R. P., Andrews, G., Hadzi-Pavlovic, D., & Christensen, H. (1990). Treatment of panic and agoraphobia: An integrative review. *Journal of Nervous and Mental Disease, 178,* 567–576.

Max, J. E., & Rasmussen, S. A. (1986). Clonidine in the treatment of Tourette's syndrome exacerbation due to haloperidol withdrawal. *Journal of Nervous and Mental Disease, 174,* 243–246.

Mitchell, J. E., Laine, D. E., Morley, J. E., & Levine, A. S. (1986). Naloxone but not CCK-8 may attenuate binge-eating behavior in patients with the bulimia syndrome. *Biological Psychiatry, 21,* 1399–1406.

Montague, D. R., James, R. E., DeWolfe, V. G., & Martin, L. M. (1979). Diagnostic, evaluation, classification, and treatment of men with sexual dysfunction. *Urology, 14,* 545–565.

Montgomery, E. B. (1992). Pharmacokinetics and pharmacodynamics of levodopa. *Neurology, 42* (suppl. 1), 17–22.

Musch, B., Cambier, J., Loiseau, P., et al. (1987). Long-term treatment of epilepsy: Open multicenter trial with progabide in epileptic patients. *European Neuroscience, 26,* 113–119.

Nelson, J. C. (1991). Current status of tricyclic antidepressants in psychiatry: Their pharmacology and clinical applications. *Journal of Clinical Psychiatry, 52,* 193–200.

Olney, J. W. (1990). Excitotoxic amino acids and neuropsychiatric disorders. *Annual Review of Pharmacology and Toxicology, 30,* 47–71.

Pincus, J. H., & Kiss, A. (1986). Phenytoin reduces early acetylcholine release after depolarization. *Brain Research, 397,* 103–107.

Poewe, W. H., Lees, A. J., & Stern, G. M. (1986). Low-dose L-dopa therapy in Parkinson's disease: A 6-year follow-up study. *Neurology, 36,* 1528–1530.

Pope, H. G., Hudson, J. I., Jonas, J. M., & Yurgelen-Todd, D. (1983). Bulimia treated with imipramine: A placebo-controlled, double-blind study. *American Journal of Psychiatry, 140,* 554–558.

Rall, T. W., & Schleifer, L. S. (1985). Drugs effective in the therapy of the epilepsies. In A. G. Gilman, L. S. Goodman, T. W. Rall, & F. Murad (Eds.), *The pharmacological basis of therapeutics* (pp. 446–472). New York: Macmillan.

Rapoport, J. L., Buchsbaum, M. S., Weingartner, H., Zahn, T. P., Ludlow, C., & Mikkelsen, E. J. (1980). Dextroamphetamine: Its cognitive and behavioral effects in normal and hyperactive boys and normal men. *Archives of General Psychiatry, 37,* 933–943.

Rapport, M. D., & Kelly, K. L. (1991). Psychostimulant effects on learning and cognitive function: Findings and implications for children with attention deficit hyperactivity disorder. *Clinical Psychology, 11,* 61–92.

Ratey, J. J., Mikkelsen, E., Sorgi, P., Zucherman, H. S., Polakoff, S., Bemporad, J., Bick, P., & Kadish, W. (1987). Autism: The treatment of aggressive behaviors. *Journal of Clinical Psychopharmacology, 7,* 35–41.

Regeur, L., Pakkenberg, B., Fog, R., & Pakkenburg, H. (1986). Clinical features and long-term treatment with pimozide in 65 patients with Gilles de la Tourette's syndrome. *Journal of Neurology, Neurosurgery, and Psychiatry, 49,* 791–795.

Reid, K., Surridge, D. H. C., Morales, A., Condra, M., Harris, C., Owen, J., & Fenemore, J. (1987). Double-blind trial of yohimbine in treatment of psychogenic impotence. *The Lancet, 8556,* 421–423.

Ritvo, E. R., & Freeman, B. S. (1984). A medical model of autism: Etiology, pathology and treatment. *Pediatric Annals, 13,* 298–305.

Sahley, T. L., & Panksepp, J. (1987). Brain opioids and autism: An updated analysis of possible linkages. *Journal of Autism and Developmental Disorders, 17,* 201–216.

Salzman, C. (1985). Geriatric psychopharmacology. *Annual Review of Medicine, 36,* 217–228.

Salzman, C. (1988). Treatment of agitation, anxiety, and depression. *Psychopharmacology Bulletin, 24,* 39–42.

Schneider, L. S., & Sobin, P. B. (1992). Non-neuroleptic treatment of behavioral symptoms and agitation in Alzheimer's disease and other dementia. *Psychopharmacology Bulletin, 28,* 71–79.

Shapiro, A. K., & Shapiro, E. S. (1980). *Tics, Tourette syndrome and other movement disorders.* New York: Tourette Syndrome Association, Inc.

Sherwin, B. B. (1988). A comparative analysis of the role of androgen in human male and female sexual behavior: Behavioral specificity, critical thresholds, and sensitivity. *Psychobiology, 16,* 416–425.

Sloman, L. (1991). Use of medication in pervasive developmental disorders. *Psychiatric Clinics of North America, 14,* 165–182.

Spring, B., Chiodo, J., & Bowen, D. J. (1987). Carbohydrates, tryptophan, and behavior: A methodological review. *Psychological Bulletin, 102,* 234–256.

Swanson, J. M., & Kinsbourne, M. (1976). Stimulant-related state-dependent learning in hyperactive children. *Science, 192,* 1354–1356.

Taberner, P. V. (1985). Sex and drugs—Aphrodite's legacy. *Trends in the Pharmacological Sciences, 6,* 49–54.

Tartara, A., Manni, R., Galimberti, C. A., Hardenberg, J., Orwin, J., & Perucca, E. (1986). Vigabatrin in the treatment of epilepsy: A double-blind, placebo-controlled study. *Epilepsia, 27,* 717–723.

Telch, M. J., Agras, S., Taylor, C. B., Roth, W. T., & Gallen, C. C. (1985). Combined pharmacological and behavioral treatment for agoraphobia. *Behavioral Research Therapy, 23,* 325–335.

Tetrud, J. W., & Langston, J. W. (1989). The effect of deprenyl (selegiline) on the natural history of Parkinson's disease. *Science, 245,* 519–522.

Thienhaus, O. J., Wheeler, B. G., Simon, S., Zemlan, F. P., & Hartford, J. T. (1987). A controlled double-blind study of high-dose dihydroergotoxine mesylate (Hydergine) in mild dementia. *Journal of the American Geriatrics Society, 35,* 219–223.

Walsh, B. T., Stewart, J. W., Roose, S. P., Gladis, M., & Glassman, A. H. (1984). Treatment of bulimia with phenelzine. *Archives of General Psychiatry, 41,* 1105–1109.

Walsh, T. L., Lavenstein, B., Licamele, W. L., Bronheim, S., & O'Leary, J. (1986). Calcium antagonists in the treatment of Tourette's disorder. *American Journal of Psychiatry, 143,* 1467–1468.

Weiss, G., & Hechtman, L. (1979). The hyperactive child syndrome. *Science, 205,* 1348–1354.

Wender, P. H. (1978). Minimal brain dysfunction: An overview. In M. A. Lipton, A. DiMascio, & K. F. Killman (Eds.), *Psychopharmacology* (pp. 1429–1436). New York: Raven Press.

Yong, V. W., & Perry, T. L. (1986). Monoamine oxidase B, smoking, and Parkinson's disease. *Journal of the Neurological Sciences, 72,* 265–272.

Drug Name Index

BRAND NAME	GENERIC NAME	BRAND NAME	GENERIC NAME
Anafranil	clomipramine	Mysoline	primidone
Antabuse	disulfiram	Narcan	naloxone
Artane	trihexyphenidyl	Nardil	phenelzine
Asendin	amoxapine	Navane	thiothixene
Ativan	lorazepam	Nootropil	piracetam
Benadryl	diphenhydramine	Norpramin	desipramine
Benzedrine	amphetamine	Novocain	procaine
Buprenex	buprenorphine	Orap	pimozide
BuSpar	buspirone	Pamelor	nortriptyline
Catapres	clonidine	Parlodel	bromocriptine
Centrax	prazepam	Parnate	tranylcypromine
Clozaril	clozapine	Paxipam	halazepam
Cogentin	benztropine	Pondimin	fenfluramine
Cylert	magnesium pemoline	Preludin	phenmetrazine
Dalmane	flurazepam	Prolixin Decanoate	fluphenazine decanoate
Darvon	propoxyphene	Prozac	fluoxetine
Demerol	meperidine	Quaalude	methaqualone
Depokene	valproic acid	Quide	piperacetazine
Desoxyn	methamphetamine	Restoril	temazepam
Desyrel	trazodone	Ritalin	methylphenidate
Dexedrine	d-amphetamine	Serax	oxazepam
Dilantin	phenytoin	Serentil	mesoridazine
Dilaudid	hydromorphone	Serpasil	reserpine
Dolophine	methadone	Sinequan	doxepin
Doriden	glutethimide	Stelazine	trifluoperazine
Elavil	amitriptyline	Surmontil	trimipramine
Eldepryl	selegiline	Symmetrel	amantadine
Halcion	triazolam	Talwin	pentazocine
Haldol	haloperidol	Taractan	chlorprothixene
Hydergine	ergoloid mesylates	Tegretol	carbamazepine
Inderal	propranolol	Thorazine	chlorpromazine
Innovar	fentanyl	Tindal	acetaphenazine
Ionamin	phentermine	Tofranil	imipramine
Ketalar	ketamine	Tranxene	chlorazepate
Klonopin	clonazepam	Trexan	naltrexone
Librium	chlordiazepoxide	Trilafon	perphenazine
Loxitane	loxapine	Valium	diazepam
Ludiomil	maprotiline	Vesprin	triflupromazine
Marplan	isocarboxazid	Vivactil	protriptyline
Mazicon	flumazenil	Wellbutrin	bupropion
Mellaril	thioridazine	Xanax	alprazolam
Miltown	meprobamate	Zarontin	ethosuximide
Moban	molindone	Zoloft	sertraline

Most of the drugs in this list are those cited in this book that have been approved (or were approved at one time) by the Food and Drug Administration (FDA) for marketing in the United States. Some of these drugs are only marketed outside the United States. Other drugs that have been cited in this text, but for which a brand name has not been provided, are under investigation or have not been approved by the FDA.

Index

Boldface page numbers indicate definitions.